Using Computers in Clinical Practice

Psychotherapy and Mental Health Applications

Marc D. Schwartz, MD, is editor of the newsletter *Computers in Psychiatry/Psychology*. He also serves as president of Cavri Interactive Video Systems, an educational technology firm. He has written extensively on the use of computers for clinical and educational purposes.

Using Computers in Clinical Practice

Psychotherapy and Mental Health Applications

Marc D. Schwartz, MD, Editor

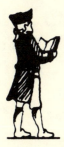

THE HAWORTH PRESS
NEW YORK

The Haworth Press, Inc.
28 East 22 Street
New York, New York 10010

Designed by Sandra Jones

Library of Congress Cataloging in Publication Data
Main entry under title:

Using computers in clinical practice.

   Bibliography: p.
   Includes index.
   1. Psychotherapy—Data processing. 2. Mental health
services—Data processing. I. Schwartz, Marc D.
[DNLM: 1. Computers. 2. Psychotherapy. 3. Mental health.
4. Information systems. WM 26.5 U85]
RC455.2.D38U85 1983 616.89'14'02854   83-18648
ISBN 0-86656-208-7

Printed in the United States of America

To my wife Anne and my sons Ted, Nick, and Jordan
in appreciation for their good humor, kind understanding,
and warm support.

Contents

Part III
Office Accounting Systems for the Psychotherapist

Part IV
Word Processing for the Clinician

Part V
Psychological Testing

Part VI
Psychological Reports

Part VII
Clinical Assessment and Interviewing by Computer

Part VIII
Computer-Based Diagnosis

Part IX
Computers in Neuropsychology

Part XII
Education as Therapy

Part XIII
Choosing a Computer

Part XIV
Other Issues

Contributors

Fred A. Alberts, Jr., PhD. Dr. Alberts is Coordinator of Psychological Assessment Services at Northside Community Mental Health Center in Tampa, Florida. He received the PhD degree from the University of Southern Mississippi and completed an internship in clinical psychology at the Devereux Foundation, Devon, Pennsylvania. His current interests include psychodiagnostics, clinical child psychology, neuropsychology, and computer applications in the social sciences. He has published numerous articles in the area of clinical neuropsychology. He is a member of the American Psychological Association and the Pennsylvania Psychological Association. *Mailing address*: P.O. Box 10414, Tampa, FL 33679.

David H. Allen, MD. Dr. Allen received his MD degree from Washington University in St. Louis. He interned at University Hospital in Ann Arbor, Michigan, and served in the US Army as a Preventive Medicine Officer. He trained in psychiatry at Duke University and is in private practice in Winston-Salem, North Carolina. *Mailing address*: P.O. Box 5141, Winston-Salem, NC 27103.

G. Octo Barnett, MD. Dr. Barnett is a Professor of Medicine at Harvard Medical School and a physician at the Massachusetts General Hospital in the Department of Medical Services. Dr. Barnett has been a medical resident at the Peter Bent Brigham Hospital and clinical associate at the National Health Institute, as well as an established investigator at the American Health Association and a lecturer in the Department of Electrical Engineering at the Massachusetts Institute of Technology. He is also a fellow at the American College of Physicians. Dr. Barnett's interests in computers in medicine include medical information systems, computer-assisted medical education, and clinical decision-making. *Mailing address*: Department of Medical Services, Massachusetts General Hospital, Boston, MA 02115.

Bruce Beebe, BS (deceased). Bruce Beebe received a BS degree from the University of California at Riverside and an MS in computer science from UCLA. He was affiliated with the Salt Lake VAMC from 1978 till 1981 and with the VA Medical District Office in San Francisco in 1981. *Mailing address*: c/o Douglas K. Gottfredson, PhD.

Dick J. Bierman, PhD. Dr. Bierman is a physicist doing research on Artificial Intelligence, with a special interest in the random processes of the brain, at the University of Amsterdam, the Netherlands. He is also doing experimental parapsychological research at the Research Institute for Psi Phenomena and Physics, Amsterdam, the Netherlands. *Mailing address*: Research Institute for Psi Research and Physics, Alexanderkade 1, 1018 CH Amsterdam, The Netherlands.

Odie L. Bracy, III, PhD. Dr. Bracy interned at the Albuquerque VA Medical Center and subsequently became a clinical neuropsychologist at Community Hospital of Indianapolis. He is a consultant to the hospital's neurology and neurosurgery services and the brain-injury rehabilitation unit, and also has a private practice in neuropsychological and cognitive rehabilitation. He has formed his own software company, Psychological Software Service, in Indianapolis and is the editor of *Cognitive Rehabilitation* magazine. *Mailing address*: 3157 Stillmeadow Drive, Indianapolis, IN 46224.

James A. Buss, MA. Mr. Buss is a private consultant specializing in computer services in Tacoma, Washington. *Mailing address*: c/o Herman Resnick, PhD.

Kathy Chin. Kathy Chin is a senior staff writer at *InfoWorld*, a major newsweekly for microcomputer users. Prior to joining the *InfoWorld* staff, she worked on a labor union newspaper, a community weekly, and a growing daily legal publication. She holds a BA degree in journalism from San Jose State University. *Mailing address*: c/o *InfoWorld*, 530 Lytton Avenue, Palo Alto, CA 94301.

Phillip W. Christensen, PhD. Dr. Christensen received a BA in psychology and humanities from the Interamerican University of Puerto Rico in 1963 and the PhD in clinical psychology from Texas Tech University in 1979. He is a staff psychologist at the Salt Lake VA Medical Center, where he is involved in developing computer applications for mental health. His work ranges from computerization of patient tracking and treatment documentation for speed and efficiency to interactive strategies for computer-assisted cognitive restructuring as adjuncts to psychotherapy. *Mailing address*: c/o Douglas K. Gottfredson.

Jerry Cinani, MSc. Jerry Cinani is Coordinator of Program Evaluation for Rural Clinics CMHC in Nevada and holds an MSc in psychology from the University of Alberta. He has been developing information systems in mental health and human services for seven years and has conducted projects both as a consultant and as a project director with consultants under contract. As Director of Research and Evaluation for an urban CMHC in Nebraska, he developed an MIS with an original design for use in a DEC minicomputer. *Mailing address*: 1336 Goshute Way, Carson City, NV 89701.

Betty Clarke, MSSW, CSW. Ms. Clarke is a psychological assistant with the Child and Family Services Outpatient Clinic of the Tarrant County Mental Health Mental Retardation Community Services Clinic, Fort Worth, Texas. *Mailing address*: 2305 Chapel Hill Lane, Arlington, TX 76014.

Daniel Cohen, CSW. Daniel Cohen is a social worker who has served as an administrator in various human-services settings, where he integrated microcomputers into his work. He also sells microcomputers for The Computer Factory of Garden City, New York. *Mailing address*: The Computer Factory, Inc., 1301 Franklin Avenue, Garden City, NY 11530.

David E. Comings, MD. Dr. Comings is Director of the Department of Medical Genetics, City of Hope National Medical Center, Duarte, California, and is also presently editor of the *American Journal of Human Genetics*. At City of Hope he runs a genetics and Tourette Syndrome clinic. His interests include the genetics of psychiatric disorders, including depression, Tourette Syndrome, and schizophrenia. *Mailing address*: Department of Medical Genetics, City of Hope National Medical Center, 1500 East Duarte Road, Duarte, CA 91010.

Philip DeMuth, PhD. Dr. DeMuth received his BA and MA in Speech Communications from the University of California at Santa Barbara, and his PhD in Clinical Psychology from the Fielding Institute of Santa Barbara. At present he is in private practice in Cleveland, Ohio. *Mailing address*: 1519 Burlington Road, Cleveland Heights, OH 44118.

Bruce Duthie, PhD. Dr. Duthie is a psychologist in private practice in Richland, Washington. He also is the director and founder of Psychological Software Specialists, a firm dedicated to the development and marketing of software relevant to the mental health field. He was first introduced to the use of computers as a research assistant while in graduate school at Texas A & M University. He acquired his first microcomputer in 1978 and founded Psychological Software Specialists in 1981. He is a frequent contributor to *Computers in Psychiatry/Psychology*. *Mailing address*: 1776 Fowler, Suite 7, Columbia Center North, Richland, WA 99352.

Marvin W. Eidinger, Jr., PhD. Dr. Eidinger is a licensed counseling psychologist in private practice in Kennewick, Washington. He received his bachelor's degree from the University of Washington and his doctorate from Washington State University. He is also a team leader for a data processing group within Rockwell Hanford Operations using microcomputers to evaluate the environmental impacts of proposed nuclear waste management practices. Dr. Eidinger taught himself computer programming, and he has been programming microcomputers for more than six years. *Mailing address*: 608 North Montana, Kennewick, WA 99336.

Albert D. Farrell, PhD. Dr. Farrell is currently an assistant professor of psychology at Virginia Commonwealth University in Richmond. He received his PhD in psychology from Purdue University. He has written extensively on behavioral assessment and social skills training. Recently, he has been involved in the development of a microcomputer-based system for use in psychotherapy evaluation. *Mailing address*: Department of Psychology, Virginia Commonwealth University, 806 West Franklin Street, Richmond, VA 23284.

John P. Flynn, PhD. Dr. Flynn received his PhD in social work from the University of Denver. He is Professor of Social Work at Western Michigan University, where he teaches social welfare policy. His current research activities involve the licensing and regulation of out-of-home care for vulnerable children and adults, computerized decision support systems in licensing decisions, and computer-assisted instruction. *Mailing address*: School of Social Work, Western Michigan University, Kalamazoo, MI 49008.

Robert Wally Fort, BS. Robert Wally Fort received a BS in systems analysis from Miami University. Subsequently, he has worked as a computer systems analyst at the LDS Hospital and the VA Medical Center in Salt Lake City, Utah. He was instrumental in setting up the current computer system in the VA Medical Center. *Mailing address*: c/o Douglas K. Gottfredson, PhD.

Gregory Freiherr. Mr. Freiherr received his BS from the University of Wisconsin-Madison and is currently a medical writer working on contract to the National Institutes of Health through the Research Resources Information Center, a private company. His interests include biotechnology and all aspects of bioresearch. Mr. Freiherr is assistant director of the Research Resources Information Center, which produces a monthly newsletter and special publications for the Division of Research Resources of the National Institutes of Health. *Mailing address*: Research Resources Information Center, 1776 East Jefferson Street, Rockville, MD 20852.

Frank Gallo, PhD. Dr. Gallo is president of Gallo Associates, Inc., of Lowell, Massachusetts, a research and consulting firm for health and human-service organizations, specializing in the application of computers. *Mailing address*: Gallo Associates, Inc., 45 Merrimack Street, Lowell, MA 01852.

Stephen M. Gee, BS. At present Mr. Gee is Programmer Analyst at On Lok Senior Health Services, a nonprofit, community-based service program in San Francisco. At On Lok, Mr. Gee has written, tested, debugged, and documented software for administrative, service-delivery, and research applications. He also designed and implemented an in-service training program in the use of the computer system. *Mailing address*: c/o Rick T. Zawadski, PhD.

Michael S. Geffen, PhD. Dr. Geffen received his PhD in clinical psychology from the California School of Professional Psychology in Fresno. He is an instructor in Parent Effectiveness Training and also the founder of the Geffen Center for Psychological Growth, in Upland, California. He also was founder and director of the adolescent program at Horizon Psychiatric Hospital in Pomona. *Mailing address*: Geffen Center for Psychological Growth, 1150 North Mountain Avenue, Suite 203, Upland, CA 91786.

Ann E. Glang, MA. Ms. Glang is a graduate student in special education at the University of Oregon. She is currently working on a project adapting special-education teaching procedures for use with head-injury victims. *Mailing address*: 1940 Jackson, Eugene, OR 97405.

Richard L. Gorsuch, PhD. Dr. Gorsuch is Professor and Director of Research at the Fuller Graduate School of Psychology, Pasadena, California, as well as an advisor to the clinical and counseling program. He is the author of *Factor Analysis* (2nd ed., Erlbaum, 1983), coauthor of *State-Trait Anxiety Scale*, and developer of numerous statistical programs for computers and several new test-interpretative programs for microcomputers. *Mailing address*: Western Psychological Services, 12031 Wilshire Boulevard, Los Angeles, CA 90025.

Douglas K. Gottfredson, PhD. Douglas K. Gottfredson had his initial experience with computers in the Air Force with an IBM FSQ–7 Sage Computer in the Air Defense Command. Subsequently he received his PhD in psychology from Brigham Young University. He assisted the computer staff in setting up the mental health computer system at the Salt Lake VA Medical Center. *Mailing address*: 9932 South 2270 East, Sandy, UT 84092.

R. Charles Gould, BA. Mr. Gould is a graduate student in counseling and psychology at the New York Institute for Technology and also works at the Behavioral Counseling Center, Whitestone, Queens, New York, with Dr. Victor Krynicki. *Mailing address*: c/o Victor Krynicki, PhD.

John H. Greist, MD. Dr. Greist is a professor of psychiatry at the University of Wisconsin Medical School, Madison. Dr. Greist received his MD from Indiana University in 1965 and completed residencies in internal medicine and psychiatry at the University of Wisconsin. He received the Distinguished Teaching Award from the University of Wisconsin Medical School in 1967, and since 1974 he has held a Research Scientist Development Award from the National Institutes of Mental Health for development of computer applications in psychiatry. He is the author and coauthor of seven books and more than 70 professional papers. *Mailing address*: Department of Psychiatry, University of Wisconsin, Madison, WI 53706.

James L. Hedlund, PhD. Dr. Hedlund received his PhD in clinical psychology from the State University of Iowa and is a Professor of Psychiatry (Medical Psychology) of the School of Medicine, University of Missouri-Columbia, and Director of the Missouri Institute of Psychiatry in St. Louis, Missouri. He is also director of the Institute's Mental Health Systems Research Unit, which conducts research, development, and advanced (Post Doctoral Fellow) training programs concerning clinical computer applications in mental health. Dr. Hedlund was responsible for the development of the Department of Defense's first major clinical computer applications project, Computer Support in Military Psychiatry (COMPSY), at the Walter Reed Army Medical Center, and he has been involved since late 1971 with the Missouri Department of Mental Health's statewide automated information system, especially its clinical components. He has consulted and published extensively in the area of mental health information systems and is a primary author of the recently NIMH-published monograph, "Computers in Mental Health: A Review and Annotated Bibliography." *Mailing address*: School of Medicine, University of Missouri-Columbia, 5400 Arsenal Street, St. Louis, MO 63139.

Vernon K. Jacobs, CPA. Vernon K. Jacobs is both a Certified Public Accountant and a Chartered Life Underwriter. He is the Editor of *Tax Angles*, a monthly tax-planning newsletter for the general public that is published by Kephard Communications in Arlington, Virginia. *Mailing address*: Research Press, Inc., Bos 8317, Prairie Village, KS 66208.

James H. Johnson, PhD. Dr. Johnson is Professor and Director of Clinical Psychology at the Illinois Institute of Technology. He has been an active researcher on the use of computers in psychology since he received the PhD in Clinical Psychology from the University of Minnesota in 1972. He is the author of nearly 100 books and papers on the uses of computers in mental health. *Mailing address*: Department of Psychology, Illinois Institute of Technology, Chicago, IL 60616.

Peter A. Keller, PhD. Dr. Keller is a practicing clinician and associate professor of psychology at Mansfield State College, Mansfield, Pennsylvania. He is co-editor of *Innovations in Clinical Practice: A Source Book*, which is published by the Professional Resource Exchange, Inc. He uses word processing in both his clinical and academic work. *Mailing address*: Professional Resource Exchange, P.O. Box 453, Mansfield, PA 16933.

Michael A. King, DSW. Dr. King is the Director of the Department of Social Work Services, Staten Island Hospital, Staten Island, New York. He is president-elect of the New York Metropolitan Chapter of the Society for Hospital Social Work Directors. His consulting firm, King Associates, has written programs for hospitals in social work and mental health and specialized programs for hospital risk managers. Dr. King has also led workshops on understanding and maximizing the use of computers. *Mailing address*: 215 Shoreward Drive, Great Neck, NY 11021.

Terry Kuczeruk, MSW. Terry Kuczeruk obtained his MSW at the School of Social Work, Western Michigan University, where he was an administrative intern in a hospital-based mental health center. He specializes in social welfare policy, planning, and administration; he also has an interest in computerized management information systems. *Mailing address*: c/o John P. Flynn, PhD.

Robert T. Kurlychek, PhD. Dr. Kurlychek received his PhD from the University of Oregon in 1977 and is currently on the staff of Sacred Heart General Hospital in Eugene, Oregon. He also maintains a private practice. Dr. Kurlychek is a Diplomate of the American Academy of Behavioral Medicine. His main interests include neuropsychological assessment and cognitive rehabilitation. *Mailing address*: Sacred Heart Medical Center, 1200 Alder Street, Eugene, OR 97440.

Victor Krynicki, PhD. Dr. Krynicki received his doctorate degree in psychology from Columbia University and completed his psychoanalytic training at Washington Square Institute in New York. While he was on the faculty of New York Medical College, he worked with Dr. Turan Itil in developing computerized assessment procedures for children with learning and behavioral problems. Dr. Krynicki is currently director of program evaluation at Queens Children's Psychiatric Center and also director of the Behavioral Counseling Center in Queens. *Mailing address*: 28 Hollis Lane, Croton-on-Hudson, NY 10520.

Lawrence M. Lanes, MD. Dr. Lanes completed his internship, psychiatric residency, and child fellowship studies at Mount Zion Hospital and Medical Center in San Francisco. He is currently completing his fifth year as candidate at the San Francisco Psychoanalytic Institute. In addition he is director of an adolescent in-patient unit at McAluley Neuropsychiatric Institute of St. Mary's Hospital in San Francisco. He also has a private psychotherapy practice. He is interested in applications of microcomputers with severely disturbed children, among other things. *Mailing address*: 3605 Sacramento Street, San Francisco, CA 94118.

Richard Longabaugh, EdD. Dr. Longabaugh is Director of the Department of Evaluation at Butler Hospital and Professor of Psychiatry and Human Behavior at Brown University. He received his undergraduate degree from Dartmouth College and his doctorate in Education from Harvard University and trained as a clinical psychologist at the Langley Porter Neuropsychiatric Institute, San Francisco. He has authored and coauthored approximately 60 papers and books on a variety of mental health topics. Dr. Longabaugh received the 1981 Certificate of Recognition by the Division of Psychologists in Public Service of the American Psychological Association for his work in the development of a series of innovative programs for treating patients with alcohol problems at Butler Hospital. *Mailing address*: c/o Leigh McCullough, PhD.

Charlene Matheson, PhD. Dr. Matheson is a director of the Kwachee Counseling Center in Tacoma, Washington. *Mailing address*: c/o Herman Resnick, PhD.

Leigh McCullough, PhD. Dr. McCullough received her MA and PhD in Psychology from Boston College. She completed her clinical internship at Brown University. She is presently working on two research projects as Project Coordinator of Problem-Oriented Systems and Treatment (NIMH 26012) at Butler Hospital and as Behavioral Consultant to the "Study of Adult Development" at Harvard University. Her primary interest is clinical research, and she has developed a brief and efficient computerized system for psychotherapy evaluation and research which is presently being tested in 30 sites nationwide. She serves on an APA committee (Division 12, Section 3) on "Science and Clinical Psychology." *Mailing address*: Department of Evaluation and Research, Butler Hospital, 345 Blackstone Boulevard, Providence, RI 02906.

Marvin J. Miller, MD. Dr. Miller is Assistant Professor of Psychiatry at the Indiana University School of Medicine and directs the junior clerkship in psychiatry. He is a staff psychiatrist at Larue D. Carter Memorial Hospital and is Director of the Computer Laboratory. His special interest is in computerized self-administered tests, and he has devised or adapted a number of tests for this purpose. *Mailing address*: Department of Psychiatry, Indiana University School of Medicine, 1315 West 10th Street, Indianapolis, IN 46202.

Richard A. Murray, PhD. Dr. Murray received his PhD in rehabilitation counseling psychology from Syracuse University in New York. He has served as a rehabilitation counselor in the New York State Education Department and as a counseling psychologist in the United States Veterans Administration. He taught at Syracuse University and has served as a consultant with Cornell University, Stanford Research Institute International, and Arthur Young and Company. He has his own Counseling Software Development service in Augusta, Maine. *Mailing address*: Counseling Software and Consulting Services, 36 Malta Street, Apt. 1, Augusta, ME 04330.

Jim Newkham, ACSW. Mr. Newkham is a social worker and Director of Mental Health Outpatient Programs for the Heart of Texas Region MHMR Center. He has worked in community mental health centers since 1971 after receiving his MSW from Tulane University and working in the Army as a Social Work Officer. He has been involved in the development and utilization of the automated community health and record treatment system since its implementation six years ago at the HOT Region MHMR Center. *Mailing address*: Heart of Texas MHMR Center, Box 1277, Waco, TX 76703.

Gary L. Pinkerton, MSW. Mr. Pinkerton received his MSW from the University of Houston, and is director of a private social service agency in Beaumont, Texas. In addition, he is owner of Shiloh Systems, which provides consultation and training in development, fundraising, and use of microcomputers to social agencies, churches, civic groups, etc. *Mailing address*: Shiloh Systems, P.O. Box 1983, Beaumont, TX 77704.

Kenneth S. Pope, PhD. Dr. Pope received an MA in English literature from Harvard and a PhD in psychology from Yale. He is co-editor of the *Journal of Imagination, Cognition and Personality: The Scientific Study of Consciousness*, a member of the clinical faculty of CCLA, and he has a private practice in Los Angeles. His books include *On Love and Loving*, *The Stream of Consciousness*, and *The Power of Human Imagination*. *Mailing address*: c/o Robert A. Zachary, PhD.

Paul R. Raffoul, PhD, ACSW. Dr. Raffoul received his MSW from Florida State University in Tallahassee and his doctorate degree in social work from Washington University in St. Louis, Missouri. He is an assistant professor in the Graduate School of Social Work at the University of Houston, Texas. He has written in the areas of substance abuse, drug misuse (noncompliance) among older persons, and social work career status among BSW social workers. *Mailing address*: c/o Gary L. Pinkerton.

Robert Reitman, PhD. Dr. Reitman is the founder and staff director of the Valley Center for Marital and Sexual Therapy in Woodland Hills, California. He is a charter-certified sex educator, counselor, and therapist (AASECT), a clinical member of the American Association of Marriage and Family Therapists, the National Council on Family Relations, the Association for Humanistic Psychology, and other professional organizations. He is a national board member of the Society for the Scientific Study of Sex and also its current executive director. He is also on the advisory boards of the Center for Sex Research, Cal State University, the L.A. Institute for Rational Living, and *Forum* magazine. *Mailing address*: Valley Center, 22055 Clarendon—101, Woodland Hills, CA 91367.

Herman Resnick, PhD. Dr. Resnick is a professor of social work at the University of Washington, School of Social Work, in Seattle, Washington. *Mailing address*: 18320 204 Avenue NE, Woodinville, WA 98072.

Lawrence G. Ritt, PhD. Dr. Ritt is a psychologist in private practice and is also an adjunct associate professor in the Department of Clinical Psychology at the University of Florida. In addition, Dr. Ritt is the publisher of the Professional Resource Exchange, Inc. He holds a doctoral degree in clinical psychology. *Mailing address*: Suite 4, 635 South Orange Avenue, Sarasota, FL 33577.

Gale H. Roid, PhD. Dr. Roid is Director of Research in Test Development and Computer Applications for Western Psychological Services, one of the largest publishers of psychological tests. He is author of *A Technology for Test-Item Writing* (Academic Press, 1982) and coauthor of computer programs for interpreting two recently published tests, the

Vocational Interest Inventory and the Barclay Classroom Assessment System. *Mailing address*: Western Psychological Services, 12031 Wilshire Boulevard, Los Angeles, CA 90025.

John A. Schinka, PhD. Dr. Schinka received his doctorate from the University of Iowa in 1974. Since that time he has been Director of the Neuropsychology Lab at the Tampa VA Hospital and a faculty member of the College of Medicine at the University of South Florida. He has most recently been involved in the development of a comprehensive information system for rehabilitation services. In addition, he is senior editor of Psychological Assessment Resources, Inc. *Mailing address*: c/o R. Bob Smith, III, PhD.

L. J. Schmidt, MD. Dr. Schmidt is Associate Professor of Psychiatry at the University of Utah College of Medicine and Chief of Psychiatry Service at the Salt Lake VA Medical Center and was Clinical Director of the Salt Lake Community Mental Health Center from 1971 till 1975. He has authored many articles on community mental health services and the use of computers in mental health settings. *Mailing address*: c/o Douglas K. Gottfredson, PhD.

Sid J. Schneider, Ph.D. Dr. Schneider was born in New York City in 1950. He studied engineering at Carnegie-Mellon University and psychology at the University of Michigan and the State University of New York at Buffalo, where he earned his doctorate in 1975. He presently is on the faculty of New York Medical College and the research staff of the VA Hospital in Montrose, New York. *Mailing address*: 44 Belleview Avenue, Ossining, NY 10562.

Dick Schoech, PhD. Dr. Schoech is an assistant professor at the Graduate School of Social Work, University of Texas at Arlington. He is also coordinator of the Computer Use in Social Services (CUSS) Network and editor of the *CUSS Newsletter*. *Mailing address*: Graduate School of Social Work, University of Texas at Arlington, Box 19129, Arlington, TX 76019.

Larry L. Searcy, MA. Mr. Searcy received his master's degree in Speech Communication from the University of Missouri at Kansas City. He has served on state-wide and city-wide task forces dealing with youth services, delinquencies, and alternative education. He is the Director of Act Together of Kansas City, a project creating an automated information clearinghouse for public and private organizations working with high-risk youth, under the auspices of the Heart of America United Way. *Mailing address*: 609E 72nd Street, Kansas City, MO 64131.

Tom Shea. Tom Shea is a senior staff writer for *InfoWorld*, a leading newsmagazine for people who use small computers. A former news reporter for the *Sun-Sentinel* daily newspaper in Fort Lauderdale, Florida, he has also worked as a hybrid computer operator, working on computerized experimental flight-simulation equipment at the NASA-Ames research facility in Mountain View, California. *Mailing address*: c/o *InfoWorld*, 530 Lytton Avenue, Palo Alto, CA 94301.

R. Bob Smith, III, PhD. Dr. Smith received his doctorate from the State University of New York at Albany in 1973. He is president of Psychological Assessment Resources, Inc., publishers and distributors of software for use by mental health professionals. *Mailing address*: Psychological Assessment Resources, Inc., P.O. Box 98, Odessa, FL 33556.

Sydney Z. Spiesel, PhD, MD. Dr. Spiesel is a pediatrician in private practice and President of Clinical Analytics, Inc., a software firm which specializes in the application of Artificial Intelligence methods to business, scientific, and medical information and data management systems. He is a former full-time faculty member of the Department of Pediatrics at Yale University and continues to hold a clinical teaching appointment. His special interests include behavioral and psychosocial issues, adolescent medicine, immunologically mediated disease, pharmacokinetics, the application of computers to medical practice, and medical education. *Mailing address*: 77 Everit Street, New Haven, CT 06511.

Zebulon Taintor, MD. Dr. Taintor is a research professor of psychiatry at New York University and he is currently living in Sri Lanka. He was director of the Multi-State Information System, Rockland Research Institute, Orangeburg, New York. *Mailing address*: c/o Administration Officer, American Embassy (Colombo), U.S. Department of State, Washington, DC 20520.

Bruce W. Vieweg, MS. Mr. Vieweg is a Research Associate of the Department of Psychiatry, School of Medicine, University of Missouri-Columbia, at the Missouri Institute of Psychiatry in St. Louis, Missouri. He received his Master of Science degree from Southern Illinois University in 1975 and has worked with MIP's Mental Health Systems Research Unit since that time. He has been responsible for conducting scientific literature searches, for organizing and preparing summaries of the literature involved, and for helping to prepare critical reviews for publication. He is editor of an extensive automated bibliographic data base for computer applications in mental health, coauthor of the *Computers in Psychiatry/Psychology* bibliographic column, and a primary author of the recently NIMH-published monograph, "Computers in Mental Health: A Review and Annotated Bibliography." Mr. Vieweg has also assisted in designing and implementing a mini-computer laboratory and has been responsible for training and providing support to post-doctoral fellows and faculty in the use of the system. *Mailing address*: Department of Psychiatry, School of Medicine, University of Missouri-Columbia, 5400 Arsenal Street, St. Louis, MO 63139.

Ken R. Vincent, EdD. Dr. Vincent is staff psychologist at the Hauser Clinic and Associates in Houston, Texas. He received his EdD degree in counseling psychology from the University of Northern Colorado. His post-doctoral training was with the Texas Rehabilitation Commission's accelerated diagnostic services project, Project Expedite. Dr. Vincent is a senior author of the *MMPI-168 Codebook* as well as numerous other publications in the area of psychological diagnosis and assessment and the computerization of psychological testing, including the *Fully Automated Rorschach*, the *Holtzman Content Analysis Technique*, and the *Computerized Holtzman Interpretation*. *Mailing address*: 11507 Chevy Chase, Houston, TX 77077.

Danny Wedding, PhD. Dr. Wedding is an assistant professor of psychology and medical psychology at East Tennessee State University. He received his PhD in clinical psychology from the University of Hawaii and completed his post-doctoral residency year in behavioral medicine at the University of Mississippi Medical Center. He is coeditor of *Great Cases in Psychotherapy* (Peacock, 1979) and coauthor of *Clinical and Behavioral Neuropsychology* (Praeger, 1983). His current interests are in computerized dietary assessment as an intervention in treating obesity and nutrition-related diseases. *Mailing address*: Department of Psychiatry and Behavioral Science, East Tennessee State University, Box 1950A, Johnson City, TN 37614.

Robert A. Zachary, PhD. Dr. Zachary received his PhD from Yale University in clinical psychology, and did postdoctoral clinical and research training at Mount Zion Hospital and University of California, San Francisco. His publications span a number of areas including program evaluation, mental imagery, coping behavior in children, and psychological assessment. He is currently Director of Clinical Research at Western Psychological Services in Los Angeles, and is a member of the clinical faculty at the UCLA Neuropsychiatric Institute. *Mailing address*: Western Psychological Services, 12031 Wilshire Boulevard, Los Angeles, CA 90025.

Rick T. Zawadski, PhD. Dr. Zawadski received his PhD in social-organizational psychology from the University of California at Berkeley. He is Research Director of On Lok Senior Health Services, a non-profit, community-based service program in San Francisco. He served as Chairman of the Western Gerontological Society's Research Utilization and Dissemination Committee, and currently he is a member of the Research, Demonstration and Evaluation Committee of the National Council on the Aging. He is also a member of the Steering Committee of the National Institute on Adult Daycare and the chairman of its Publication and Research Committee. *Mailing address*: On Lok, 1441 Powell Street, San Francisco, CA 94133.

Joseph Zefran, MSW. Mr. Zefran is a former social work practitioner who is now specializing as a researcher and information system consultant in Chicago. In addition to his full-time employment in a large midwestern juvenile court, he is currently employed part-time as the Human Services Project Manager for Synergistic Office Systems in Mundelein, Illinois, a microcomputer hardware/software vendor. *Mailing address*: 4918 North Hamilton, Chicago, IL 60625.

Foreword

U*sing Computers in Clinical Practice* is a most timely and helpful book. While only a small number of clinicians have begun to use computers, most are interested in learning how to learn how to use them. Until now, too little had been accomplished to justify serious inquiry by clinicians. Even financial and insurance matters were literally best handled by hand. Hardware, while quite reliable, was also very expensive. Software, while often idiosyncratic, unreliable, and inflexible, was both expensive and seldom worth the money. Bringing hardware and software together into a useable computer system was a task for computer science departments or masochistic individuals with a morbid curiosity to start things up to see why they wouldn't work. Spellbinding salesmen used computerspeak to tout meaningless hardware performance data because they could not present viable computer systems for clinical practice.

The last decade has brought a growing number of clinical computing experiments, and the field has witnessed the gradual emergence of some programs of proven usefulness. Marc Schwartz has assembled an amazingly comprehensive set of papers touching all important aspects of clinical computing. The contributors are pioneers in the field, and each describes a particular part of the clinical computing enterprise. None of these contributors is so bold as to offer a comprehensive system. That goal awaits the second edition of this book. Yet, the elements of the comprehensive systems clinicians will come to use and depend on are all described in this volume.

It is clear that enough good work has now been done that careful clinicians can acquire a computer system that will help more than it hinders. How to assess hardware and software (and the prior question of whether a computer system is needed at all); the strengths and limitations of financial and other business programs, word processing, data base management systems for clinical record keeping, interview construction programs, specific patient interviews, consultation programs, bibliographic programs; steps in acquiring a computer system down to the details of contract writing; and effects on office and clinical procedures and on clinicians and staff are all presented from a number of points of vantage.

As editor of *Computers in Psychiatry/Psychology*, as well as developer of an innovative microcomputer-based clinical education system, Marc Schwartz has been at the center of the rapidly expanding field of clinical computing. The best articles from *Computers in Psychiatry/Psychology* have been reprinted here along with many new pieces. The diversity of clinical practice is reflected in the variety of perspectives and writing styles contained in this book. Some may perceive this diversity as unevenness, but it is, in my view, an honest and helpful representation of the reality of this moment in clinical computing.

Using Computers in Clinical Practice is the most helpful and authoritative source book for clinicians interested in using computers. Clinicians can "work up" the problem of clinical computing and proceed with at least as much confidence as we often have in treating our patients.

John H. Greist, MD
Professor of Psychiatry
University of Wisconsin Medical School
Madison, Wisconsin

Using Computers in Clinical Practice

Psychotherapy and Mental Health Applications

Introduction

If you are a mental health clinician or administrator; if you are thinking of buying a computer or are presently using one; and if you would like to know about the real experiences—failures and successes—of others like you who have used computers in mental health over the past decade, then this book is for you.

A thread that runs through the chapters of this book is the desire of the authors to share with you their personal experiences in developing computer systems. This book contains practical, applicable information. It is meant to help you take advantage of the extraordinary capabilities the computer offers, while avoiding painful errors and blind alleys many have stumbled into.

You will find very little in the book about wonderful pie-in-the-sky promises that "the next generation of computers" will deliver. Regardless of the particular application, be it administration, diagnosis, psychological testing, or therapy, the promise of computers can be awesome. The neophyte must guard very carefully against the temptation to confuse this promise with current reality. In general, the more experience people have with computers, the more modest are their expectations of them, and the more willing are they to tolerate the series of frustrating and confusing incidents that may occur in the course of implementing and learning to use them.

It is very important in evaluating how you wish to use your computer for you to decide what you really want the computer to do for you and to weigh carefully the benefits and costs of those uses. There is a temptation to implement computer programs because you have every reason to believe they should be able to carry out particular tasks, and it seems tempting to automate those tasks. As an example of the consequences of this kind of misguided thinking, you need only look at the unbelievable amounts of time, money, and effort that have gone into attempts to computerize the medical or psychiatric record, with rather meager results.

The information in a psychiatric record, particularly as it relates to psychotherapy, is often written in a highly individual and subjective style and therefore does not lend itself well to the storage and retrieval capabilities of the computer, which require more organized input to generate useful output. On the other hand, well-structured notes about incident reports or about patients' use of medication, which can be much more easily organized into categories (e.g., type of medication, dose, frequency, side effects), lend themselves very well to computerization.

1

Know what you want to accomplish, and study whether, given your present record-keeping system, the computer can help you. You may decide you must change your system in order to adapt to the computer's need. That may be fine, but be sure that is what you want to do.

The poster on the wall asks, "Why is there always time to do it right the second time?" This is a question that anyone planning to buy a computer or computer program should ask. Only after the awful realization dawns that the computer will NEVER do what it was purchased to do, that the program will NEVER do what you believed it should, do the consequences of too rapid acceptance of a system become vividly clear. Impelled by enthusiasm to join the crowd, nurtured by high expectations and advertising hype, the naive computer user can find it too easy to accept the recommendations of the last "expert" to be consulted. (Anyone with two weeks' more experience than you have can appear very expert indeed as you are just getting started.) It seems so self-evident that all billing systems are basically the same, you tell yourself, and it's so time-consuming to check them out. They must all work or they wouldn't be on the market, you say. (They don't.) They could never destroy all your files. (They could.)

Some chapters of this book contain poignant anecdotes told by brave pioneers. The chapters also contain many heroic tales of innovative and persevering clinicians who explored a terra incognita and came back to provide us with a clear map to the new-found land. Their experiences are invaluable to anyone considering the use of computers in mental health.

The book starts with an overview of the use of computers in the clinical setting, presenting material that should make it easier to evaluate your need for a computer. Part II of the book then presents a series of perspectives on how the use of a computer will affect various people in your professional environment and how you can most constructively deal with them.

Two of the most common uses of the computer in the clinical setting are not specifically clinical in nature. They are billing and word processing. Parts III and IV of the book are designed to help you decide whether these uses of the computer will be of value to you.

Next, a variety of clinical uses are examined, starting with the most common application, psychological testing. The nature of tests, how they are constructed, the legalities and ethics of their use are explored from various points of view. Then the book looks at the computer's role in clinical assessment, interviewing, and diagnosis. These functions have not achieved the degree of acceptance that was predicted for them. Many believe they are grossly underutilized; others think they will never realize the promise they were early believed to hold. Parts VII and VIII of the book give you an opportunity to examine both sides of the issue and make your own decision.

The computer's place in psychotherapy remains a controversial subject. While some studies suggest a beneficial role for the machine, humanistic and other considerations must be taken into account in assessing how the computer can and should function in this area. Two sections of the book, one on the computer as a therapy adjunct (Part XI) and the other on the computer-assisted instruction in therapy (Part XII), provide a wide-ranging overview of the current state of the art.

Just when you thought the book would never get around to discussing computers and computer programs, comes Part XIII, presenting clinicians' reviews of a selection of hardware (computers) and software (programs). The products reviewed are not presented because they are better or worse than others. The intention is to present reviews that give you a better understanding of the issues clinicians have found to be of importance in their selection process. The issues are more important than the products.

The book concludes with a group of chapters each touching on an interesting aspect of the use of computers. Many other such chapters were not included because there just was not enough space.

The field of computers in psychotherapy and mental health is growing rapidly, and it is difficult to keep up with all the new ideas being generated. It is an exciting time for anyone who is becoming involved in it. I hope this book will help you to more quickly and successfully join others in developing applications that will make the work you do more effective and more enjoyable.

PART I

An Overview

In Part I of this book, a number of authors give an introductory overview to the use of computers in mental health. In the first chapter, John Schinka and Bob Smith survey the applications of the computer in the psychotherapist's office. Then, going into more specific detail, Joe Zephran helps you organize and analyze the information needs of your practice or organization and decide whether you really need a computer.

Larry Lanes then takes a wry look at the somewhat less than scientific nature of his own decision-making process in buying a computer. Finally, Doug Gottfredson and his colleagues at the Salt Lake City VA Medical Hospital describe the information needs of the hospital's psychiatry service and how they have been met by a computer-based system. The emphasis in all these chapters is on what has been done and what can now be done . . . by you.

1

The Computer in the Psychotherapist's Office: Present and Future Applications

John A. Schinka, PhD
R. Bob Smith, III, PhD

The last decade has seen a number of professional, economic, and social changes that have had a significant cumulative effect on the practice of the clinical therapist. Many professional journals have documented the continuing increase in scientific knowledge that must be digested by the clinician. In addition, with the development of specialized skills in the areas of behavioral medicine, forensic evaluation, neuropsychology, and biofeedback, traditional clinical activities have evolved into a multi-assessment, multi-treatment service-delivery situation. The therapist now assumes the responsibility of providing specialized treatment and evaluation procedures to a much wider variety of treatment populations. These responsibilities not only require the monitoring of larger bodies of scientific literature, but also place a burden on the clinician to maintain required continuing education units for an increasing number of clinical skills.

The instability of the national economic situation has also had an impact on the practice of the therapist. The use of money management techniques is virtually required today in order to maintain an adequate level of compensation for the therapist's professional endeavors. An indirect effect of this instability has been an increasing paperwork burden as governmental agencies attempt to regulate the flow of tax monies in a more productive manner. This paperwork burden is also accentuated by the demands of licensing boards and agencies for tighter documentation of clinical skills.

Efficiency of the clinician's office practice is also made necessary by the advent of the consumers' movement and the accelerating incidence of litigation against all health professionals. These factors force the clinician to maintain not only data pertinent to the delivery of service, but also data that are defensive in nature and protect against potential legal challenge.

These facts are not unknown to the practicing therapist. This review, however, focuses on two primary aspects of the clinician's work. The first is that the therapist, in his professional and business roles, is primarily a manipulator of information. In this sense, the clinician's activity is information-intensive. Secondly, since the clinician is the sole source of managing the collection and manipulation of information, the work is time- and labor-intensive. There is a limit to the absolute amount of work that can be done in a given time period.

A small but growing number of clinicians have looked to technological solutions to deal more effectively with demands of therapy practice. For these clinicians, the advances in computer applications and increasingly attractive cost-performance ratios of computers make this solution worthy of consideration.

CURRENT COMPUTER CAPABILITY

Hardware

At this time there are well over 100 manufacturers of small computers, generally referred to as *microcomputers*. While there is no strict definition of a microcomputer, for the most part they encompass an 8- or 16-bit microprocessor with a single video monitor (CRT) and keyboard. Main memory (RAM) is generally in the 48-Kb (kilobyte) to 128-Kb range, although expansion boards can take this capacity up to 512 Kb with some models. Peripheral storage is typically provided via floppy disk systems or Winchester hard disk systems. For professional use, a dual floppy disk system with 200-Kb storage capacity is considered minimal. Winchester disk systems allow for storage of up to 80 Mb (megabyte). Generally, these microcomputers provide reasonable clarity in text presentation on a monochrome or color monitor; several offer the ability to present data in a graphic format. Hard-copy output is available through the use of dot-matrix printers, which produce type suitable for internal office use, and daisy wheel printers, which provide letter-quality print. A microcomputer fitting the above description is currently available in the price range of $2,000 to $10,000. With the major brand names, repair and equipment upgrades are available locally, and these systems will perform adequately for several software applications.

An important point to note with these microcomputers is that they are single-user, single-task computers; that is, only one person can perform one job with the microcomputer at any given time. In the office situation, this dictates that users will bring their jobs to the microcomputer rather than having access at their own work locations. A further implication is that, as uses for the microcomputer increase in any given office setting, the number of microcomputers will necessarily have to increase to meet demand by the users. Thus, the single-user, single-task microcomputer technology requires large increases in investment as the number of uses and concurrent users increases.

Software

While the selection of a microcomputer system might appear to be the primary task in applying this technology to the office practice, it is actually the case that software applications must be evaluated first. The reason for this is that different microcomputers will accommodate only specific operating systems and languages. The key issue, therefore, is the selection of software programs for specific applications and subsequently the matching of an appropriate microcomputer, which will run the software programs. An important point here is the fact that even commercially available software requires training time to gain full use of software capability. Many users are surprised to find that user manuals of up to 200 pages in length accompany a software program. Learning to write software programs is also a time-consuming task and is unlikely to be cost-effective for the clinician, given the current cost of carefully selected software packages.

The following is a list of software programs that have potential applications in the therapist's office.

Word Processing. This is basically a program that allows the user to create and edit a document on a CRT (cathode ray tube or video tube) and subsequently print the document for formal use if required. The document may be saved on disk for further modification or for additional copies. Most higher-order typing and editing functions such as corrections, centering, pagination, insertions, and deletions can be performed with several simple key strokes. Master documents can be created for reports or letters that are repetitive and have a standard format, allowing the user to simply fill in blanks to create the printed document. Word-processing programs differ greatly in the number of features offered, and it is likely that the therapist who produces much in the way of formal reports would be required to run a fairly sophisticated program, which would cost in the higher price ranges ($100 to $500) for this type of application.

Psychological Testing. Two publishers now distribute software programs that will administer and score some of the more frequently used personality tests, for example, the Minnesota Multiphasic Personality Inventory (MMPI). These programs are generally sold for an initial leasing fee plus a fixed cost for each test administered. The number of tests available at this time is quite limited and programs are currently available for only a small number of microcomputers. Two companies currently offer a bundled package of hardware and software dedicated to psychological testing. While some therapists may doubt the acceptability of this technology to patients, users routinely report that patient compliance with automated testing is at least as high as with paper-and-pencil administration. The automated scoring of test data is a positive feature in promoting accuracy of scoring and rapid feedback of test results.

Biofeedback. Many clinicians are familiar with single-measure biofeedback instruments such as EMG (electromyogram) or thermal devices. Two companies currently offer laboratory configurations that marry the full range of biofeedback instrumentation to microprocessors, giving the clinician programmable control over simultaneous multiple-measurement techniques. The use of the microcomputer allows for the presetting of treatment parameters across the full range of physiological measures, recording and reduction of data, hard-copy output, and the ability to save data on disk for further reference or research. In addition, the microcomputer can run any other compatible software when not driving the biofeedback modules. The cost of these systems runs in the $12,000 to $30,000 range.

Billing/Office Accounts. Although not specifically designed for the therapists' office practice, a number of software companies offer billing, accounts receivable, and master insurance programs. These programs vary greatly in features and in price. The best programs will maintain patient ledger cards and provide accounting statistics by the day, week, month, or year. File data for patient accounts can be printed on a universal insurance form in an appropriate format. Full accounting packages, which generate formatted data for accounts receivable, accounts payable, general ledger, payroll, billing, and insurance, are also available, but at greatly increased expense. These total packages generally also require consultation by the office accountant. Given the relatively small number of patient accounts, personnel, and payable items of the typical therapist's office, these software packages are not likely to be cost-effective unless used in a group practice. They also require substantial training to fully utilize the extensive features.

COMMENTS REGARDING CURRENT CAPABILITY

The review of potential computer applications for microcomputer-based systems reveals few current uses that are applicable to the therapist's office practice. In addition, several comments are warranted for those considering implementation of such a system. It is important to note that there are no cost-effectiveness studies that relate the cost of evaluation, installation, maintenance, and service contracts for a micro-computer system to the potential time savings for the therapist. While it may appear that the hourly therapist's fee is substantial enough such that a relatively small time saving would justify the cost, it should be noted that most of the potential applications do not involve tasks that are performed by the therapist. A more appropriate factor to enter into the cost-effectiveness analysis would be secretarial or technician time, since these support personnel would likely be the major users of avail-able application software.

Training time is also a factor that should not be ignored in the de-cision to implement a microcomputer system in the office setting. Al-though most professionals and resource personnel have the capability of becoming successful users, current applications require the develop-ment of a fairly thorough knowledge of the hardware, operating sys-tem, and software. Lack of motivation is a virtual guarantee that the cost of implementation will not be met by sufficient return of invest-ment. To maximize the potential of this technology requires a substan-tial investment in training time, which should also be entered into the cost analysis.

A final point addresses an inherent problem of the single-user, single-tasking systems. It is inevitable that, as the use of such a system proves successful, demand for use will increase to the point where purchase of a second system is required. An example of this might be the case in which an office secretary employs one system virtually full-time for word processing and billing purposes, leaving no access time for psychological testing. This presents a situation in which the cost of a second system can be justified only on the basis of a single appli-cation.

The decision to implement computer technology, given the current status of hardware and software configurations, is a complicated one. It would appear that those therapists who simply see this technology as a panacea for increasing the organizational and managerial sophisti-cation of their offices will meet with no small amount of frustration. For the therapist with a need for a specific application or an interest in the technology of microcomputers and the patience to develop a modi-cum of expertise, the investment in this technology will likely be re-turned with satisfaction.

FUTURE COMPUTER CAPABILITY

Integrated Systems

The review of current computer applications to the therapist's office demonstrated that the market is characterized by piecemeal software programs running on single-user, single-tasking microcomputers. Several shortcomings of this situation have been delineated, but this is an area of technology that sees tremendous changes in very brief periods of time. There are several factors that appear likely to have significant impact on computer applications in the areas of therapists' professional and business activities.

Probably the most important factor lies in the fairly rapid decrease in the cost of multi-user, multi-tasking systems, which have been generally associated with extremely large business and manufacturing settings. Engineering advances have progressed to the point where these systems are now packaged as desk-top minicomputers. As a general description, these are typically 16-bit computers with anywhere from 256 Kb to 4 Mb of main memory and up to 200 Mb of peripheral storage, typically in a Winchester disk format with streamer tape back-up systems. The minicomputer commonly allows 4 to 12 active terminals and 1 to 4 printers to operate simultaneously; thus, it provides a multi-user environment. In addition, the operating systems of minicomputers allow several programs to run simultaneously; that is, these computers are multi-tasking. The obvious advantage to this format is that several different office activities can be supported concurrently with the single computer. Prices for minicomputers have dropped to the range of $12,000 to $20,000. These are not small sums but, for the office with several applications, the cost is quite competitive when measured against the expense of several single-user, single-task microcomputers.

Concomitant with the price and engineering changes that make minicomputers a viable office computer have been attempts to down-size larger operating systems and software packages to fit the office environment. Most of this development has occurred within the larger computer manufacturer's own software development divisions, but significant work has also been accomplished in several public-health settings.

The promise of these software packages is very great since the developmental design of the software has been to look at the total information flow throughout the setting, rather than designing for specific functions within the setting. One obvious advantage of this approach is that it allows complete interaction of all software programs running under the package. These larger systems make it feasible to seriously discuss the suitability of an office information system as opposed to a collection of software programs that address only specific office practice functions.

Finally, advances in telecommunications and the development of large, national data bases mean that access to information of either a professional or business nature will be available via the office computer system. Recent changes in normative data, research advances, continu-

ing education, and electronic mailboxes will provide efficient and essentially effortless access to information that is now gathered only at
the expense of office resources.

In an attempt to describe the full range of features that will be
available in future systems, a large office operation consisting of therapists, secretaries, and technicians is envisioned. Figure 1–1 portrays
the typical applications that would be used by each of the office personnel. The following section details these applications.

Software

Psychological Testing. As opposed to single tests or a limited
number of tests, this software package will contain a full armamen-
tarium of personality, vocational, and intelligence tests as well as specialized interviews. Test "driver" programs will allow the creation of
custom-tailored interviews without requiring knowledge of the
programming language. Algorithms within the package will focus on
key symptoms of the initial intake to generate a comprehensive test/
interview battery for each individual patient. In addition to outputting
raw scores, standard scores, and profiles, the package will generate appropriate normative comparison data, given the patient's demographic
statistics; provide a rough-draft interpretive report for therapist review;
list diagnostic options and treatment plans; and suggest appropriate
tests and time schedules for evaluation of treatment effectiveness. In
addition, programs for projective techniques will allow the technician
to enter raw score data and obtain the same types of output as normative and predictive comparison data. Neuropsychological evaluations
will be administered directly via patient interaction with terminals designed specifically for this task.

Biofeedback. Current technology will be expanded to provide capability to run multiple patients concurrently with the full range of
physiological measures. This program will automatically set and adjust
treatment parameters in an ongoing fashion, present within-session
and across-session statistics, generate group statistics for research purposes, and relate physiological changes to other patient data to assist in
analyzing treatment failures.

Audiovisual Aids. Computer-controlled optical disc recorders will
allow a full range of informational and educational data to be provided,
based on the patient's level of knowledge or skill. These programs
essentially survey the patient's knowledge base, via continuing questionnaire items, and provide audiovisual presentations on material
requiring training. Examples of this application would be programs ex-
plaining vocational opportunities to the job-seeking client or providing
information on the effects of stress on physical symptomatology for the

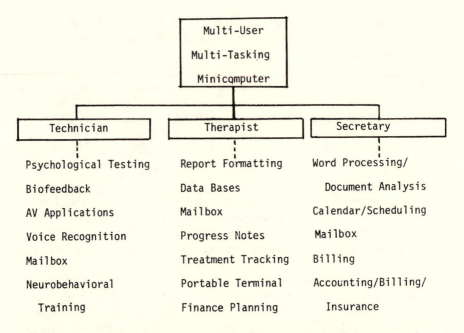

FIGURE 1–1. Typical Computer Applications, by Job, of Office Personnel

patient with a psychosomatic disorder. This technology also has potential interface with systematic desensitization, relaxation training, and biofeedback treatment programs by way of audiovisual information contingent on physiological parameters.

Voice Recognition. A large segment of the population is moving into the older age ranges, which means that therapists will see increasing numbers of physically disabled patients, many of whom will be unable to operate standard terminal keyboards. Voice recognition technology allows the patient to simply provide a verbal response to any item of inquiry on the terminal screen. Applications for blind patients can be programmed by interfacing with a computer-controlled video disc recorder for oral presentation of tests and interviews.

Neurobehavioral Training. One substantial shortcoming of retraining the brain-damaged patient is the arduous, repetitive nature of task drills, which make the manpower cost of this intervention extremely expensive. Programs that control presentation of text and graphic stimuli and record oral and manual responses allow for thorough and inexpensive treatment and provide for sophisticated drill exercises, which bear a close behavioral similarity to real-life requirements. Again, performance data for each session and across sessions are provided, and the program automatically adjusts rate of presentation and rate of movement of stimuli to guarantee a success rate that maintains patient motivation.

Report Formatting. The package will present "report shells," which will automatically insert patient referral data and present sentence and paragraph elements for therapist insertion via single-keystroke commands. The program will contain a format dictionary for common referral problems and high-base-rate diagnostic impressions. An example would be a report summarizing the results of an intellectual evaluation of a client referred by a state agency for disability assessment. For more complex reports, this program presents a "shell" which essentially guides the therapist's dictation to insure a comprehensive and detailed answer to the referral question.

Data Bases. Most therapists are familiar with computer-generated library searches, such as Med Line, which are basically bibliographic data bases. The office computer will allow access via telemodem to a wide variety of data bases, which will provide information to support several different office activities. Access to normative data for special populations will allow more precise diagnostic conclusions. Literature searches and monthly review of journal releases will be able to be accomplished directly from office terminals. Listings of continuing education activities and even continuing education course-work will be available. Management of office finances will be facilitated by constant availability of interest rate and finance market information.

Financial Planning. Spreadsheet programs, which access the office accounting data and data bases for financial information, will allow sophisticated control of cash flow and produce detailed alternatives for solutions to questions involving short- and long-term investments and their tax consequences for both office and personal fiscal planning.

Progress Notes. This program provides a format for therapist dictation of therapy progress notes. Key indicators derived from the initial evaluation provide treatment progress indicators, which can be addressed in the progress notes.

Treatment Tracking. This program interacts with the initial evaluation and progress notes to schedule routine assessment with formal tests in order to provide reliable measures of change as a result of therapy. In one sense, this is a computer-generated audit system, which informs the therapist of the efficacy of the treatment plan in a reliable manner and facilitates knowledgeable changes in treatment strategy.

Portable Terminal. The advent of small, lightweight terminals that include a flat-panel CRT will provide a terminal that is portable and can be used by the therapist at home via a simple telemodem hookup. These terminals will also allow the therapist to extend the office applications program to settings outside the office. One example of this capability is hospital consultation. In the hospital setting, the therapist can obtain the same intake, interview, and test data as in the office. Data analyses are then completed by telemodem hookup through a hospital phone to the office. The therapist obtains reduced data immediately and is able to provide more sophisticated hospital consultations without returning to the office. Consultation with office attorneys and accountants can also be facilitated by the portable terminal. Business meetings in the practice accountant's office can be much more productive with instant access to the therapist's accounting information.

Word Processing/Document Analysis. In addition to providing the features of word-processing programs that are currently available, these programs will provide full editorial capability to allow deletion and insertion of sections of documents from existing ones. A program that verifies each word of a document will insure spelling accuracy and also provide synonyms for often-repeated words to avoid stilted flow of phrasing within the document. A communication analysis program will review documents for clarity and ease of readability to maximize the communication to the intended reader.

Calendar/Scheduling. This program operates as an automated month-at-a-glance calendar. It allows the workday to be designated by hourly appointments or by any fraction of an hour for each member of the office. Scheduling is accomplished by single-keystroke commands for next available appointment, appointments for specific days and time of day, and automatic scheduling of repeated appointments. The program provides analyses to examine workload flow through the office so that the most efficient scheduling of office staff and space can be accomplished.

Accounting. This program organizes and maintains all financial data for the office. It operates a ledger card for each patient, which instantly updates all services delivered by type and amount of fee and it records all credits to the patient account. Account balances are therefore always current. Office payables are tracked by individual payees, and outstanding balances, due dates, and payment histories are maintained. Office payroll is automatically computed, with maintenance of all data pertaining to deductions. The program maintains a daily ledger and cumulative ledger so that transactions can be analyzed by any time period requested. Statistics and graphics components of the program allow for detailed analysis of workload and financial return against specific clinical activities by source of referral, type of patient, and type of treatment. This program interacts with the financial spreadsheet program to allow the therapist to examine options for reallocation of office resources or determine investment strategies. The program provides automated bills, generates completed master insurance forms, and generates monthly statements for all patients.

Mailbox. This program operates a mail system within the office environment. At the touch of a key, an office staff member has access not only to his calendar, but also to a terminal "message board," which displays telephone messages, interoffice notes, and changes in the daily schedule. The mailbox program provides a log for office communications for future recapture and works to increase office efficiency.

CONCLUSION

The impact of developments in computer technology on the practice of psychotherapy is likely to occur more quickly and in a more significant fashion than is widely appreciated by the community of clinicians today. It is probably the case that, while this technology provides a solution to the increasing variety of skills required of the therapist, it also requires to some extent another area of knowledge that the therapist will need to acquire. Even though the office information system of the future will be substantially easier to manage from the user's standpoint, it can be anticipated that there will be some resistance on the part of the clinician to use these highly technical tools to support the very private and complex activity of assessment and therapy. A key question in this regard is the unknown effect of this technology on the practice of therapy per se. From the standpoint that this technology provides a solution to the routine, repetitive activities of the therapist and to the reduction of raw data into interpretable form, it offers the potential to free the therapist to focus even more intensely on those endeavors for which the therapist is uniquely trained: the treatment and care of the patient's psychological self.

2 Analysis of the Information Needs of a Private Practice

Joseph Zefran, MSW

In 1902 Sigmund Freud began a minor revolution in the science of human behavior; in 1974, the small computer began a minor revolution in the science of information management. Just as psychotherapy was made possible through the work of Dr. Freud, the small computer was made possible through development of a technology that is one of the world's oldest: ceramics. The silicon chip, made from sand, has quite literally allowed computers to be sold "dirt cheap." The revolutionary aspect of Freud's work did not arise so much from a new burst of knowledge; knowledge of human behavior existed before Freud. Rather, the Freudian revolution arose from the fact that knowledge of human behavior could be used in new ways and for a wider group of people. In the same way, the revolutionary aspect of the small computer is that the power of the computer is now available to be used in new ways and for a wider group of people: the individual in the home, the small business owner, and professionals including those in the private practice of psychotherapy.

The small computer may be ready for a whole new group of users, but are the new users ready for the small computer? For most of the new group of users, owning and using a computer will be a new experience; this may be especially true for the human-services professionals. Nevertheless, virtually everyone today has had some form of experience with computers. Widespread use of computers, primarily by large organizations, has been the norm for the past two decades. For many, experience with computers has had negative connotations— bills received are computerized, getting a computer error corrected may have been difficult, and the volume of computerized junk mail may have been overwhelming. For those in the human services, computers may seem too impersonal and lacking in creativity and humanness. For psychotherapists considering the purchase and use of the computer, there is fear of the unknown and perhaps a fear of "getting burned"; these are feelings similar to those of the first-time home buyer or of a reluctant client entering therapy.

BENEFITS OF THE SMALL COMPUTER

In spite of the negatives, thousands of new users have "taken the plunge" and purchased a small computer, including psychotherapists and others in the human-services professions. Evidence of this phenomenon is seen in the recent publication of a newsletter for human service professionals, the *CUSS (Computer Users in the Social Services) Network Newsletter*. The newsletter was established to provide a way to network the new group of human services professionals who are now using computers. The humorous acronym CUSS was chosen to describe the response of human-service computer users to those occasions when things do not quite work as planned.

There is a reason why the small computer industry has grown from one which grossed only a few thousand dollars eight years ago to one which grossed nearly $2 billion this year. The reason is simply because the small computer can do it better. Information can be handled more easily and at less cost. A small computer can help to meet the increasing demand for information; one small computer that costs approximately the same per month as the salary of a clerical person can handle the work of three to five people. With the aid of a computer, a person can more readily provide information that is complete (all that is needed for management and planning); accurate (information free of random error); timely (information when it is most needed); concise (only that information which is needed); and relevant (only the information which is most vital and necessary). Furthermore, the use of the small computer for gathering and processing information has unique advantages over manual methods of information management. Not only does the computer handle tasks that people find repetitive and boring, but it can also perform tasks that simply cannot be done without a computer. Some of these complex uses are exotic, such as guiding a spacecraft; most, however, are more down to earth, such as the simultaneous analysis of multiple characteristics of human behavior and human interaction.

The reason one would use a computer for gathering and processing information is much like the reason one would choose a jet plane to travel across the United States. Although several modes of transportation are available (hiking, biking, traveling by car), it makes little sense to walk when one can fly—unless, of course, one wants the trip to be an adventure and not just a trip. So too with the gathering and processing of information; when one needs to know more than was known before, it makes little sense to "walk when one can fly."

For the psychotherapist in private practice, the benefits of the small computer are enticing. The information needs of the typical private psychotherapy practice are increasing. Information is needed for third-party insurance payments, for taxes and payroll, for liability matters, for individual and collective client records, for scoring of test results, for planning future personnel needs, and so on.

As one who is foreign to the world of computers and information technology, the psychotherapist may feel bewildered, confused, and may need to know the answers to many questions. How can a small computer help my private practice? How do I decide what computer to buy? How do I make the computer gather and produce the information I need? Where do I begin?

Answers to these questions can be arrived at through a process not unlike psychotherapy itself—the information system development process. Just as psychotherapy begins with an analysis and assessment of the client's psychological needs, the system development process begins with an analysis of information needs. The psychotherapy process proceeds to helping the client discover and design new ways to meet his or her psychological needs; the information system development process proceeds to the design of a system of gathering, processing, and producing information. Psychotherapy concludes with the successful integration of new attitudes and patterns of behavior; information system development concludes with the installation of a new, successful information system.

ROLE, PURPOSE, AND NATURE OF INFORMATION

Before describing the information system development process, some basic concepts concerning the role, purpose, and nature of information should be understood.

There are three elements essential to all human activity: energy, materials, and information. People need information to operate some sort of enterprise (household, club, small business, or a private practice) and to make decisions necessary to achieve the goals of the enterprise. The quality of operations and decisions is dependent upon the quality of the information used to inform those operations and decisions. Quality information is that which is accurate, timely, complete, concise, and relevant.

All information consists of data. Data are unorganized bits of knowledge. For data to be transformed into information, data must be arranged (or processed) in an ordered, meaningful, and useful way; hence, the term *data processing*. The purpose of data processing is to evaluate and organize data so that useful information is produced, information that is needed to operate an enterprise and to make decisions to achieve the goals of the enterprise. An information system is nothing more than a specific data-processing application; that is, a systematic way to collect and process data to produce needed information. Information systems can be entirely manual, as are nearly all systems in private psychotherapy practice. However, as some psychotherapists have already discovered, computers can be very beneficial in processing data to produce information needed in their practice.

The typical office of a private psychotherapy practice is a good example of how an information system works. In this office is a secretary, a desk with a calculator and telephone, and a file cabinet containing drawers, file folders, and paper. In this typical office, data elements (client name, address, phone, presenting problem) are received through the telephone and entered by the secretary onto a sheet of paper. The secretary stores the paper in a labeled file folder, which is stored in a labeled file drawer. In some cases, the secretary may use the calculator to produce other data elements (number of visits, balance due). When information is needed for a report, the secretary searches through the file drawers and file folders, finds the relevant papers with the help of the drawer and folder labels, and rearranges the data elements into useful information produced on the report. Thus, it can be seen that an information system, whether manual or computerized, is simply a way of gathering data (input), storing and/or manipulating data (processing), and producing information (output).

Another important information concept is that of the *data base*. In the same way that a file cabinet serves as an integral part of the office described above, a data base serves as an integral part of a computerized information system. A data base is a collection of stored data used for an application of some particular enterprise. Both data base and file cabinet provide an organized way to store data; that is, they have a *storage structure*. Both are organized to provide a means of retrieving data to produce useful information; that is, they have an *access strategy*. The file cabinet contains data items written on pieces of paper placed into labeled file folders, which are placed into labeled file drawers. A data base consists of *data fields*, which are groups of alphabetic and/or numeric characters comprising a data item (for example, a client's phone number consists of 10 numeric characters). The data fields are organized into *data records*, which are a collection of data fields (for example, all data specific to one client). Data records are organized into *data files*, which are a collection of data records (for example, all records for all clients). A collection of several data files is organized and comprises the data base (for example, all the data needed to operate the private practice).

Just as the secretary may use the data in the file cabinet for many purposes, a data base is described as *integrated* because it contains data for many uses and, at times, involving many users. The term *integrated data base* has three basic implications: (1) One user or application may be concerned with only a small portion of the data base (for example, the caseload of a particular therapist); (2) There are parts of the data base (for example, client file, billing file, accounts payable file); and (3) There is a relationship among those parts (for example, accounts payable relates to the general ledger book).

One of the primary advantages in developing a computerized information system is that it allows one to structure a computerized data base. A computerized data base has many advantages over a manual data base (that is, a file cabinet). Since the computer operates by means of electronic impulses, which travel at the speed of light, electronic processing of data is much quicker than manual processing. This speed enhances the ability of a data base to provide centralized control of the data used to produce information. For example, the computer can search several different files to produce whatever information is desired by the manager of the private practice. With a computerized data base, redundancy is reduced: one entry of certain data elements can be copied to different files. Inconsistency can be avoided: similar data items can be standardized for easier processing. Data can be shared while privacy and security can be more easily maintained. For example, individual therapists can be allowed access only to their particular cases; however, a supervisor can be allowed access to the cases of all supervisees. Finally, greater accuracy can be maintained. For example, the computer can be instructed to accept only correctly formatted information and to notify the user of errors.

INFORMATION SYSTEM DEVELOPMENT PROCESS

The information system development process is a logical, step-by-step method of analyzing, designing, and installing any information system—manual or computerized. The steps described below apply to the development of any information system; however, they will be discussed in terms of developing an information system in a private psychotherapy practice that would incorporate the use of a small computer.

The information system development process consists of seven major phases:

1. Analysis of goals and operations;
2. Analysis of information needs;

3. Design of the new information system;
4. Identification of data items and reports;
5. Design of the data base;
6. Installation of the new system; and
7. Evaluation of the system.

Within each of the seven phases, there are certain tasks that need to be done before proceeding to the next phase. These tasks are described below; we include examples useful in a typical private psychotherapy practice.

Before describing the actual phases and tasks involved in the information system development process, there are four important points that pertain to the process as a whole. First, as the phases and tasks of the process are described, it will become evident that the process does require some work. But the work need only be as simple or as complex as the information needs of the private practice itself. Developing an information system for a small practice will be easier and simpler than for a larger, multiservice practice. On the other hand, according to the proverb, "a stitch in time saves nine," the work spent in development of the information system will usually save a greater amount of wasted effort once the information system is operating. Whether the practice be small or large, it is suggested that written notes be made on the results of all the tasks completed for each phase; sample formats for notes on some of the phases will be provided below. Second, it should be noted that the information system development process applies to all aspects of the information system for any private practice; that is, the process applies to both manual and computerized aspects. Third, in a private practice where more than one person is involved in some aspect of the information system, it is strongly suggested that ideas and input be solicited from all employees involved. This is especially important, because the new information system will affect those employees in some way and because failure to involve employees increases the likelihood of later problems. Employees who are asked to do the work of collecting, storing, or processing data and producing information are far more likely to do a better job of it if they receive and perceive benefits from it. Finally, it is very important that *all* steps in each phase be completed. The reason for this is quite simple. Information systems are successful when all tasks are completed; systems are usually failures when some tasks are omitted.

Phase 1: Analysis of the Goals and Operations

If the goals and operations of the practice have already been carefully considered, the four tasks involved in Phase 1 should be easily completed. The four tasks are described below.

1. Description of the current goals of the practice and the goals for the near future. As a helpful first step in formulating the goals, a listing could be made of all specific services provided by the practice as well as the operations involved in their performance. For example, a goal of service might be to provide therapy to families with acting-out teenagers. An operational goal might be to provide service by appointment only, in the office, and on a regular schedule. Another goal, one that is obvious but often overlooked, would be to provide an income for the employees of the practice.

2. Description of the internal structure of the practice; that is, a description of the employees (including credentials, titles, duties, functions, and hours of employment) and the manner in which they interact. This type of information may be gathered from job descriptions, funding proposals, and possibly from an organizational chart.

3. Description of the external relationships of the practice. This includes descriptions of specific clientele being served; sources of referral; consulting professionals; association memberships; licensing agencies; insurance companies; office equipment suppliers; advertising (phone directory, information and referral directories); and so on. Even in a one-person practice, these external relationships can be very extensive.

4. Analysis of specific requirements and constraints, both from within and without, which have impact on the practice. Examples of these include legal requirements (licensing, liability coverage); financial constraints (overhead, tax laws, timing of payment); and time limitations (service time, case planning time, business hours).

After arriving at a basic understanding of the goals and operations of the practice, the information needs of the practice can be more easily determined.

Phase 2: Analysis of Information Needs

The analysis of information needs can be accomplished by answering five basic questions. They are listed below. The results of this analysis can be listed on a 5-column form similar to the sample form presented in Table 2–1.

1. What kinds of information are needed to achieve the goals of the practice and to maintain its operations? To answer the question, it is helpful to begin by identifying and listing the different functional areas of the practice and the specific kinds of information needed in each area. For example, intake information would include client demographic information, source and manner of referral, psychological characteristics, source of payment, and so on. The personnel area would require employee demographic information, qualifications, salary information, and so on.

TABLE 2–1. Sample List of Information Needs

Type of Information	Who Needs It	Why Needed	When Needed	Requirements/ Constraints
Client Info.				
Demographic	Practice manager	Planning	Monthly	None
	Therapist	Treatment	As needed	None
Psychological characteristics	Therapist and supervisor	Treatment	Weekly	Confidential to therapist
Payment info.	Secretary	Billing	On demand, monthly	Confidential to client and practice
	Accountant	Accounting	Monthly, yearly	IRS, state tax laws
Personnel Info.	Manager	Personnel relations	On demand	Manager only
	Payroll clerk	Payroll	Twice monthly	Required deductions

2. Who needs the information? Those needing information would include the employees within the practice, listed by title or duties (that is, manager, supervisor, therapists, secretary), as well as persons or organizations outside the practice (referring therapists, insurance companies, accountant, etc.).

3. Why is the information needed? The reason a particular kind of information is needed forms the justification for collecting and producing that information. Information may be needed to perform a specific function, to make a vital decision, or to plan for the future. For example, information on client characteristics is needed to formulate an individualized treatment plan; source-of-payment information is needed for billing, accounting, and tax purposes.

4. When is the information needed? The timeliness of the information is important in determining how the information should be collected and processed. Billing information may be needed immediately for producing a statement following a session, or it may be needed monthly for insurance reimbursement.

5. Are there any constraints or requirements regarding the information? What degree of security is necessary? Considerations about information constraints and requirements are necessary to ensure that vital, required information is collected and to avoid potential legal difficulties. For example, certain kinds of information may be required for accrediting bodies, licensing agencies, or liability insurance companies. Listing information governed by therapist-client confidentiality laws may help to avoid lawsuits from clients or may help to limit those offi-

cials trying to force disclosure of confidential information. Because confidentiality issues are important in the private practice of psychotherapy, security needs must be specifically addressed. This involves the level of security necessary and the manner in which security will be maintained. Security can be handled procedurally (that is, procedures to limit dispersal of information), or it can be handled physically (that is, physical restraints to limit access to information). When a computer is used, security can be maintained by limiting access through the use of secret passwords. The monitoring of security procedures, and other security issues regarding sanctions for violation of security must be considered.

Once the analysis of information needs is completed, the work of designing a new, more useful information system can begin.

Phase 3: Design of the New Information System

The next step in the information system development process is to construct a conceptual, systematic design of the flow of information that will adequately meet the needs of the practice. There are four tasks involved in Phase 3. They are discussed below.

1. Determine the performance criteria of the new system; that is, how accurate, timely, complete, concise, and relevant does the information need to be and what are the procedures for identifying and correcting errors? Drawing upon the work done in Phase 2, each of the above criteria can be determined by reviewing the list of the type of information needed. For example, accuracy of accounting and payroll information is very important, timeliness of client progress reports and billing is important, completeness of diagnostic reports is important, and so on.

2. Identify alternative ways to maximize the flow of information (that is, the collection, storage, processing, and retrieval of information). Ideas for several alternative designs may be obtained through discussions with other psychotherapists in private practice who have well-developed information systems; through attendance at human-service information-system seminars; or through reading articles and books. Perhaps the best way to construct alternative designs is through the hiring of a human-service/information-system consultant who has been recommended by others. Indeed, this is the first point in the information system development process where an expert may be helpful not only with the task itself, but also as a consultant on the information system work done by the staff of the private practice.

After the various alternative designs are identified, each alternative should then be evaluated, using the performance criteria that were decided upon in the preceding step. The decision on the best alternative is then made on the criterion of cost-effectiveness. First, the costs of the current system should be tallied; that is, what is being spent for supplies, equipment, and the proportion of professional and secretarial staff time spent in information system work. Table 2–2 is a worksheet for figuring the cost of items that are commonly incurred in a manual information system. Second, general cost estimates (not actual, specific costs) of all alternative information systems should be gathered. Table 2–3 contains a worksheet for recording the general cost estimates of at least three new alternatives that would include the use of a small computer. The choice of the best alternative is made in favor of the one that would be better able to meet the current and near-future needs of the practice while, at the same time, being the one that

TABLE 2–2. Worksheet for Figuring Monthly Costs of a Manual Information System

Item Description	Costs per month	
	Item Costs	Total Costs
1. Staff Time (for clerical work)		
(a) Professional Staff Time		
Staff Salary x % Clerical Work Time =	$_____	
($_____ x __._____ = $_____)		
(b) Clerical Staff Time	$_____	
(c) Other Staff Time Costs	$_____	
Subtotal Staff Costs		$_____
2. Office Equipment*		
(a) Typewriter(s)	$_____	
(b) Copy Machine(s)	$_____	
(c) Dictating Machines	$_____	
(d) Calculators	$_____	
(e) File Cabinets, etc.	$_____	
(f) Other Equipment Costs (insurance, maintenance, other equipment)	$_____	
Subtotal Equipment Costs		$_____
3. Office Supplies		
(a) Desk Supplies (staplers, pens, calendars)	$_____	
(b) Machine Supplies (ribbons, recording tapes, batteries, etc.)	$_____	
(c) Paper Supplies (paper, cards, folders)	$_____	
(d) Printing	$_____	
(e) Other Supply Costs	$_____	
Subtotal Supply Costs		$_____
TOTAL INFORMATION SYSTEM COSTS (per month)		$_____

*Monthly costs of equipment can be figured by using the monthly leasing payment amount or by using 1/60 of the purchase price (assuming 5-year equipment life) and adding monthly maintenance costs.

TABLE 2–3. Worksheet for Estimating Costs of Information System Alternatives

Item Description	Sample Figures*	Alternative A	Alternative B	Alternative C
Hardware Costs				
Computer	$7,000			
Printer	3,000			
Other (Modem, Terminals)	200			
(Less tax savings,				
5-year depreciation)	−5,916			
Subtotal (after-tax)				
hardware costs	($4,284)			
Software Costs				
System software,				
program language	-0-			
Application software	3,000			
Modifications	200			
Subtotal software costs	($3,200)			
Other Costs				
Consultant	3,000			
Installation (site				
preparation, training)	200			
Insurance	400			
Subtotal other costs	($3,600)			
TOTAL INITIAL COSTS OF AUTOMATED PART OF SYSTEM	($11,084)			
Total Monthly Costs				
over 5 years (÷ by 60)	185			
Monthly Maintenance	60			
Automation Supplies	50			
TOTAL MONTHLY COST OF AUTOMATED SYSTEM	$ 295			
Total Monthly Cost of Manual Part of New System**	$3,240			
TOTAL MONTHLY COST OF ENTIRE NEW SYSTEM	$3,535			
Difference in Costs of New System vs. Old System (savings [−] added costs [+])	−$65			

*The sample figures are rough estimates of a highly automated system for a small practice (4 therapists, 2 clerical staff, 100 clients).
**Monthly cost of manual part of new system includes the cost of the current system plus/minus costs of staff, equipment, and supplies required/replaced by the automated part of the entire new information system. In this example, it was estimated that monthly cost of current system was $3,600; savings were 10% ($360); ($3,600 − $360 = $3,240).

would be lower, the same, or slightly higher in cost than the current system.

3. Draw a diagram of the new information system. The diagram should identify the sources of each kind of information (input from clients, referral source, employees, etc.); the actions performed with the information (processing by employees and others); and the form in which the information will be used (output of information and reports). The diagram can be in rough-sketch form or in a formal flow chart. Before constructing the diagram or flow chart, the listing completed in Phase 2 should be reviewed for what output is needed and then for what input and processing is needed to produce that output. For example, the diagram, or flow chart, would begin with the actions involved when a client is first referred and first visits the office. After intake information is taken, the diagram would show the resulting actions and flow of intake information (client's assignment to a therapist, data entries to the billing system, formulation of the treatment plan, and so on).

4. Determine the parts of the new information system that will be handled manually and the parts that will be handled by the computer. In order to maximize the computer's unique capabilities (speed, memory capacity, interactional data base), those parts of the information system that involve the structure and storage of larger amounts of data, the searching and sorting of records, and other tasks involving repetition or requiring speedy response should be considered to have the most potential for computerization. For example, in a private practice employing 3 therapists each serving 20 clients, it may be best to do the personnel/payroll functions manually but to computerize the client information and accounts receivable areas. In the first instance, since there are only three employees, computerizing payroll has very little advantage over manual methods. In the second instance, the large amount of data for clients and family members, repetitiveness of billing procedures, and the need to search records for compiling reports can be more efficiently handled by the computer.

After the design of the overall information system is completed, the next phase involves the completion of detailed work in listing data items and designing the formats of forms and reports.

Phase 4: Identification of Data Items and Reports

Although the work of compiling a detailed list of data items is about as enjoyable as doing a process recording, it is an important task because the data items comprise the raw materials necessary to produce information. The listing of data items is most easily accomplished by filling out a "Data Item Description Form," like the one presented in Table 2–4. The form contains thirteen categories, each category providing some information about the data item and its relationship to other parts of the information system. The thirteen categories are explained below.

1. *ID Number*: an arbitrarily assigned number that provides a useful way to identify data items, especially for cross-referencing.
2. *Name*: a title that is descriptive of the data item.
3. *Description*: a brief description of what the data item represents.
4. *Purpose*: an explanation of all the ways the item is used, including the title of the person(s) using it and whether the item is used as input (designated with an "I"), for processing ("P"), or as output ("O"). If it is an input item, the source, form, and manner of input will be noted in the next category, "Source." If a processing item, the type of processing (that is, arithmetic, sorting, etc.) should be

TABLE 2–4. Sample Data Item Description Form

ID Number	1	2	3
Name			
Description			
Purpose			
Source			
Processing			
Reporting			
Values			
Edit Criteria			
Length			
Relationships			
Volatility			
History Requirements			

noted in Category 6, Processing. If an output item, the report or output form on which it will appear will be noted in Category 7, Reporting.

5. *Source*: the source, form, and manner of input of the item is listed along with the person(s) responsible for the entry and updating of the item.

6. *Processing*: the type of process that is used to create the item or the processing for which the item is used. It is also helpful to record the ID numbers of the other items that this item is processed with as well as the person(s) who will do the processing.

7. *Reporting*: a listing of the reports or output forms on which the item will appear and the person responsible for compiling the report. It is helpful to record the identifying number of each report on which the item appears, as explained in the report description section below.

8. *Values*: a list of the codes used for the item. These may be descriptive words or characters; the characters can be either alphabetic or numeric. If the values of the item are to be entered into the computer, it is recommended that the values be numeric; the use of numeric values, instead of alphabetic ones, helps increase the computer's efficiency in terms of storage space and searching speed.

9. *Edit Criteria*: usually used for items entered into the computer. The term *edit criteria* refers to the criteria (or rules, instructions) given to the computer to "edit" the item. That is, it may be desirable, in the interests of greater accuracy, to specify a certain range of values or type of characters that are the only ones possible for this item; the computer can then be instructed to indicate to the user when any unspecified values occur. For example, if the edit criteria for the item "Client Sex" are specified as only *M* or *F*, the computer will prevent the attempt to enter any other erroneous characters; it will only allow a correct value to be entered.

10. *Length*: the exact number, or maximum number, of characters to be used for the item. This is especially important for items to be computerized, because the computer must be instructed as to the exact amount of storage space to be used for a record or file.

11. *Relationships*: the way in which this item is affected by or affects other items, reports, or general types of information. The use of item and report ID numbers is helpful here.

12. *Volatility*: the frequency of the data item's usage. When necessary, some note should be made about how often the item is used, updated, or entered. For example, an item that is used frequently may be more prone to error; this may be important if the accuracy of the item is important.

13. *History Requirements*: the length of retention of the item. The data

associated with the item may only need to be kept for a certain length of time. Whether the item is handled manually or by the computer, this item is helpful in the elimination or differential handling of outdated information.

Following the completion of the detailed listing of data items, the next step is to complete a similar listing of the reports generated by the information system. Each report should be described separately; a sample "Report Description Form" is presented in Table 2–5. There are fourteen descriptive categories relating to each report or each form containing output as follows:

1. *ID Number*: an arbitrarily assigned identifying number.
2. *Name*: the title of the report or output form.
3. *Purpose*: the reasons why the report is produced and/or the ways in which the report is to be used.
4. *Writer*: the person(s) responsible for compiling the report.
5. *Users*: the person(s) who will be receiving and using the report.
6. *Medium*: the medium on which the report will be produced; that is, whether the report will be on paper, special forms, computer paper, computer screen, and so on.

TABLE 2–5. Sample Report Description Form

ID Number:
Name:
Purpose:
Writer:
Users:
Medium:
Number of Copies:
Frequency:
Content:
Sources:
Priority:
Sample Format (see attached):
Accuracy Requirements:
Consequences of No Report:

7. *Number of Copies*: the number of total copies to be made as well as the specific number of copies to each report user.
8. *Frequency*: the frequency, dates, or time of day when the reports should be delivered. For some reports, it may be helpful to indicate when the compilation of the report should begin.
9. *Content*: a list of the data items (by ID numbers) that are to appear on the report. The list should also indicate how the data items are to be organized on the report.
10. *Sources*: a list of the sources from which the data items will be gathered.
11. *Priority*: a note to indicate the relative importance of the report in the overall information system of the practice. For example, the billing "report" may be listed as "Top Priority" because the practice would go bankrupt without it.
12. *Sample Format*: graphic design of what the report should look like. Some considerations in the graphic design of the report are: a) size of report (size of paper, number of pages); b) readability (reader's eye can easily follow items in correct order); c) spacing (not too crowded); d) self-evident items (requested information for item requires little or no supplementary instruction); and e) flexibility (items can easily be added, changed, or deleted to meet future demands).
13. *Accuracy Requirements*: some notes on the importance of accuracy of the report as a whole or of specific data items on the report.
14. *Consequences of No Report*: some notes about what would happen if the report is not produced. This may include notes on the effect on operations and decisions, on sanctions against those failing to produce the report, or on alternative actions that will need to be taken until the report can be completed.

Following the completion of the detailed listing of data items and reports, the final phase in the design of the new information system can be performed.

Phase 5: Design of the Data Base

The importance of data base design arises from the important, crucial role that a data base occupies in an information system. As previously defined, a data base is a collection of stored data used in one or more applications; it is the central part of the information system, relating to all the other parts. The two main features of the data base (its storage structure and its access strategy) suggest the two major tasks involved in the design of the data base.

The first major task is determination of the storage structure of the data base. This task involves the grouping together of each and every file that will be part of the new system; for example, the personnel file, the payroll file, and the accounts-payable file are grouped together because they share data items. After all the files are grouped together, specific data items are then grouped under each file that they are connected to. This can be easily done by reviewing the Data Item Description List. When a data item is found to be common to more than one file, it is likely that the item can be entered once and recorded by the computer in the files to which it is connected. The end result of the tasks described above will be a data base that is structured to store various data items logically grouped into files that are, in turn, logically grouped together.

The second major task involved in the design of a data base is the determination of the access strategy. In addition to the logical structuring of the contents of the data base, some decisions need to be made concerning rules and procedures for the following:

1. The timing and manner of making additions, changes, and deletions of the data (that is, considerations regarding input);
2. The use of specific data items for sorting, searching, and computational procedures (that is, considerations regarding processing);
3. The timing and manner of producing reports and other forms of output (that is, output considerations);
4. The security measures needed to control access to the data (that is, whether security should be procedural, physical, or internal to the computer, using passwords);
5. The strategy for backup and recovery of data in the event of loss of data due to computer malfunction, fire, flood, or other causes; and
6. Procedures for the correction of errors in the data.

The tasks involved in designing a data base probably seem to be the most technical part of the information system development process; data base design is the most technical phase because it is most closely related to computerization and because it is the most difficult. The most difficult part of setting up a completely manual office information system is organizing the file drawers and file folders so that the information is easily accessible.

Because a knowledge of computers is helpful in the design of the data base, it is suggested that a human-services computer expert be consulted or, at least, that several computer software products be looked at. Computer software are the prewritten computer programs that contain the actual instructions that "tell" the computer to do the tasks that one wants the computer to perform. Fortunately for the new computer user, one of the major benefits of the small computer revolution is that more and more prewritten software is available and that the software is increasingly easy to use, even by the novice user. Because a data base is a very common part of any information system, there are many easy-to-use data base management software packages available. These data base software packages may already have features that will be of great help with the tasks involved in designing the data base. For example, many data base software packages have built-in methods for input, processing, and output procedures, as well as built-in methods for security and backup procedures.

Phase 6: Installing the New Information System

The ultimate objective of the work performed during the first five phases of the information system development process is to prepare for the installation of the new information system. Just as the thorough preparation of the first five phases is essential to the success of the information system, a thorough and carefully planned installation is also essential. The major steps for the successful installation of the new information system are briefly presented in the sample timetable in Table 2–6 in the section below. The steps involved in installation will likely be performed, in whole or in part, by an expert in information systems and computers. Such an expert may be an individual consultant or an employee of the vendor (that is, the company from which the computer and/or the software was purchased).

Installing a new information system involves nine different steps:

1. Purchase of Software, Computer, and Computer Equipment. Most likely, the new information system has been designed to use a computer. But, as previously mentioned, purchasing a computer for the private practice is not quite as simple as some advertising would suggest. Although the computer itself is the major, visible component of the computer system, the software is by far the most important. Consequently, the software should be selected first.

There are three basic types of software—system software, applications software, and programming language. System software are prewritten programs that are internally stored in the computer and provide centralized control of all or several other programs. The two main types of system software are the *operating system* (usually included in the purchase price of the computer itself) and the *data base manager* (usually purchased separately). Applications software are prewritten programs that instruct the computer to perform specific kinds of tasks (for example, accounts payable/receivable, payroll, mailing lists, etc.). A programming language consists of symbols and characters whose

TABLE 2-6. Sample Installation Timetable

	Month 1	Month 2	Month 3	Month 4	Month 5	Month 6
1. Purchase Computer						
2. Design Reports						
3. Install Software						
4. Initial Testing						
5. Prepare Parallel						
6. Train Personnel						
7. Parallel Testing						
8. Notice of Installation						
9. Installed!						

use is governed by grammatical rules; it is similar to any other written or spoken language. A programming language allows a programmer to transmit instructions to the computer so that the computer can perform the tasks for which it has been designed to perform. A programming language is necessary to write individualized programs that cannot be purchased in prewritten form; some version of a language is often included with the computer.

Once the software is selected, the computer itself is chosen along with its related hardware components or, as they are called, the computer peripherals. Computer peripherals are the printers (letter-quality or dot-matrix types), additional terminals, additional storage devices (tape or disk drives not part of the computer), telephone connectors (modems), and so on.

The purchase of software and hardware can be a risky undertaking for the new computer user. In order to avoid the risks (that is, buying less than is needed at the right price or buying what is needed at too high a price), the following suggestions should be followed. First, a careful search should be made for a single vendor who is able not only to sell both software and hardware but is also able to support them for at least five years after purchase. Consultation with human-service/computer experts or with other private practitioners who have computers is recommended. Second, the purchase contract should contain, in clearly understood language, the following three items: exact costs of both hardware and software, warranties on both hardware and software (including what is not covered), and specifications of all other services to be performed by the vendor. These items are necessary in order to avoid any future unanticipated costs, should the vendor's products fail to perform in the manner desired and expected.

2. Final Design of New Forms and Reports. The design and graphic layout of any new forms for the collection and processing of information should be finalized at this point. The formats and layouts of reports and other forms of output (that is, mailing labels, form letters, billing statements) should also be finalized. These forms and reports should be designed in accordance with that specified in the previous two phases.

3. Installing Software and Writing Programs. The major task in installation is to, literally, sit down at the computer and install the software (according to the instructions provided) and, if necessary, to modify the software and/or write any special programs that may also be needed. This task will, and should, probably be performed by a person skilled in computer programming.

4. Initial Testing. After the computer programs are installed and written, they should be tested with sample data that represent all foreseeable possibilities in normal operations and exceptional situations. Completeness in the sample data should result in detecting nearly all the problems and errors that may arise in the functioning of the new information system.

5. Preparation for Parallel Testing. Following the initial testing, the new information system should be tested with real data. This means that the new information system should run in parallel to the current information system. Preparation for parallel testing includes the writing of procedures for employees to follow, the printing of a small number of forms, and the ordering of supplies.

6. Training of Personnel. The final task in preparation for parallel testing is the training of everyone involved in the operation of the new information system. Those who will collect and process data will need to learn new procedures; those who receive reports will need to learn how to use them in the most beneficial way.

7. Parallel Testing. Although parallel testing will involve a duplication of effort by those employed by the practice, it is the best method of ensuring that the new information system is working exactly as planned and producing the information desired. Parallel testing should take place over a 2- to 3-month period at least or longer if necessary. If it is discovered that some minor modifications need to be made, the parallel testing should continue for at least one month after the last change is made.

8. Notice of Installation Date. When the new information system is working satisfactorily, notice of the first date of its operation should be

given to the employees of the practice and to any persons outside the practice (clients, referral agencies, suppliers, etc.).

9. Installation of the New Information System. The information system development process is virtually over. All the work performed can now come to fruition. The only two remaining steps are to: (1) enjoy the benefits of the new, successful information system, and (2) to evaluate the performance of the system, from time to time, for any enhancements or modifications that may need to be made.

Phase 7: Evaluation of the Information System

Periodic evaluation is a simple, but often neglected, phase of the information system development process. The reason for it is simply that things change; people change (at least a therapist believes they do) and situations change.

For new information systems, evaluations should occur for the first few months of operation. After the initial period of operation, evaluations need only occur once or twice a year to ensure that the information system is meeting the information needs of the practice. Not only do information needs change, but advances in computer technology also are made. Improvements in the information system that are now impossible may become possible.

Evaluation of the information system is simply a process of measuring its performance against the goals and criteria developed in the earlier phases of the information system development process. That is, does the information system produce the desired information? Is the information complete, concise, accurate, timely, and relevant?

Applications of the Microcomputer in the Private Practice of Psychotherapy (or How to Rationalize the Purchase of Your New Toy)

Lawrence M. Lanes, MD

Perhaps you are like me—a psychiatrist in private practice, doing mostly individual psychotherapy, with occasional hospitalized patients. You have a mixture of private and publicly funded patients and participate part-time in teaching and supervision. You're experiencing a mushrooming amount of paperwork, evaluations, reports, and correspondence, and an increasingly complex financial situation. You've watched as your hospital, insurance company, and grocery store have become computerized. And you have observed with heightened interest as the initial swell of microcomputer use has enlarged to a virtual tidal wave, with an exponential increase in the amount of advertising and the number of stores hawking this Wave of the Future. Occasionally, you meet someone who owns or uses a micro, and you've found yourself saying, "No kidding? I've been thinking of getting one."

At least, that was the point I was at that day nearly two years ago when I first set foot in my brother-in-law's computer room. As both a real estate investor and an academician, he had extensive need of and uses for the computer, and I stared in awe at the screens full of text and data displays, the printers buzzing efficiently, and the calm and purposeful humming of the disk drives. A few demonstrations later, I was hooked. I had seen the future and recognized the power and potential of this marvelous new tool.

Within days I was setting up my own microcomputer; within

weeks I was well immersed in learning BASIC (a programming language). I tackled my first project, writing a checkbook-balancing and record-keeping program. After several weeks of using this program, I discovered that it required considerably more time to enter and use the program than to balance my checkbook manually. No matter. I had begun to tame the power and potential of the microcomputer, or so I thought. It became my guiding principle, which was fortunate, because over the last months and years I have begun to discover that my diligent and innovative applications of this powerful new tool have needlessly complicated just about every aspect of my life.

I read about uses of the microcomputer in patient history and record-keeping. Advertisements for commercial programs boast capacities for up to 10,000 patients and multidoctor practices. This seemed excessive for my 20- to 30-patient solo practice. I began to create my own files using my word-processor program. Instead of being able to jot down my records spontaneously, I now had to wait for the end of the day when I could sit down, fire up my micro, and type in the information. This resulted in a net increase in the time I was now required to devote to my records.

I noticed that the billing forms for many of my privately and publicly insured patients were similar and would lend themselves to computerized billing. Commercial programs were available for several hundred dollars and up. I devised a way to use my word processor to format and fill out the forms. However, by the time I set up the printer for these forms and then made the changes necessary for different insurers, and checked that the correct information was printed in exactly the right little box, it resulted in a net increase in the time necessary to complete my billing.

I was impressed by the versatility of the mathematical spreadsheet programs that can be used to maintain financial records. I immediately set about devising a format that would provide automatic updating and aging of accounts to keep track of my billing. After several days of effort I attained this goal with only a small net increase in the amount of time necessary to record my billing.

The advantages of a word processor over a conventional typewriter were transparently clear, and I immediately began using a word processor program for all correspondence and reports. Unfortunately, until this time I had not used even a conventional typewriter in my practice. My touch-typing skills, barely acquired in high school, took months to sharpen. This resulted in a significant increase in the amount of time required for correspondence and reports. No matter, at least I had a professional-looking document, or so I thought until I received a letter from the first company I sent a report to complimenting me on the content but complaining that "trying to read those little dots drove us crazy."

More recently, I have noticed a plethora of devices, both hardware and software, created to enhance, speed up, or simplify the computer and my use of it. Unfortunately, trying to decipher the instructions or become familiar with quirks of the programs or hardware, which I gather should be self-evident to anybody with at least an engineering degree, often consumes vast amounts of time. The result is a net increase in the amount of time for any task performed on my micro.

Well, you get the idea. By now, my wife is beginning to wonder about the utility of a device that allows me to perform in two hours what used to require one. Inevitably, in my frequent attempts to demonstrate the purpose or usefulness of a program or piece of hardware, I run into some problem that demonstrates clearly my lack of mastery of the computer or the software, and my position seems to be eroded yet further. Untold hours are spent in the pursuit of some procedure which may, at best, shave minutes.

Perhaps you've already considered these initial stumbling blocks and begun to read the magazines and specialty journals to see what others were doing with their micros. More discouragement. These people really seem to *need* the computer. Computerizing psychological testing or patient assessments. Interfacing computers to biofeedback devices. Software developed by professionals for professionals. Research projects that acquire massive amounts of data from patient surveys. You think to yourself, the only biofeedback you use in your practice is when your stomach's growling tells you it's time for lunch. Your confidence is beginning to falter. By now, there are small, but unmistakable signs that your environment is growing hostile. You notice your wife repeatedly "by mistake" throws out the computer journals you've begun to accumulate. Perhaps your analyst seems a mite less sympathetic to your financial concerns since you expressed an interest in acquiring a computer. You become downright worried. How are you going to rationalize, uh, justify the purchase of a microcomputer?

This is the part you've been waiting for. It is important that your responses be graduated according to the sophistication of your inquisitor.

For those around you who are not yet familiar with the nature of the beast, stating your intention to use the computer to "keep records," "streamline tax preparation," "automate billing," or "word-process" that article you've been meaning to write should be sufficiently impressive.

For those who may recognize the absurdity of using a computer for such limited applications, the cause of Computer Literacy can always be invoked. This is a good time for the Wave of the Future, Power and Potential stuff. Get into "C.A.L." (Computer Assisted Learning) and how our kids will be exposed to this practically from birth, and we may become anachronisms before our time unless . . . O.K. Now you have them reeling. Time to pin them to the ropes with the importance of understanding the principles of programming. You may point out that while "hardware" has attained a high level of sophistication and reliability, "software" is still in its "infancy" and that "user-friendly" programs for a practically unlimited number of applications are eagerly, even frantically sought after. After launching this salvo, you can administer the coup-de-grace by slyly intimating that, in fact, you have a few ideas about applications in your own professional area of expertise. No dilettante, you. Now, you may walk away triumphant, just as long as you really do know the score about programming.

Learning to program is indeed best done "hands on." However, be aware that writing a commercial-grade program after just starting out is somewhat akin to taking up a musical instrument and immediately writing and orchestrating a hit song. Not impossible, but certainly difficult and relatively rare. As I found out, even if software is still in its infancy, there are already approximately one trillion commercial programs available to balance a checkbook. It is true, however (and I admit I haven't quite tried all of them) that none I have used takes less time than balancing it manually. But that's not quite all there is to it, actually.

You see, it is also true that my patient records have never been better organized or more detailed (I can now type quite rapidly). My billing records are crystal clear and my bills and correspondence now look quite professional, as I have upgraded my printer (at least it's deductible). And seemingly trivial but practically epic in its lack of precedence, my checkbook now balances, every month, *to the penny*. And these benefits are for real. Being able to see my accounts aging has made me stay on top of overdue accounts with an improvement in my percentage of collection and cash flow. Using budget categories has enabled me to collect my total and deductible expenses in more detail than I ever used to, with benefits to me both in terms of reduced taxes and less time with my accountant. In the long run, I may yet realize time and financial advantages to using my micro. So, while it may not yet represent the arrival of the millennium, my use of the microcomputer, as evaluated two years later, has actually been a boon. By the way, while software is improving dramatically, by and large you still need some familiarity with the basics of how your computer works in order to successfully use most software and hardware. For the most part, it's not yet to the point of "heat and serve."

Ultimately, I have stumbled upon the best answer of all to those who question or ridicule. I have discovered that I don't have to rationalize my microcomputer, not to anyone else, and most of all, not to myself. I have discovered a fascinating new discipline, which has excited my own sense of exploration and discovery. I have become not just computer-literate, but computer-sophisticated. The computer, wherever it may occur, no longer generates the anxiety or the sense of helplessness that it used to. When I see or hear about possible applications of the computer, I am able to assess how realistic they are based on my own familiarity with software and hardware, what it can do and, even more importantly, what it cannot do. In the final analysis, understanding computers and their limitations has transformed me from feeling a victim to feeling I am an active participant. For those who question or even ridicule, I no longer defend myself. I invite them to join me. Some do, increasingly so. And, since you have read this far, I have a sneaking suspicion you will too.

The Salt Lake VA Medical Center Experience

Douglas K. Gottfredson, PhD
L. J. Schmidt, MD
Phillip W. Christensen, PhD
Bruce Beebe
Robert Wally Fort

From 1972 to the present, the Salt Lake City VAMC [Veterans Administration Medical Center] has designed, developed, and upgraded a computer system for increased capability in the diagnosis and treatment of veterans with mental health problems. Initially the computer system was developed under the direction of Thomas A. Williams, MD (1975), assisted by James H. Johnson, PhD, and others, using a CDC 3200 computer. A psychiatric assessment procedure was designed to use interactive computerized self-report information along with data gathered by a paraprofessional interviewer for the purpose of making psychiatric diagnoses and triage/admission decisions. A total of seven psychological tests were programmed for computer administration and scoring. These tests included: a validity scale, three intellectual screening instruments, two affect tests, and a personality test. Interviewers were able to enter: a physical examination, History–Part 1, Current and Past Psychopathology Scales (CAPPS), and an initial problem list. These computer applications were developed from 1973 to mid-1977. Twenty-five journal articles and chapters in two books describe the computer system with the CDC computer. A list of references of the publications is available on request. Dr. Williams and those associated with him in the computer project left Salt Lake VAMC in 1977.

In 1977 and 1978 a computerized Day Hospital Client Monitoring System was developed by one of the authors (Dr. Gottfredson) to improve efficiency in managing programs for mental health care and vo-

"The Salt Lake VA Medical Center Experience" originally appeared in *Computers in Psychiatry/Psychology*, 1980, 3(2), 5–8, and is reprinted by permission.

cational rehabilitation for veterans participating in the Day Hospital Programs. The innovative computer programs developed on the CDC 3200 computer had considerable utility, but were plagued with problems, such as computer down time, slow interactive CRT terminals, long programming times to make changes, no editing capability in the event of errors, high maintenance and utility costs, etc.

Because of computer problems and limited capability for additional computer applications, we changed from the CDC 3200 to a new Digital Equipment Corporation 11/70 Computer System with 256K bytes memory and two disks, each with 67 megabytes of storage. The 11/70 uses the MUMPS* programming language. At present the computer system has 22 Lear Siegler ADM–3A CRT terminals and 5 matrix printers. The computer was installed late in January 1979. Conversion of some programs from the CDC 3200 computer into MUMPS for use on the DEC 11/70 computer and development of the current Mental Health Treatment Computer System was accomplished by the authors of this article, working as a team. After conversion of the desired routines from the old system, we developed many new mental health computer applications. We also worked with other MUMPS users in the VA system in a cooperative effort to increase computer capabilities at different sites. We are especially indebted to Robert Lushene, PhD of Bay Pines, Florida, VAMC for programming numerous psychological tests and interviews and to George Timson at San Francisco VAMC for file manager routines. This cooperative effort greatly accelerated the development of the current computer system.

A brief summary of the Mental Health Treatment Service computer applications is given here. A more complete description of the computer programs is contained in a users' manual dated 1 June 1980 (Gottfredson, 1980). Copies of the manual are available on request.

Initial information on veteran patients is generated in the Psychiatric Assessment Unit (PAU). Additional information is added on inpatient wards and outpatient programs. The information entered at the PAU includes the following:

Pau-Generated Computer Information

1. Demographic Information
2. Q1—Validity Scale
3. Psychological Tests
4. Vocational Tests
5. History–Part 1 (HX1, History of Present Illness)

---

*[MUMPS is an acronym for Massachusetts General Hospital Utility Multi-Programming System—*Ed.*]

6. History–Part 2 (HX2, Past History, Health History)
7. History–Part 3 (HX3, System Review)
8. Physical Examination
9. Diagnostic and Statistical Manual (DSM-III)—Decision Tree
10. DSM-III—Diagnosis
11. Mental Status Examination (MSE)
12. Problem List
13. Referral Sheet
14. Bed Census—Admit Team Selection
15. Patient Disposition

At the present time there are approximately 60 psychological and vocational tests and 20 histories and questionnaires in the computer system. Psychological tests which are commonly used include: the MMPI, Shipley-Hartford, Beck Depression Scale, Strong-Campbell Interest Inventory. The histories and questionnaires include: an alcohol history, medical histories, anger and pain questionnaires, etc. A complete listing of the tests and sample printouts, including interpretations, are included in the Salt Lake Users Manual (Gottfredson, 1980).*

The process of computer administration and scoring of psychological tests has created some interesting issues. Obtaining permission agreements or licenses from copyright holders has been time-consuming and challenging. We have spent considerable time during the last 6 months negotiating with 15 different copyright holders. Although we are in substantial agreement with the terms required by all of them, we presently have signed contracts or agreements with approximately half of the copyright holders. Consequently, we are currently not using some of the texts that are available.

A second issue related to automated testing concerns ethical standards of psychologists in the utilization of assessment techniques. Though this issue cannot be thoroughly discussed here, we have established procedures with a level of computer security to allow access to psychological testing results only to psychologists or mental health professionals directly supervised by psychologists.

In addition to doing psychological testing on veterans applying for treatment or on consultation from other services in this VA medical center, we also provide automated testing services to other VA medical centers. VA sites with some type of printing terminal and an acoustic coupler can dial our computer directly and enter test answers through a quick-entry procedure from locally completed answer sheets and then immediately get a computer-scored printout. The MMPI, for ex-

---

*Further information on the Salt Lake Users Manual may be obtained by writing to the Salt Lake VAMC, Mental Health Treatment Service, Salt Lake City, UT 84148.

ample, requires approximately 8 minutes to enter and then 5 minutes to generate a 5- or 6-page printed report, including a standard profile, several paragraphs of automated interpretation, a listing of critical items, and 67 special scales. Some of these scales are: the Harris and Lingoes scales, the Wiggins Content items, the subtle-obvious scales, and other scales, some commonly used and some added because of interest by Salt Lake VA staff. With this very flexible computer system, it is simple to add special scales or other tests as needed or desired. At the present time we are providing testing services to approximately 15 remote users.

After admission to an outpatient program or an inpatient ward, staff may enter additional information into the computer. Outpatient programs maintain information on participant activity in individual therapy, group therapy, vocational programs, educational modules, etc. Management information system reports are available on a monthly or quarterly basis to summarize all program and participant activities. Computerized discharge summaries and treatment histories are currently being developed for all mental health patients.

One of the significant clinical applications has been in the area of dissemination of critical patient information in a timely manner. This has been accomplished through the message and crisis-progress notes routines. Messages are entered into the patient's file by date. The routine dictates that any current clinical and/or crisis information about a patient will be displayed on the CRT whenever a user calls up that patient's name. In this way, staff are made aware of critical information at the time of their interaction with the patient. This has proven to be very valuable at the admitting office during off-duty times when the patient may be seen by the officer of the day.

An effort to standardize diagnoses by using the Diagnostic and Statistical Manual of Mental Disorders (DSM-III) has also produced some interesting issues, such as how to handle "rule-out," "provisional" and "by history." Additionally, how can diagnostic disagreements by different clinicians be handled? Again, space precludes a complete discussion. We currently are storing DSM-III diagnoses along with modifiers such as "provisional," when appropriate, and the date, name, and title of the individual making the diagnosis. Through computer security, others cannot change existing diagnoses. They may, however, enter a different diagnosis and express disagreement in progress notes. The same general principles apply to other information entered into the computer, such as History–Part 1 information or items on the problem list.

User acceptance remains an important aspect of the Salt Lake VAMC Computer experience. Williams and associates addressed this issue in three articles (Johnson, Williams, Klingler, & Giannetti, 1977;

Johnson, Williams, Giannetti, & Schmidt, 1977; Johnson, Williams, Giannetti, Klingler, & Nakashima, 1978). Aware of resistance to computer-assisted approaches by staff in the Mental Health Treatment Service, they discussed "organizational preparedness for change," "the problem of change," and "concepts for improvement of clinician acceptance." These feelings of resistance toward the computer appeared to linger after we received and began to program our new computer. We noted that users did not feel they had an opportunity to guide the development of the programs they were expected to use. Whereas in the past program changes were slow or never occurred, we now have the capability of quickly achieving alterations in format. Likewise, in the past, some computer-assisted approaches appeared to increase clinicians' effort rather than save time and improve efficiency. With the enhanced flexibility and ease of programming of the new system, essential modifications were now more achievable. With the advent of conversion to the new system, we commenced a weekly meeting of program developers, computer programmers, and clinician users, wherein problems were mutually discussed. With this emphasis on dialogue between users and providers, the problem of "resistance to change" has been substantially reduced. Frequently, the user-suggested changes are incorporated into the computer system within an hour or so after the conclusion of the meeting. Even major changes are usually completed and operational within a week. We now notice the resistance only where there has been insufficient interaction between users, developers, and computer personnel. Providing opportunities for interaction with all users and continuing education concerning changes and new developments is a continuing challenge.

At this point we believe the Mental Health Treatment Service Computer System is on a solid foundation. We currently have a good data base and are continuing to add to it. Although the research potential of the system has not been fully developed, its benefits for program-evaluation are being widely used. In the future we anticipate developing ways of using the data for research and further evaluation to improve patient care.

REFERENCES

Gottfredson, D. K. *Mental Health Treatment Service Computer System Users Manual*. Salt Lake City: VA Medical Center, June 1, 1980.

Johnson, J. H., Williams, T. A., Giannetti, R. A., & Schmidt, L. J. Strategies for the successful introduction of computer technology in a mental health care setting—the problem of change. In R. R. Korfhage (Ed.), *AFIPS Conference Proceedings: 1977 National Computer Conference* (Vol. 46). Montvale, N.J.: AFIPS Press, pp. 55–58.

Johnson, J. H., Williams, T. A., Giannetti, R. A., Klingler, D. E., & Naka-
    shima, S. R. Organizational preparedness for change: Staff acceptance of
    an on-line computer-assisted assessment system. *Behavior Research Meth-
    ods and Instrumentation*, 1978, *10*, 186–190.

Johnson, J. H., Williams, T. A., Klingler, D. E., & Giannetti, R. A. Inter-
    ventional relevance and retrofit programming: Concepts for the improve-
    ment of clinician acceptance of computer-generated reports. *Behavior Re-
    search Methods and Instrumentation*, 1977, *9*(2), 123–132.

Williams, T. A., Johnson, J. H., & Bliss, E. L. A computer-assisted psychiatric
    assessment unit. *The American Journal of Psychiatry*, 1975, *132*(10),
    1074–1076.

PART II

Dealing with People

This is a book about computers, not people. Why then is one of the first parts of the book about people and one of the last about computers? Why not start off with a part telling what computer to buy, what software to use? The reason is that some of the best computer systems have failed and some of the best software has gathered dust, because the people for whom it was bought didn't use it or misused it. Part II is the first of many in this book to address the issues related to the people who are critical to making your computer system a success or failure.

The introduction of a computer into a clinical setting is a very special event, for which there are few parallels in modern clinical practice. Regarding this event as a technical one similar to the introduction of a typewriter or copy machine rather than a cultural event that will have wide-ranging consequences for virtually every individual in your organization can lead to major problems that may finally preclude the use of the computer at all.

Many people will be involved in the implementation of your computer system. Within the clinical setting: you; perhaps professional colleagues; clients or patients; secretarial or office staff; employees; employers; and members of a board. Important people outside your organization may include a salesperson, a dealer, a programmer, a hardware specialist, and members of your community. Even the solo practitioner must deal with many of these people if he or she wishes to develop a functional computer system. Part II begins with a review of a study of the effect of computer-mediated work on individuals and organizations. Five authors then present their perspectives on the role of professional colleagues, office personnel, programmers, and computer salespeople in the introduction of a computer system into a mental health setting. Each author states what he believes to be important for you to know, based on his years of experience with computers in mental health.

5

People in the Organization: The Effects of Computer-Mediated Work on Individuals and Organizations (A Review)

Marc D. Schwartz, MD

Information technology is rapidly transforming the kind of work people do. Clerical workers are affected by word processing, electronic mail, and the automation of the office. Blue-collar workers are increasingly required to interact with computers to monitor and control a wide variety of manufacturing operations. Managers are making greater use of computer conferencing, decision-support systems, modeling procedures, and on-line information management systems.

Funded in part by a grant from the NIMH Center for Work and Mental Health, S. Zuboff has been studying the subtle effects of this technology on people and the issues that are likely to affect how it will be used in the coming decade. Over the past few years, she has interviewed approximately 200 employees, supervisors, professionals, and managers from several organizations to find out how people respond to their work when it has been fundamentally reorganized by the introduction of information technology. In "New Worlds of Computer Mediated Work," she outlines the principal themes that emerged from her interviews and observations.

One issue that stood out clearly was the reluctance many managers felt at having the computer de-skill them. Certain judgments can be

"New Worlds of Computer Mediated Work," by S. Zuboff, appeared in the *Harvard Business Review* of September–October 1982 (pages 142–152). The present review by Marc D. Schwartz of that article originally appeared in *Computers in Psychiatry/Psychology*, 1983, 5 (1), 6–8, and is reprinted by permission.

reduced to algorithms or decision rules. As these rules become more explicit, they require less and less human activity. "For some jobs, the word 'decision' no longer implies an act of human judgment but an information-processing activity that occurs according to rules embedded in a computer program," Zuboff noted.

How do people respond to this? In one bank, all twenty credit analysts refused to use a decision-support system that was supposed to free them from the most mechanical and boring aspects of their job. One stated, ". . . with this system, I am supposed to type into the machine and let it think. Why should I let it do my thinking for me?"

Another kind of de-skilling takes place when the logic and procedures of one person are incorporated into a computer program that makes decisions for many people. Although the methods of the person on whom the system was modeled may have worked excellently for him or her, others may resent the method of decision-making into which they are forced by a program that "thinks" differently from the way they do.

Another issue that emerged was people's difficulty in accepting the computer's interposing itself between them and their work. Rather than directly experiencing and sensing their relation to the materials with which they were dealing, they found themselves manipulating ephemeral computer symbols and abstractions. It can become very frustrating when you want to get some basic information out of an information system and there is no way to obtain it, when there is no way to even get to the raw data upon which you could make some calculations. The comptroller of a bank noted: "People become more technical and sophisticated, but they have an inferior understanding of the banking business. New people become 'system people'; they can program instructions that don't necessarily reflect the spirit of the operation." Anyone in the mental health field who has worked with a computer specialist who was not a clinician can understand the implications of this observation to information systems in psychiatry and psychology. Making the mental connection between data describing people and the reality of real human beings requires imagination and an unusual ability to relate abstract data to human activity.

The abstraction of computer-mediated data leaves many workers feeling frustrated and insecure. The absence of a tangible piece of paper on which information is printed, which can be held, is difficult for many to accept. The transient nature of information, displayed on the screen one moment and gone the next, is problematic for many. Major obstacles can be encountered in getting the computer to correct an error made. Creative, active interventions are hard to implement in a fixed system.

Computer work requires focused attention and abstract comprehension. It is not really known what effect adaptation of large numbers of workers to this kind of work will have on them and their mental health in the long run.

Computer work not only affects the individual. It also affects the social structure in which she or he works. The terminal can become the employee's primary focus of interaction, leading to feelings of isolation and impersonality. (Of course the terminal can also become a buffer against unwanted social intrusions.) On the other hand, with computer conferencing, the individual can greatly extend the range of possible interactions, initiate dialogues, and form coalitions with people in other parts of the organization.

A much greater degree of control and oversight of people's work is possible with computer-mediated work. The computer system that is so helpful in carrying out the work can also keep track of the amount and kind of work done. "In some cases, these capabilities are an explicit objective, but too often management employs them without sufficiently considering the potential human and organizational consequences," Zuboff notes. Risk-taking behavior and innovation are minimized by those who know they are being scrutinized.

Even those who would like to engage in more creative work find this difficult once a computer system has been put in place. Exploratory deviations from standard practice stand out and can be difficult to justify, even though they may represent a better way of doing something. If an innovator cannot identify and explicitly state his/her model of thought as clearly and logically as the model on which the computer system was built, it is likely to be rejected. Since many person-years may go into the development of the system, it becomes more and more difficult to present an alternative system having the current system's breadth and coherence. Superior or alternative methods may therefore be easily rejected.

The computer system comes to be seen as a kind of authority in itself, not merely a representation of the authority of the supervisor. Transference feelings can be evoked by wires and bits that are as real and heartfelt as those generated by flesh and blood. This may become an especially troublesome problem when any degree of artificial intelligence is built into the system or the system is "user-friendly" to the point where it imitates human responses.

Information is power. The diffusion of information in computer-based systems can affect the distribution of power. For example, it is more difficult for individuals to control parts of the organization by withholding or feeding information as they wish. While some managers can become almost corrupted by the power that information gives them, others gain a new sense of orderliness and competence. Still others are overwhelmed by the amount of raw data that inundates them.

Work can become more regimented, as electronic mail systems and scheduling systems keep careful track of tasks done and not done. Nothing slips through the cracks. Everything planned and not completed is up there on the screen as a reminder, for better or for worse. The perception of whether a system provides orderliness or regimentation exists in the mind of the beholder.

The completeness of information available from the computer can also be regarded as a blessing or a curse. Some see it as a way of reducing uncertainty and errors of judgment based on insufficient data. Others see it as reducing the room for intuition, artistry, and even inspiration. These people tend to feel increasingly cramped as the time and volume of work increase to fill their available (and computer-clocked) time. Subterfuge and subversion are sometimes used by employees who wish to maintain a sense of mastery over their work environment. Reports of employees keying in fictitious accounts or records are not unheard of. Zuboff is convinced that the more managers attempt to control the process, the more employees will find ways to subvert that control. In fact, outsmarting the system can become a new way in which employees can demonstrate to themselves their mastery over their work. In what appears to be a political rather than strictly scientific assessment of this phenomena, Zuboff notes that "managers may dismiss these subversive activities as 'resistance to change,' but in many cases this resistance is the only way employees can respond to the changes they face. Such resistance can also be understood as a positive phenomenon—it is evidence of an employee's identification with the job."

Although technology may be regarded as neutral, its implementation and use are not. The computer will affect the workplace and the individuals in it for better or for worse, depending on how it is used. Dealing with the computer in a strictly "rational" manner, ignoring human needs and human feelings, will often result in a system that satisfies neither its users or the organization it is intended to serve. Managers of computer systems need to understand the effect of computerization on skill demands of work and to develop educational programs that allow employees to develop new competencies, including theoretical comprehension of the task and how the computer system organizes it. Employees must be given the knowledge and authority to capitalize on the vaunted potential of the new information resources, or the systems will be undermined or under-used.

The effects of control on the pleasurable boundaries of work must be carefully watched. Daydreaming and bantering are universal and probably essential parts of most jobs. To the extent that managerial control over attention eliminates these, this control may have unexpected and unwanted effects on workers' mental health. Zuboff has found that imposing traditional supervisory approaches to the computer-mediated environment can create considerable dysfunction.

What is the effect of computer-mediated work on people's perceptions of themselves? "When a person's primary work consists of monitoring or interacting with a computer screen, it may become more difficult to answer the questions 'Who am I?' and 'What do I do?'" Zuboff concluded. Work no longer needs to be done at the same time others do it, or even at the same place. The individual's commitment to the job may decrease as his or her skills become more transferable, and social interactions at work decrease. This could have major implications for organizations and for the relative importance of work and nonwork activities.

Zuboff's study makes it clear that the introduction of a computer to an organization involves more than purchasing another new office device. It can change the nature of human relationships and the definitions of tasks. It is a significant cultural transition. The need for a thoughtful response to this transition goes far beyond designing a user-friendly interface or even insuring user involvement in the planning for and implementation of the system. Habitual and basic assumptions about the role of the individual, the job, and the organization must be looked at and new solutions found to significant new problems. Resistance to computerization should not be regarded as petty conservatism that will be swept aside by the march of progress. Perhaps the real reactionaries are those who do not recognize the deep nature of the change that computerization brings both to the individual worker and to the organization.

Professional Colleagues: Confronting the Attitudes of Professionals toward Microcomputers

Gary L. Pinkerton, MSW
Paul R. Raffoul, PhD, ACSW

If you are a professional considering using a microcomputer in an office where you have no staff and no clients, then this article is not for you. However, if your decision to computerize will affect anyone else, then reading on may be helpful, because during that computerization effort, it is likely that you will confront attitudes that are not as positive as your own. In this article, we will outline some of the attitudes that human-services professionals hold towards computers and ways that these attitudes can be confronted, in order to help insure a successful computerization effort.

BACKGROUND

Computers, as we know them today, formally celebrated their 30th anniversary in 1981 (Davis, 1977). During that 30-year period, computer technology has undergone a rapid evolution from room-size collections of vacuum tubes and wires to fingernail-size *chips*, or microprocessors, with the same capacity. These chips form the basis for the current evolution and revolution in microelectronics.

Whether we are completely aware of it or not, computer technology has become pervasive in our society. A "computer" may be in the wristwatch we wear, the microwave oven in our kitchen, or inside the video game that we so willingly plunk our quarters into, but the technology is so broadly based that one may use a computer-based system

61

of one kind or another many times daily and never even be aware of its intervention.

The point of interest for professionals reading this book regarding computers is probably not the video game, however, but rather the "personal" microcomputer or small business computer being considered for use in an individual or group mental health practice. At the point of consideration of a microcomputer for the professional's office, there are many factors that can affect the success or failure of the implementation of the decision to computerize. This article will attempt to call attention to one human factor that is often overlooked when assessing the need for a microcomputer-based system and its chances for successful use in the office setting. The specific factor that this article will consider is the attitudes of human-service professionals toward computers and their use in human-services settings.

A SCENARIO

For an example, let's consider the following hypothetical situation:

> You are a clinician in a group practice that includes a psychiatrist, two psychologists, and an office manager. Being aware of current trends, you recommend to your colleagues that the group consider the use of a microcomputer to assist in maintaining case records, help with word processing, operate a client billing system, and be used for client interviews, testing, and psychological evaluation. In the staff meeting you called to discuss this, you are surprised when confronted with strong resistance to the idea. The office manager says that the current manual billing system works fine and that a computer would only make it more impersonal. The psychiatrist and psychologists ask about the use of the microcomputer for evaluation purposes and wonder how the office manager will be able to perform that task (assuming that since the computer is "office equipment" that she will be in charge). When you try to explain that everyone in the office would be expected to be able to use the computer, you encounter even more questions and resistance. The psychiatrist says that he hasn't got time to learn anything else. One psychologist comments that his values won't allow him to be involved in a practice that uses a machine to do what humans should do. The other psychologist is interested, but comments, under his breath, that if he had wanted to learn about computers he wouldn't have become a psychologist.

Faced with this situation or a similar one, you might begin to question the possible success of an attempt to use a microcomputer in this office. Much has been written in professional and popular literature about microcomputers, but there is still a general uneasiness about being confronted with the necessity of using one directly. In a recent newspaper article ("Get vertigo?," 1982), it was noted that a medical phenomenon called *cyberphobia*, which is indicated by nausea, hysteria, vertigo, stomach aches, and cold sweats when the afflicted person is confronted with a computer terminal, may affect one-third of the workforce studied. The study at St. Joseph's University by Sanford B. Weinberg found that at least 30% of the nation's office workers suffer some kind of discomfort in the presence of video display terminals. With these kinds of problems to face, the attitudes of staff toward computers may quickly become the first "surprise" factor in considering the use of microcomputers in a professional office.

MORE ABOUT ATTITUDES

In a study of human-services professionals in administrative positions conducted by one of the authors (Pinkerton, 1982), varying attitudes toward computers were noted. Pinkerton's survey of the attitudes of 56 human-services professionals toward computers reveals some attitude trends that may be helpful in planning for the use of microcomputer systems in private practice.

In the survey, an attitude scale of 25 items was developed by the researcher. Based on responses to these items, a total attitude score was computed. Respondents were then divided into those with negative attitudes toward computers and those with positive attitudes. Following this grouping procedure, a series of variables were examined for their influence on attitudes. The results of the analysis are presented briefly for consideration.

1. Administrators of smaller agencies (20 or fewer staff) tended to have a more positive attitude toward computers; 59% of the administrators of smaller agencies had positive attitudes, versus 31.8% of the administrators of larger agencies. The study found a statistically significant association between the size of the agency and the attitude of the administrator toward computers ($r = -0.3226$, $p < 0.010$).

2. The longer the administrator was employed in human services, the more significantly negative the attitude. A larger group (62.9%) of the administrators with 12 years' experience or less had positive attitudes, while only 33.3% of the administrators with 12 years or more experience had a positive attitude toward computers. Study results also found a significant difference between the mean attitude scores of

these two groups, based on length of employment (t = 2.88, p < .0035), as well as a statistically significant negative association between length of employment and attitude (r = −0.4234, p < .001).

3. Administrators of private agencies had more positive attitudes than those in publicly funded agencies (62.5% positive attitudes in private agencies and 43.5% positive in public agencies).

4. Administrators with no computer training had a significantly more positive attitude than those with some training; 36% of the administrators with computer training had positive attitudes, while 64.5% of those with no training had positive attitudes. A statistically significant difference between the mean attitude scores of administrators with some training and those with no training was noted (t = 2.85, p < .003).

Among the other variables that were examined and found to have little or no distinguishing effect on attitudes were: (a) administrator use of a computer outside the work setting; (b) prior experience with use of computers; (c) educational level of administrator; and (d) sex of administrator.

Some of the unsolicited comments made on survey items provide additional information about the feelings of human-service professionals toward computers and their use. One administrator, commenting that "human services and medical care have no relation to computers," expressed very succinctly the feelings of many human-services professionals toward computers. Many others, whose perceptions of computers may include only those "monsters" we are frequently at odds with, commented that their agencies were too small or their staff not sophisticated enough to operate a computer.

SUGGESTIONS AND HINTS

Faced with situations and attitudes such as these, there are some things that can be done to help insure the success of a computerization effort in the professional's office and to confront the attitudes held by professional staff. Many guides to developing microcomputer-based systems mention general concerns, but specific, practical considerations are often omitted. The following guidelines may be helpful to consider in confronting such negative attitudes toward computers:

1. Involve staff in every step of the decision-making and implementation process. In larger offices, this could be with an appointed committee; in smaller offices the entire staff should be included.

2. Make sure that the system is oriented toward solving specific needs in the office and not performing unneeded or entirely new functions. Beginning the process with simple applications, or even games, which will allow the staff to become comfortable with the com-

puter and more familiar with its use, will permit the staff to learn to accept the microcomputer as an aid and not a threat. Control over the applications, use, and development of the computer system may be the discriminator in the attitudes of smaller vs. larger agencies found in the survey. Make it your advantage!

3. Use the successful efforts of other offices as examples, either by reports and articles or by visiting an operating system. In our experience, speeches and visits by computer retailers can do more harm than good when the audience is composed of computer novices. An explanation by a professional peer is undeniably more helpful in demonstrating the use of the microcomputer system than one by a computer salesman, no matter how glib he may be. This would hold true for training in the use of the microcomputer as well.

4. Make training available to all staff and allow free time during the business day for learning and practice on their own. This will allow each staff member to pursue particular interests and to develop skills at his or her own pace.

5. Identify the skeptic. Despite all your efforts there may be someone in your office who refuses to accept the system and may even attempt to frustrate the computerization effort. Based on the survey results, this may be someone who has been around a long time. Identify the person as someone with valid concerns and either provide more support and training to encourage his acceptance of the system or allow him time to be uninvolved. (Remember, you may be dealing with a *"cyberphobe"*!) Sometimes, a few months of peripheral involvement will give the person enough time to see the usefulness of the microcomputer.

6. Avoid philosophical and ethical issues about computer use. The computer is a tool that can help make the office more efficient and help professionals spend more time helping. Computers are to typewriters what typewriters are to pencils, simply an improvement on the standard way of doing things. It's been said that when mechanical typewriters were first introduced, much discussion and anger focused on the issue that a letter that wasn't handwritten just wasn't the same as one produced on an "impersonal" machine. (Sound familiar?) Concerns about issues such as those raised by our hypothetical psychologist must be discussed, but should not become major contentions that prevent the consideration of using a microcomputer in the office.

7. Make sure that the hardware and software are "user-friendly"—that is, that they tolerate errors, are easy to understand, and do not require extensive technical knowledge. This will help insure that the "too-busy-to-learn" person in your office won't have to spend too much time in learning about the computer and can just learn about the particular application for your office.

8. Protect each staff member's position in the office. Computer lit-

eracy brings its own special power and control and may upset the usual balance in the office. Also, if staff feel that their jobs or positions in the office are threatened, deliberate frustration of the computerization effort is more likely.

9. Be patient! Allow time for your office's system to adapt to the microcomputer. It will quite often take a year or more to see the real benefits, so try to schedule in some more immediate, visible benefits without pressuring the staff or the system to overperform.

CONCLUSIONS

The human factor of professional attitudes toward computers is one that is easy to overlook or downplay, even for human-service professionals. Nevertheless, for any professional considering computerization of his professional office, an awareness of the attitudes of other professionals and office staff is essential in developing a successful computerization effort. Although the attitudes of professionals in the human services have been particularly negative towards innovation and computerization in the past, the survey findings reported here indicate that there may be some easing of these negative attitudes as computers become simpler to use, less expensive, and their adoption even more inevitable. Statistically significant study findings indicate that paying attention to the impact of number of staff of the agency or office, age and length of employment of co-workers, and the computer training provided for staff may assist in developing more positive attitudes toward computers.

Even when negative attitudes are found, however, there are several steps that can be taken to help ease the resistance and allow those with negative feelings toward computers to become more familiar with their use and accept them as tools for more efficient service to clients. Who knows, maybe soon a professional in private practice will use a microcomputer to develop a treatment program for desensitization of cyberphobia!

REFERENCES

Davis, Ruth M. Evolution of computers and computing. *Science*, March 18, 1977, *195*, 1096–1101.

Get vertigo over video displays? Maybe it's a case of cyberphobia. *Wall Street Journal*, June 8, 1982, p. 29.

Pinkerton, Gary L. Computers and the attitudes of human services administrators. Graduate research report, Graduate School of Social Work, University of Houston, 1982.

Why Do Psychiatrists Avoid Using the Computer?

Marc D. Schwartz, MD

Ever wonder why psychiatrists do not like to use a CRT terminal? Monte Meldman, at Forest Hospital in Des Plaines, Illinois, carried out a survey of this phenomenon and found a number of explanations. Most important, he found there is a role model conflict between the psychiatrist's view of himself as a professional (philosopher-king) and himself as a computer user (common technician). Highly valued interpersonal skills were seen as being exchanged for the simple (and lower status) exercise of data collection/manipulation. Psychiatrists also felt that the use of a computer implies they lack humanity.

Many mental health professionals believe (correctly for the most part) that accurate measures in the field tend to be irrelevant, and relevant measures tend to be inaccurate. In addition, higher echelon professionals don't like to acknowledge, let alone demonstrate, their lack of skill in using a keyboard and CRT. Now you know why psychiatrists don't like to use CRTs.

Dr. Meldman cautions that with the increase in computerization of records, more and more standardized paperwork will be demanded of psychiatrists by the government, by insurance companies, by PSROs, etc. Psychiatrists don't want to do this paperwork and believe much of it is meaningless. When psychiatrists feel they are being forced to "play games" to optimize insurance benefits or justify treatment decisions, they fear the result may be dishonesty and corruption.

"Why Do Psychiatrists Avoid Using the Computer?" originally appeared as "Why Do Psychiatrists Avoid Using the CRT?" in *Computers in Psychiatry/Psychology* 1978, 1(4), 10, and is reprinted by permission.

8

Microcomputers in Clinical Practice: Preparing and Involving Office Personnel

Fred L. Alberts, Jr., PhD

During the past several years, much has been written regarding computer applications in a wide variety of settings. This information has been available in special-application journals, through computer groups, and in professional computer journals. Considerable attention has been given to hardware factors, software factors, "how-to" instructions, special applications, and product evaluations. Individual manufacturers have addressed some of the human factor issues such as color of screen, dot-matrix size, glare, screen size, computer table size, special chairs, and ease of operation. These factors are often cited in advertisements to attract potential buyers. However, there has been a paucity of available information in the popular computer literature regarding human factors in computer applications. It appears that even members of the mental health profession overlook critical human factors in their zest to automate their practices. Greater consideration should be given to these factors. More specifically, there remains a dearth of information regarding how to best prepare staff members in the practice (e.g., clerks, secretary, accounting clerk, and other associates) for the eventual automation of the psychotherapy practitioner's office.

With the advent of computers and automation in small business practice, it appears that a goodly number of unprepared and untrained staff become anxious, even fearful, and often resistive when engaging in discussions regarding possible utilization of the computer in the practice. The staff's proper preparation, in a systematic and collaborative manner, is essential. This chapter describes some effective preparation guidelines to be used in independent clinical practice. Systematic preparation of the staff should be an ongoing process. Thus, these guidelines include details to be considered both before and after the computer arrives.

INITIAL PREPARATION

Explain to the staff the intention of exploring computer utilization in the practice. Initially, offer in a general manner the basic intention and how the computer may assist them in doing their jobs. Help them to understand what a computer is capable of doing and what a computer is not capable of doing. Much anxiety often evolves from the notion that computers will replace humans. Reinforce the fact that computers are only capable of doing what they are "told" (programmed, instructed) to do by humans. If a computer is to be used to "replace" major job responsibilities of an individual, reinforce for those employees the implications of the change. Explain that most employees are overloaded with detailed responsibilities, and that the computer is a way to alleviate the overload and to free the individual to do more human-oriented work. Specifically, it is not the job or the person that the computer replaces, only the manner in which the work is completed.

Case History: Part I

Mrs. Campbell, the office manager, was informed by her employers that they were considering the use of computers. Mrs. Campbell responded rather typically to this news and immediately questioned, "How will the computer affect my job or the jobs of others?" Her employer told her that he could think of several ways in which the computer would assist in many of the job functions, but assured her that no one's position was in jeopardy. Mrs. Campbell was somewhat relieved but understandably anxious as they continued discussing computers. Her employer continued to explain that he could think of a few ways in which computers could actually free her in order to do more human-oriented work. It was at this point that he got her attention. Mrs. Campbell had worked in this practice for many years and had continued to take on more and more responsibilities. As a result, the time available for performing more human-oriented functions was limited. Mrs. Campbell reflected, "I used to enjoy the initial patient intakes but, because of the workload, they have become too automatic." As she considered this, she said, "If the computer will be able to reduce the time I spend on payroll, then I might be able to spend more time talking to the patients on initial appointments." In a short period of time, Mrs. Campbell had become aligned with the movement to use computers in the practice. After the initial preparation of the office manager, the employer was then better able to begin discussing the same considerations with other staff members. Since Mrs. Campbell supervised the secretary and clerk typists, she was of considerable assistance in initially introducing the idea to the other staff.

INVOLVEMENT

Once the staff is comfortable with the idea of computers and have been duly briefed, it is important to involve them and to solicit their input, including their feelings, attitudes, and recommendations for usage. Involve the staff in determining the various needs and the ways in which a computer could be of benefit to the practice. Even experienced practitioners may find that, much to their surprise, the clerical staff are very much attuned to the subtleties of their job responsibilities and requirements and thus are in an excellent position to brainstorm and to develop a list of potential uses of a computer in the practice.

After the staff have had an opportunity to delineate various needs and potential computer applications, allow them an opportunity to view the equipment and sample available software. It may be necessary to travel to local computer stores to see the various types of equipment. Regardless, the staff should be able to see, first-hand, what the computer looks like and "how" it works. If time is not a critical factor, then attendance at a local computer show (Expo) is an excellent way to see the various products available and to talk with those who use them.

Allow the staff to assess the desired equipment and peripheral equipment in terms of overall suitability (aside from technical considerations). The staff will be in an excellent position to address the human factor concerns if they first have an opportunity to use several of the potential systems. Allow them to "try out" the keyboards of various units, for example. Solicit input regarding desired furniture to accommodate the equipment. Also, remember that office space utilization will be a concern, and it is their space, typically, that is invaded. Their input for planning for the equipment is essential.

Case History: Part II

A second illustration describes the manner in which one office staff was involved in the computerization of the office. Both formal and informal meetings proved to be excellent ways to brainstorm the possible ways a computer might be of assistance. A meeting was arranged to solicit input from the staff. At this particular meeting, Mrs. Campbell was extremely interested in the use of computers in payroll. The office secretary, Mrs. Lobstein, indicated that she had heard of word processing, but had never had an opportunity to use the equipment or, in fact, see the equipment operate. Computers began to be the talk of the office. Mrs. Lobstein pointed out that she had a friend who used word processing and arranged for a time to talk with her friend regarding her experiences with computers. Much of the initial fear was now subsiding, and there was an active involvement, almost excitement, among the staff regarding the project.

EDUCATION

Education, of course, is a critical and ongoing concern for computer utilization in the practice. Some preparatory educational effort is necessary in order to alleviate excess anxiety associated with the computer's eventual arrival. For an example, one can circulate various popular computer magazines that describe and illustrate popular systems. Becoming familiar with the basic vocabulary and language is also helpful in reducing the apprehensiveness of staff. Some introductory texts that are not technical in nature are available. A joint effort in reviewing and reading the texts will lessen staff fearfulness and eventual resistiveness. Basic computer vocabulary is essential to being able to converse at a comfortable level (e.g., differentiating hardware and software; micro, mini, and mainframe; hard disk and floppy disk).

As part of the education process, solicit assistance from individuals familiar with computers. Trained persons in staff positions similar to those of the staff in the practice would be ideal. Identification with the trainers and opportunity to ask questions facilitates receptiveness and reduces the anxiety. Emphasize the difference between programming and utilizing software programs. Much of the fear often associated with computers evolves from a misunderstanding that each time a computer is used it must be programmed. The potential users should become familiar with software capabilities.

Offer some type of continuing education to foster more independent and self-starting interests in computers. Topical seminars, presented in Expos or by computer groups or stores, are available from time to time for special applications (e.g., accounting, medical practice, word processing).

Case History: Part III

The therapists had been distributing pamphlets, short articles, etc., to the staff. The staff became familiar with some of the computer jargon and initially, when not fully comfortable with the language, made humorous statements when using the jargon. The staff enjoyed reading the various magazines, catalogues, and booklets that had been distributed. After a short while, without any formal education, some of the staff were able to make very astute statements regarding computers. In fact, Mrs. Lobstein's interest was best exemplified by her clipping newspaper articles on the use of computers. She became the office "librarian" for computer information.

A much larger clinical practice nearby had been using computers for over a year. The therapists arranged for the office staff of both practices to get together to discuss the computers in an attempt to acquaint the staff, in a hands-on manner, with computers. The therapists arranged for an in-office, catered luncheon. During the extended lunchtime, the staff discussed the various functions and operations of the computer. Of particular note was Mrs. Campbell's relief when she realized that she wouldn't be expected to program the computer (although in time she may want to). The staff viewed some very sophisticated software that assumed, essentially, computer ignorance, and found its operation quite simple. Mrs. Campbell learned of a local word-processors' association and inquired about membership. Mrs. Lobstein enrolled in a local community course on microcomputers. It appeared that the involvement, continuing education, and resultant office personnel cooperation yielded an extremely successful venture.

In summary, the practitioner has many decisions that must be made regarding the utilization of computers in a psychotherapy practice. It becomes increasingly complex when the computer must interface with the process and products of an individual's job. It then becomes the responsibility of the practitioner to prepare the staff in a systematic way in an effort to guard against staff fearfulness and resistiveness. Involvement and education are very critical considerations. While the guidelines presented above are general, they are provided in order to illustrate how very subtle, inexpensive attention to some human responses to computers can actually facilitate a successful implementation of computers in an independent practice.

The Computer Professional: The Relationship between User and Computer Professional in System Development

Jerry Cinani, MSc

The installation of any automated information system is a complex enterprise and usually is approached with a focus on the computer and the functions it will perform. In the following discussion I hope to persuade the reader to look at another dimension of computer projects with attention equal to that given the computer. Since the primary "deliverables" of a system are the hardware and software, it is natural to allow the computer to become the focus of attention. This natural tendency, however, is misleading and often the cause of extensive delays in project completion and expensive cost overruns. The computer, at least initially, distracts a consumer's or user's attention from the computer professionals involved in the system development. Unfortunately, the success or failure of the system rests largely with the computer professionals, and seldom with the system itself.

Although the college curriculum for computer training is usually found under the rubric *computer science* and the discipline itself requires great attention to detail, logic, and realistic assessments of problems, a user should not expect his or her project to be conducted with scientific precision. It is not uncommon for the computer professional to display the type of projections associated with government forecasts of spending. For example, a computer professional such as a system analyst might evaluate the volume of mass storage (hard disk or tape) in the following manner. First, he or she will consider the volume of transactions in an environment, i.e., number of records generated, and calculate the precise length of each record (e.g., name, date, and social security number might require 47 characters or 47 bytes). From this information, the analyst might then proceed to calculate the number of bytes of disk space needed for data. The analyst might then consider the operating system required, the amount of disk space it will occupy, and the number of bytes required for the system memory. Usually, the analyst will also consider overhead requirements for disk space. Finally, the analyst will tally all of these figures and arrive at a specific number of bytes of disk space (e.g., 20 megabytes, or 20 million bytes) necessary to support a system. When approached for the figure by a user, the analyst might discuss his or her calculations, pause, and reply "our calculations show that you need 20 megabytes of disk storage, so we better double that to be on the safe side." The analyst may support his or her conclusion by reference to past experience installing systems in similar environments.

The example above is not intended as a sarcastic comment on computer professionals. In fact, a user would be wise to listen to an analyst such as the one above. The analyst would probably be right. The example does reflect the extent, however, to which computer professionals rely on common sense as well as technical knowledge.

All of the organizational tools relied upon in projects typically focus on either the computer or system design and the flow of money as regulated by the contract. Little attention is devoted to the relationship between the user and the computer consultant. Although some information projects, such as those required for a small psychiatric clinic or office, may appear a relatively simple affair and the apparent simplicity may be reinforced by computer professionals' claims that the task can be done easily, there are no simple installations of automated information systems. Therein lies the deceptive magic of computer applications. A well-developed computer system along with good organizational tools mislead computer professionals and users to expect straightforward or simple installations. There are seldom simple installations.

The difficulties involved in the installation of a system are not eliminated by planning or system design and definition. The success of the installation of a system relies heavily on the relationship between the user and computer professional. Without an effective relationship, any project is destined for failure or excessive delays and unexpected cost overruns.

The relationship between user and computer professional and the role that relationship plays in a project is clearly reflected by the issue of completeness vs. modification. The issue of completeness as opposed to modification comes up frequently in system development projects. It may create lengthy delays while the user and computer professional attempt to negotiate their way through the issue. On occasion, the negotiations end in a lawsuit instead of a return to the project. The issue is suggested in the following quote:

> The Contract should specify very carefully and completely what shall constitute the completed system. The agency should negotiate for an "operational" system, that is, one which is in proven, productive use at contract completion. The vendor, on the other hand, may negotiate for an "operable" system, one which has been tested successfully but is not necessarily in full operation at contract completion. Both stands are valid and defensible (Paton & D'huyvetter, 1980).

Ordinarily, the user and computer professional begin a project with the assumption that both understand what is meant by a "completed" program and a "modified" program. Further, they assume each has the same meaning for these two terms. The user, however, typically believes a program specified in the system design is completed when he or she is satisfied with its performance. The computer professional's view is frequently quite different. The computer professional regards completion in terms of programming tasks and the routine followed by a programmer. When a programmer has written a program that conforms to the steps indicated by the design, tested the program's performance, and found it operational, the computer professional considers the program completed. Although the program may not perform as expected by the user, the computer professional will usually treat any changes as modification.

The statement quoted above contains a distinction between *operational* and *operable*. The difference between these terms does not adequately represent the contrast between a user's viewpoint and that of a computer professional. The terms *operational* and *functional* are more descriptive of that difference. The term *operational* describes the status of a program acceptable to the computer professional, while *functional* describes the condition for the user. A completed program might be defined as that which is both operational and functional. A program that meets only one condition is incomplete as far as the user is concerned.

The conflict regarding completeness is created because of the assumption of similar meanings and an expectation that as long as the system design is sufficiently specific it will be clear when a program has been completed. In fact, it is not possible for a system design to reach the level of specificity required for unquestionable agreement and completeness. For, if the design were to reach such a level, it would cease being a design and become the source code statement of a program. Therefore the organizational tool of system design cannot eliminate the problem.

The issue of completeness may appear as a complaint during the course of a project. The following dialogue depicts such a complaint.

Background. Mental Health Organization staff and a computer firm's system analyst have been working on installation of a system driven by a DEC PDP 11/23 computer. The applications programming is approximately 50% complete (*complete* being defined, as above, as operational and functional). A number of input programs have been written and they are running on a daily basis. The analyst and the mental health organization's evaluator are developing programs for processing data into accounts receivable reports. The report they are working on at the particular moment is the Aging Accounts Report. The system design contained a specification for the production of an Aging Accounts Report on a monthly schedule and indicated the report should show each client account in terms of 30-, 60-, 90-, 120-, and 360-day intervals, with the sum of across columns equal to the total amount owed by the client. The purpose of the report is to provide the accounting staff with a means of identifying past-due accounts owed the organization. The complaint is expressed in the following dialogue:

EVALUATOR: Jane (the systems analyst) says that the aging report program is complete and any changes will be treated as a modification and billed for time and materials at the rate of $40.00 per hour.

SENIOR SYSTEMS ANALYST: Jane is probably correct. What is the problem?

EVALUATOR: The current form of the aging report is unacceptable, and I do not think the program is complete. The accounting staff claim they cannot read the report. They say the numbers do not appear to make any sense. There are too many different sources of payment with aging accounts for a single client. Furthermore, the column values for many accounts do not add to the correct total, and the accounting staff cannot determine whether the 30-day interval represents 30 days past due or the current amount owed.

SENIOR ANALYST: Does the program contain all of the elements specified in the written contract?

EVALUATOR: I believe so.

SENIOR ANALYST: Can you call-up the program and produce a report?

EVALUATOR: Yes, we can produce a report, but it contains errors.

SENIOR ANALYST: Does the report comply with the specifications in the design?

EVALUATOR: Yes, the report in general conforms to the design requirements.

SENIOR ANALYST: The program for the aging report then appears to be complete. We need to fix the sums across columns, but otherwise the program is complete.

EVALUATOR: The report does not adequately serve its intended function as specified in the design. Therefore, the program is not complete and changes in the format must be viewed as corrections rather than modifications.

SENIOR ANALYST: I'll talk to Jane.

The most likely result of the above conversation is that the analyst (Jane) will continue to resist any request for a correction. A major change in the report format would probably require extensive alteration of the program and a good deal of programming time.

There are three types of conditions under which a computer professional and user might disagree about the completion of a program. The conditions are described below.

Condition 1. A program is partially functional and the existing portions are operational. For example, a program has been written to generate a report of the number of units of service provided within each of four categories (outpatient, emergency, partial care, residential). The data and definition of unit has not been available for the residential service and the report does not show residential units. The program is not in need of repair because it performs tasks correctly. The program simply needs an additional element. Thus, it is partially functional and all existing parts are operational.

Condition 2. A program has been written, tested, and designated as operational, but it does not perform the specified function. For example, the system design calls for a program to produce a report on staff time by organizational unit within a clinic, e.g., about the outpatient program. There are organizational units 1, 2, 3, and 4 with a total of 10 staff. Each staff who has spent time in a unit should appear in the report as a member of that unit with his or her corresponding time. A staff person might have 6 hours of service provided under Unit 1 and 4 hours under Unit 2. The systems analyst has written the program, tested it, and found it operational. When the program is executed, however, it produces a report that shows a number of staff under Organizational Unit 0 and each staff has some service hours shown for the Unit of 0. The program obviously has a problem. However, it has calculated all of the time correctly. The problem lies in the criteria for assigning a staff to an organizational unit, i.e., clients unassigned to a therapist but provided service are tallied under a zero organizational unit instead of under the staff member's primary unit. The program is operational but not fully functional.

Condition 3. A program is found to be functional but it is not fully operational. The condition is exemplified by the following: A program has been written, according to design, to produce a summary of clients' accounts. When executed for a "live" run, the report shows values for the beginning balance, charges, payments, adjustments, and ending balance. In many cases, however, the values for the ending balance were incorrect. A check on the arithmetic across columns revealed that the beginning balance, charges, etc. all added correctly to give the ending balance. The problem in this case was a data-entry error. The beginning balances were entered incorrectly. The program was operating as designed and serving its designated function. However, the program was not fully operational because the report it produced contained many incorrect values.

Here is a second example of the condition, but with a slightly different problem: A program was designated to produce a billing statement for services rendered within the past month. In addition to listing the services, their respective charges, and showing a total charge, the statement reflected the accounts status, i.e., beginning balance, current charges and payments, adjustments, and the ending balance (balance forward). When the program was executed it produced the itemized charges and total and printed the current charges and payments in the account status section, but printed zeroes in the beginning and ending balance areas. The program was functional, i.e., it was producing a billing statement according to the function specified and the statement could be used for billing a client. However, the program was not printing the correct values for two positions on the statement and therefore it was not fully operational.

The conditions outlined above illustrate several dimensions to the issue of completeness and modification. The issue is significant and cannot be resolved by the organizational tools typically relied upon to ensure a successful project. The issue may be mentioned in the terms of a contract, but its resolution will depend upon informal arrangements developed between the user and computer professional.

CONCLUSION

The success or failure of an information project will greatly depend upon the computer professional selected to carry out the project. Technical knowledge, expertise, and experience cannot be the only criteria used in selection of a computer professional. The computer professional should also possess an understanding of the dynamics involved in system installation and an appreciation of the differences in viewpoints on issues such as completion as opposed to modification. The computer professional should exhibit flexibility in the potential problem areas and a willingness to incorporate procedural as well as contractual safeguards that are conducive to resolving such relational problems as might occur during a given project. It is essential that such issues be discussed prior to the award of a project and reaffirmed at the outset when the project is awarded and periodically thereafter.

REFERENCE

Paton, John A., & D'huyvetter, Pamela K. *Automated management information systems for mental health agencies: A planning and acquisition guide.* National Institute of Mental Health: Rockville, MD, 1980, p. 139.

10 The Computer Salesperson: Thoughts on How to Buy a Computer

Daniel Cohen, CSW

As a social worker turned computer sales representative, I have a particular orientation towards the mental health professional's purchase of computer systems. Too many mental health professionals walk into a computer store and find themselves in the position of not knowing anything about computers. By reading this, you are one big step (or more) ahead of them.

If you want to fare better than most, then educate yourself. Take advantage of the numerous publications now available on the magazine stands or in the library or articles in the daily paper that describe how to buy a micro. Don't depend solely on charts and tables for comparisons of features. (I'd bet every computer firm believes that significant facts about their products were overlooked or misrepresented.) And don't depend on company ads comparing themselves to others without finding out what features they overlooked or what drawbacks of their machine were glossed over.

Buy or borrow a paperback guide for the first-time computer owner. Then talk to present or prospective owners of micros. Don't wait until your computer arrives to start identifying what it should do and who is going to do it. Begin talking with your associates (professional and clerical) about what the computer should accomplish, about how it will change jobs, and about other adjustments that will come about as a result of its introduction.

Talking with Computer Salespeople

Most of the computer sales staff I have met are enthusiastic about their product(s) and computers in general. The question is not which product works versus which does not. The question is which does specifically what you want in the way you want at the cost you want, with the service and support you need, when you require it. When you do meet salespeople, have your questions ready.

Don't buy a computer for today's need alone. Anticipate future needs. Just around the corner are concepts that were once science fiction, which will soon become your reality (e.g., telecommunications, voice-activated office equipment and home appliances).

But don't be oversold. A 16-bit computer for small office word processing and bookkeeping is probably unnecessary. And don't undersell yourself. Too many buyers believe that the computer referred to in the ads applies to them. The implication: for a few hundred dollars almost all office functions can be computerized. . . . No way.

Choosing a Vendor

Buying a computer is not like buying a television set. Very likely you will want to develop a comfortable relationship with your vendor. Updates on programs, new programs, new peripherals, and even new computers that may be of interest to you can come along at any time. If your vendor is familiar with your needs and you, you have a better chance of keeping up with changing technology. Buy a computer from a vendor who has a track record in the community. It is predicted that the number of computer stores will actually decrease in the next five years.

Competent service is important. Your machine should be repaired within a day or two. If the machine needs to be "down" longer, your dealer should provide a "loaner" if necessary so that your work can go on. Customers who purchased equipment in a store get first priority over those who did not. Some stores offer significantly better prices than others. Also find out if the vendor provides educational services and/or seminars to help familiarize his customers (and the public) with the product.

Making the Transition

Making the transition to computer use takes time. Although the system will in all likelihood run smoothly right out of the box, it may take a year to hone the people/machine interface. It is necessary to facilitate the entry of the appropriate information in a timely fashion, as well as make full use of reports generated by your system.

Someone in the agency must be responsible for directing the system's integration into the daily flow of the office, as well as for educating others on the benefits of the computer system. Staff training should not just be given to those operating the computer but to all agency staff. A standard system for recording and entering information is required to enable output of accurate, timely reports.

Know from whom information is collected, how often, and on what forms. Which reports are to be produced? To whom are they to be directed? How often? are but some immediate questions. Full documentation of just what role a computer plays in an organization will help staff understand roles and responsibilities of all involved. When the initial orientation and training become past history, it will serve to introduce new staff members to the system.

Learn only one software package at a time, starting with the easiest. Set up a usage schedule when things get busy and it seems everyone wants access to the computer. Decisions as to what jobs receive priority may need to be made.

Learn what the machine can do for you. You have the best understanding of your practice or organization. Although the computer sales representatives may know little about the mental health field, tell them about your situation. They may be able to suggest programs that would be of special use. Recognition of the benefits and limitations of microcomputers will enable a prospective customer to take advantage of the power offered now. But keep an eye out for new generations of software that will address special needs of the mental health field.

III

Office Accounting Systems for the Psychotherapist

For most practitioners, the real payoff of an office computer system is in billing. Month after month, the same set of calculations must be carried out on the accounts of tens or hundreds of patients. Virtually every other business in which such accounting is required now uses computers. Mental health's time has come. Are you ready? Possibly not. Perhaps you wonder if your practice is large enough, if the expense of a computer system is warranted, if its introduction will slow things down, how to make the transition, or what kind of system you need.

What exactly can a billing system do for you? Well, it can provide you with monthly statements for each patient, of course. It can also give you a summary of how much is owed in the total practice; how much of the total is a month overdue, two months overdue, etc.; it can automatically type up collection letters individualized by patient name and circumstances; it can speed the processing and record-keeping for insurance claims as well as for disability and Workmen's Compensation claims; and it can even, in some circumstances, allow you to send information to insurance companies by "electronic mail," that is, over the phone lines, and thereby speed the processing of claims.

An office computer system can routinely provide annual statements to patients for tax purposes as part of the January billing process; it can provide you with a day sheet telling exactly what work you did each day of the month. And it can assist with follow-up scheduling and patient reminders and recalls.

With a computerized billing system, your office can become more orderly, efficient, and effective. On the other hand, it can become more inflexible, unresponsive, and mechanical. Through its demands for clarity and consistency, gaping holes in the fabric of your organization's financial system can be revealed. If your administrative or financial system is disorganized or inconsistent, a computerized billing program will not help. Your current noncomputerized system may therefore have to be changed. So in considering the implementation of a computerized billing system, take a long look before you leap.

Should everybody have one? No. Practice consultants unanimously agree that over half the billing systems they see installed are not right or not needed. To determine whether a system is useful for you will require some serious homework. You want to be sure you are solving some manifest problems by instituting a computer billing system. Is your billing slow, are your insurance claims piled up, is there ineffective follow-up of patients or bills, are you uncertain where your referrals are coming from, do you have inadequate information about management decisions regarding your practice? For a larger practice, the cost of a medical or psychological management consultant might well be justified in helping to answer some of these questions.

An excellent start for mental health practitioners exploring their requirements for a billing system is provided in the following chapter by Michael Geffen. Michael runs a group practice having between 600 and 700 active accounts. In this chapter, he addresses many issues he has found to be of importance in setting up the billing system for his psychological center.

11 | Selecting an Office Accounting System for Private Practice

Michael S. Geffen, PhD

When mental health professionals are in graduate school, they receive no training in the utilization of computers and computer programs to manage practices. However, when you are the director of a group practice that has over 500 accounts, it is essential that you become immersed in the world of computers to complete successfully the standard tasks such as billing, accounting, and the dreaded completion of insurance forms. I would actually expect that any practice, be it individual or group, that has more than 250 active accounts is in need of a computer.

Memory Capacity

When I began the long, drawn-out process of shopping for the right system for my practice, I quickly learned how much I didn't know. Among the tidbits I learned was that there were a few specific features that were essential. One was to have a large enough random access memory (RAM) capacity. The small computers such as the Apple may start out with as little as 16K of random access memory.

It is very easy to become lost in the information about memory and I must admit that I'm far from being an expert in this area. Suffice it to say that I bought a system with 256K bytes of disk memory and find that it is inadequate (without using multiple disks) in handling a group practice the size of ours, which has between 600 and 700 active accounts. When you are dealing with a practice this size, you need to look at the difference between hard and soft disks.

Soft versus Hard Disks

Briefly, a soft floppy disk is very similar to a 45 rpm record, while the hard disk resembles an album. The hard disks generally operate more quickly and have a much greater storage capacity. They also add $3,000 to the cost of the basic system. While the floppy disks are much cheaper to purchase, you cannot fit enough data for a group practice onto one. As a result, it may be necessary to divide your practice and have patient information stored on more than one floppy disk. This can be done either alphabetically, having all patients whose names begin A–L on Disk 1, and M–Z on Disk 2, or by the type of account. All Welfare or other government accounts, such as Medicare and Medicaid, could be on one disk, and all other patients on another disk.

There currently is one complicating factor to the use of a hard-disk system. It is essential to have a backup copy of all the data stored on a disk, in case a disaster occurs and original data become lost. It is common practice when using the soft floppy disk to make a copy of all work every day, so that the same material will be on two disks. It is also recommended that one of those disks be taken out of the office each evening so that if there is a fire or robbery and the data disks are lost or destroyed, all of the data are still available on the backup copy. This is a very simple process when using soft floppy disks; copying a disk takes less than five minutes. However, this is not the case when using a hard-disk system. At the present time, copying a hard disk is most typically done with a video cassette machine. At the end of the day, you make a video cassette tape of the information on the hard disk and then take the tape home each day. So, as with most things in life, there are pros and cons. The hard disk provides quicker speed and larger storage capacity, but it is more costly and more difficult to back up with a copy.

Dot-Matrix or Letter-Quality?

Most of the hardware systems I looked at were quite similar. Almost every system that I personally examined provided me with virtually the same capabilities. The more important question is what program to run on the computer system. However, before I leave the subject of hardware, there is one final consideration. In buying a printer, it's vital to consider whether or not you intend to use the printer for correspondence as well as data. If it is just to be used for a patient accounting system, then a dot-matrix printer would be sufficient. If you also intend to use the computer system for word processing to handle correspondence and reports, then a letter-quality printer is essential.

Most letter-quality printers are quite noisy. Unfortunately, this aspect will add $300 to $400 to the cost of the initial purchase, since it will be necessary to buy a noise cover for the printer. This additional expenditure is vital. If you intend to use the printer during the course of the normal working hours, you must be able to reduce the noise. It is extremely difficult to talk on the phone, much less accomplish any other task, with the noise that you get from the standard letter-quality printer.

Choosing the Right Patient Accounting System

After looking at ten to fifteen computer hardware systems, I also had the opportunity to view at least twice as many patient accounting systems. As a result, by the time I made my selection, I thought I knew all I needed to know about patient accounting systems. The truth is that I did not learn all I needed to know about the system until I'd been trying to use it for two to three months. There are many little considerations that you just do not have any way to be forewarned about until you have used the system and tried to get what you want out of it. Thus the main purpose of this article is to assist my professional colleagues in making their choices so that they will not have to go through the trials and tribulations that I have suffered. I also hope to describe this material in standard, everyday English language as opposed to the double-talking, rapid-speaking jargon you hear from the computer salesman.

Assigning Account Numbers. When evaluating patient accounting systems, one of the first items to consider is the process of entering patient information into the system. When first using the accounting system, you will be converting existing accounts to a computerized program. These accounts will already have balances and may also have account numbers. If these account numbers are important, then it is also important that the program allows the entry of an existing account number. Some systems will only let you enter new patients in such a way that they automatically receive the next sequentially available account number. You cannot assign numbers of your choice to them. In practical terms, this is probably advantageous if you are willing to change account numbers on all existing patients. This will make it possible to always have new patients assigned the next available account number.

Entering Different Types of Accounts. Another consideration is what type or categories of accounts you can enter into your system. For instance, the ability to enter a Medicaid account, which automatically implies a specific type of insurance claim form, is invaluable. Also you may need to enter accounts that automatically give a patient a discount from the usual fees. Other variations include accounts that have been accepted on a budget basis of x amount of dollars per month. This could be automatically printed onto a bill at the end of a month, stating that the monthly payment of x amount of dollars is now due. Some accounts may not ever receive statements. These would be people who come in and pay directly or those where special arrangements are made with another party, like an attorney, to pay the fees. Another application of this would be when a patient is treated in a hospital and the account is totally paid by insurance. You might never want to bill the patient directly, so it is important to be able to enter several types of accounts.

Entering the Responsible Party's Name. The next consideration is whether the system will allow you to enter the name of the "responsible party" as well as the patient's name. All accounts should be listed by responsible party, so that it is this person's name and address that comes out on the statements. Then, within the responsible party's account, there would be a place to enter the patient's name. It is important to be able to enter the patient's first and last name because in many cases, like stepfamilies, the responsible party's last name is different from the patient's last name.

Entering Insurance Information. You also need to be able to enter information about insurance when entering a patient into your system. You should be able to list the insurance company and all the basic information that will be needed to go on the insurance claim form.

Entering Accounts-Receivable Aging Figures. A final consideration when entering patient data into your system is the accounts receivable aging figures. When converting existing accounts to the computer, it is important to be able to enter the outstanding balance and how much of it is already 30, 60, or 90 days past due. If you are unable to do this, the aging figures in the system will be distorted. By only entering existing balances, these balances are then aged over the next four months, even though in actuality they may already be 90 days past due.

For example, you enter a patient on March 1st with an outstanding balance of $100.00 that is already 60 days past due. If the system cannot enter the aging, then on March 1st your system would show $100.00 past due and on April 1st, it would show that it is only 30 days past due. In actuality, on April 1st that $100.00 is already 90 days past due, the 60 days that had already passed when it was entered into your system on March 1st and the next 30 days from March 1st to April 1st. Therefore, it is important to be able to enter aged accounts at the time you're converting all your patients from the present system to the computer. That way it is a one-step process to enter patients with all of their information when making the conversion.

Posting Daily Activity

Entry of Diagnoses. Entering daily charges is the next item to examine. There are numerous considerations. Some accounting systems will only allow the entry of one diagnosis for a patient. With the advent of DSM-III, we now have five axes. Although most insurance companies are not interested in anything from Axis III to Axis V, it is conceivable that you could have more than one Axis-I diagnosis and possibly an Axis-II diagnosis as well. Therefore, it is extremely helpful for a system to allow the entry of several diagnoses.

It is also helpful if the system will automatically use the previous diagnosis posted for a patient when new charges are submitted. This way you do not have to repeatedly enter the diagnosis. It saves a great deal of time in trying to remember what diagnosis was actually used before and also saves the data-entry person from entering an extra line of data.

Patient's Insurance. Another consideration is entering daily charges is the patient's insurance. If treatment of this patient is covered by insurance, this needs to be entered when the daily charges are posted. The place of treatment also needs to be entered at that time. Most insurance forms require an indication of where the patient was seen.

Procedure Codes. The procedure codes must be stored in a computer system prior to entering any charges. A list of procedure code descriptions and usual fees is necessary. This makes it possible to enter *90803* and have the program say *individual psychotherapy, 45–50 minutes, $75.* When treating patients in the hospital and on a daily basis, it saves a great deal of time to enter these charges once a week. In that way the patient account may be called up just one time to enter the charges for all five days. This does, however, present another complicating factor. After entering the day's charges and receipts, a day sheet is generally printed out by the computer. The issue is whether or not the daily sheet is to consist of the charges that are entered in the computer that day or only services that were specifically provided on that specific date. For example, if a hospital patient is seen on October 11, 12, 13, 14, and 15, but entry of charges is on October 15 for all 5 days, will the day sheet for October 15 list all five charges with their correct dates, or will it only list the charge for October 15? It is obviously more helpful to have all five of the charges printed out, to have a correct document accounting of the work.

Entering Daily Receipts. Entering daily receipts is the next step in the process. The first time-saving factor to consider is whether or not the daily receipts can be entered at the same time as the entering of the charges. This makes it easier to handle an outpatient account, for example, in which the person comes to the office, is charged $75, and also pays $75 at that time. By entering the receipts at the same time the charges are entered, it saves calling up that patient's records twice, once under *charges* and once under *receipts*. Instead, simply call up a patient's account under *charges* and, after entering charges, enter the payment received.

Split Payments. The next issue is split payments. There are some patients that are seen by more than one professional in a group practice. For example, a doctor may see a patient individually and someone else may see him for group therapy. Or, one person may see the patient for psychotherapy and another person may do a psychological evaluation. This raises a question of what to do when the money is received for the services. In the receipt section, you should have the ability to divide payments by doctors. So, when a $200 payment comes in, $150 can be credited to Doctor #1 for individual therapy and $50 can be credited to Doctor #2 for group therapy. If you are unable to split payments, then the receipts must be entered as if they are two separate payments. This would require calling up the same account twice, therefore doubling the time spent on this account.

Adjustments. The ability to make adjustments on accounts is also important. This should be done at the same time as the daily receipts are entered. This means that a payment and an adjustment can be entered on the same account at the same time. The program must ask questions that provide the opportunity. These questions would take a format such as the following:

Type of payments? 1. adjustment 2. insurance 3. patient

If Option 1, for *Adjustment*, is chosen, after the amount of adjustment is entered, there should be a question about the amount of payment. This allows for the immediate entry of the amount of payment after you have entered the amount of adjustment, rather than having to indicate that the transaction on this patient is ended, and then having to recall the patient's account to enter the amount of money received. While this seems to be a minor item, it becomes quite a time-saver when dealing with a large group practice. The same holds true for government accounts. The Medicaid and Medicare accounts almost never pay the amount billed. As a result, every time you are entering a payment, there is also an adjustment. It can become quite a time-consuming process if all those patient accounts must be re-entered for payments and adjustments separately.

Further Notes about Service and Diagnosis Codes

I briefly alluded to the issue of service codes earlier. It is time to look at this in more depth. Freedom to choose the service codes to enter into the system is important. The most common are the procedure codes in the Relative Value Studies (RVS) published by the California Medical Association. These include both numbers and descriptions. Most standard insurance forms are set up to handle the procedures with both codes and descriptions.

There should be a section in the computer program where the service codes are entered exactly as desired. The codes will obviously coincide with the services provided in the practice. Although the RVS codes are the norm, there are some situations that will require different codes. For example, in California, Medi-Cal procedure codes are different from the RVS codes. As a result, the system needs to have the flexibility to enter those other codes in addition to the RVS codes. Other codes will be needed strictly for accounting purposes. For example, when a payment is received from an insurance company, you need to be able to indicate the type of payment in the receipt section. A service code indicating insurance payment would be helpful. Service code 888 could have the description *insurance payment*. Service code 999 could say *payment, thank you*, indicating patient payment.

Service codes are needed for adjustments too. The adjustment may be an accounting error within the office, an insurance disallowance, professional courtesy, or discount account. Separate service codes for each of these adjustments is helpful. A patient accounting system must provide this flexibility. A miscellaneous code is essential for things not covered elsewhere; for those who offer classes in addition to standard psychological and psychiatric services, specific codes for each class would help account for charges and payments.

A program needs to be flexible enough for choices of the diagnosis codes to be used. Whether it be DSM-III or ICD 9, the system should be able to accommodate both. The system should accept the numbers and the labels that coincide. For example: *300.40 Dysthymic Disorder*. This is a fairly straightforward and simple procedure, yet some systems lack the flexibility and storage capacity to do so.

The Benefits of Computers: Reports

Now that you have come this far—you have entered all of your patients, their insurance data, their account data, their daily charges and receipts—you should be able to begin reaping the rewards. The reports from the system on a daily basis should give a tremendously increased visibility to what's going on in your practice. There are many reports that you should be able to get from a system, and we'll review the features that need to be included in each one.

The Day Sheet. The first report is the day sheet. This should list all of the day's charges and receipts. It should include the date, the patient's name, the diagnosis, the service code, the charges, the receipts, the doctor number, and the balance of the account. As mentioned earlier, everything that was entered on this date is needed, even if some of the charges were for a previous day. So the October 15 day sheet should show charges that were entered on this date for October 11, 12, 13, and 14.

There are some other important features that need to be included on a day sheet. A month-to-date figure at the bottom of the day sheet is helpful. This should give the total of the charges for the entire practice for that month and the total of the receipts for the practice for that month. It is the fastest way to know the status of the practice. Similarly, a year-to-date figure for charges and receipts could be included.

Accounts receivable (on money due to the practitioners) would also be helpful on a day sheet. Only totals are needed. A chart that reads something like this would be handy:

1. Previous total accounts receivable	$2,000.00
2. Additional charges	+ 1,000.00
3. Additional receipts	− 500.00
4. New total accounts receivable	2,500.00

Having this information available on a daily basis gives maximum visibility of the practice.

In a group practice, there may be reasons, for example, patient confidentiality, that the total practice information should not be available to each individual doctor. This necessitates a day sheet by producer. So Doctor Number 3 could have a printout each day of all of his or her charges and receipts. The printout should include month-to-date figures for that specific doctor. This gives each member of the group accurate daily information on his or her own individual activity. This day sheet should be produced after entering all of the charges and receipts for the day. The process should not be a very lengthy one. The system should simply have to search up the most recent material entered.

A helpful hint to note well: When trying out a patient accounting system, enter twenty patients and also some charges and receipts for them. Then attempt to compile a day sheet. You need to observe how long this actually takes the computer to accomplish. Some programs are designed to search through two hundred records before stopping. As a result, it might print out all of the day's data, and then go into a long search process to make sure there is no additional data. This may waste 45 minutes or longer. Other more desirable systems can very simply and quickly print out the day's activities in 10 to 15 minutes.

Accounts Receivable Aging. The next report in order of importance is *accounts receivable aging*. This needs to be run once at the end of each month. It lists all of the patient accounts by responsible party and breaks down the outstanding balances into how much of the balances are 30, 60, or 90 days overdue. Some reports also include the date of the last payment. A total is needed at the end of the report to give you a breakdown of just how much is outstanding for the total practice. This report is especially helpful when reviewing accounts that need special attention. The date of last payment tells you whether or not a patient is at least making a payment each month. The report should be alphabetical. Again, if you enter twenty accounts into a computer to attempt to try out a program, you should be able to use these twenty accounts to print out an accounts receivable aging report for your evaluation.

Continuous Patient Ledger. Another important report I will label the *continuous patient ledger*. This is an alphabetical printout of all patients, the basic identifying information, and any payments or receipts for a certain specified period of time. This report could be run just once a month, at the end of the month, listing all of the activity on all accounts. This is especially helpful, since it gives a written copy of everything that is entered into the computer. It makes it very simple to look up an account without having to turn the computer on, enter the program disks, call up the program, and then call up the patient account. It is a valuable time-saving process, especially if you need to go back several months. If, for example, in October you want to look up the activity on an account in May, instead of having to find the May program disks, simply look it up in the continuous patient ledger for May.

Delinquent-Account Report. There are some other reports that are nice to have, but not essential. A delinquent-account report can be helpful. Although this information is on the accounts receivable aging report, the delinquent-account report specifically lists just the accounts with overdue balances and no activity. It usually lists the address and phone number of the responsible party and provides room to make notes of what activity has occurred in the attempts to get payment.

Messages on Monthly Statements. The ability to put messages on monthly statements is also helpful. Systems sometimes allow five different messages, and these can be based on how old an account is. For example, an account with no activity for 30 days can automatically have a message printed on it that payment is requested. Another message for an older account might indicate that the account will be turned over to collection if no payment is received. An additional message may state that payment is urgently needed on an account. If these messages are set up based on the amount of time the account is past due, they can automatically be printed on the statements.

New-Patient Report. A new patient report can be of assistance.

This printout at the end of each month simply lists the names of all new patients and the people who referred them. The obvious utility is the chance to be certain that all of the referral sources have received letters thanking them for sending the patients. A mailmerge feature is useful to send a letter to a large portion of the patients in the practice. Mailmerge makes it possible to put the body of a letter into the computer and then automatically type in the names and addresses of the patients or referral sources so that all of the letters look individualized.

Report Writer or Query. The last item to cover in the report section is a special program often called *report writer*. Another name for this is *query*. This program allows you to choose several specific items on which you'd like a report from among many of the variables that have been entered into the system. For example, if Doctor #3 would like to have a list of all of his patients having certain characteristics, the report-writing section would allow you to specify those variables and print out such a list. This could also be done on items such as age of patients, diagnosis, and service codes. It provides for many different ways of analyzing various aspects of a practice. You can even get percentages of time spent in different procedures if, for example, you want to know how much time was allocated to hospital work versus office work.

Billing

The next section of the accounting system to examine is billing procedures. There are numerous considerations here. First is the question of whether or not billing is to be cyclical (patients whose names start with A through E the first week, F through J the second week, etc.). A system should provide this flexibility. Yet a floppy disk system with just one month of data on a disk makes a cyclical system impossible. For example, the entire month of May would be on one disk. If patients A–E were billed after the first week, the last three weeks of their previous month's visits would be missed. So cyclical billing will not work on a floppy disk system that stores only one month's data on a disk.

One of the most important issues is the format of the bills. Some systems provide the flexibility of choosing the variables to be included and their locations on the bill. In essence, you have the opportunity to totally design the bill's format. It is my opinion that choosing bills with a flexible format offers an extremely valuable chance to prevent a system from becoming obsolete. If you choose a patient accounting system that has just one standard format for billing, it's impossible to use new billing forms. The program that allows you to design your own bill never becomes obsolete. You have opportunity to use it in many different ways. Statements that patients can submit to their insurance companies could use a form that has multiple copies, a place to list state license numbers, tax-identification numbers, and all other identifying information needed about yourself and the patient, including diagnosis.

Once the format is designed, it's time to talk with a printer to create a professional-looking piece of paper on which the bills will be printed. However, it is vital to design the format before going to the printer. I didn't—and now have 6 months' worth of billing forms I hate. You need to know how much space the form requires for the date, procedural code, description of procedure, charges, and receipts. You need to know the space needed for doctor's name and identifying information, as well as patient's name and identifying information. You need to decide whether or not billing messages are desirable. You also may want a place to indicate how much of the account is 30, 60, and 90 days past due. So make sure the computer system gives you the flexibility of including all of these variables; then lay out the variables as you want them. Then go to the printer and have a form designed for the computer system.

At the time the form is being designed, it is also helpful to purchase window envelopes. These will show your names and address as well as that of the patient and should be set up so that the statement can be folded just once and be lined up perfectly with the windows.

One last tip about statements. In laying out the form, you need to know how many rows and columns exist on the paper. The standard size of an 8½" by 11" sheet of paper is 80 spaces across. When printing statements, a shorter piece of paper is often used, so you need to measure how many rows down you have. This must be specified to the computer in the printout part of the program; for example: on row 6, column 5, the patient's name is to begin and should continue for the next 20 spaces. This can be an extremely difficult process without a special ruler that shows 80 spaces across the top and also indicates the spacing of the rows of the paper as well. These rulers are available from standard computer supply companies. They are typically called *form design rulers* and sell from $2.50 to about $8.00, depending on the type of material utilized.

Insurance Forms

It is my opinion that a program that allows you to design an insurance form is the best choice. Although there is a standard Health Insurance Claim form (HIC), various companies require different formats. In California, Medi-Cal has one setup, Medicare another, CHAMPUS a third, and then most other insurance companies accept the HIC forms. If you're not able to design the insurance forms, then the program must have several different formats built in to fit all of these needs. This is extremely rare.

The insurance form program section should allow you to design insurance forms in pretty much the same way as the previously discussed billing format program did. The variables are indicated and a decision is made as to which variable is put where on the form. Then, when the insurance companies decide that they want to change forms for some reason, you are able to change the printout format, and the program is not obsolete.

It is important to organize how to use insurance forms. It is our practice to enter hospital charges once a week and print out an insurance form the same day we enter those charges. Each insurance form has five charges for the week's work with hospital patients. It is printed out on the day the charges are submitted and sent in to the insurance company that very same day. With outpatients, the procedure is a little different. At the end of the month, a helpful feature in a computer is to be able to print out all insurance not billed. This is the time when the outpatient forms can be generated. You do not have to keep track of which outpatient forms are sent in. The computer just automatically prints out the month's work for those patients.

Miscellaneous

Now that most features of the basic billing programs have been covered, there are some additional aspects to be considered.

Accessibility of the Programmer. When buying a program, find out if it has been designed by someone who will be available for help when troubles arise. When something isn't working right, you need to have access to the person who has all the answers. For example, by being able to talk to the person who wrote the program that we currently use, we learned that we can abort the printing of a lengthy report at any time by simply striking any key on the keyboard as the computer is in the midst of printing a line. This has saved considerable time. Once we have the information we want, we are able to keep our system from going into a lengthy search process by aborting the rest of the report. We have found this type of information invaluable and are greatly relieved that, when the local dealer who sold the system can't answer our questions, we can call the person who actually wrote the program.

This becomes more important when you realize that computer programmers are not the best people at writing what is called *documentation*—that is, descriptions and explanations about the programs. Very often computer programs are revised, but the manuals that describe how to use them are not. More critically, the people who write the manuals don't take into account all the things that are going to arise when you are struggling to use their program. It's not unusual for the manuals to be incomplete. Being able to speak directly with the programmer is a tremendous help. It's also important that the local person who sells you the computer system, including both the computer equipment and the programs, is accessible. This person should know enough about computers, hardware and software, to help you through some difficult times.

Overlapping of Manual and Computer Systems. When you start to use the system, you should allow for a two-month overlap between the system currently used and the accurate functioning of the new computer system. First of all, it will probably take a week of full 8-hour days to enter all the data needed to start up the system. So, for example, if on February 1st you begin entering data on existing patients, this step could probably be completed by February 8th. This should allow enough time to enter service codes and diagnosis codes. Then, on February 8th, you are already behind on February's activity. All of the charges and receipts for the week of February 1st to 8th were being done on the old system while you were merely entering patient data to get the computer ready. So now, on February 8th, begin by entering the data of the previous week. This will also take a few days, just to get caught up. So by allowing two weeks of hard work, you should be able to have the system ready on February 15th to be current on a day-to-day basis.

You might think this is the time to stop using the old system and just use the new computer. However, your problems have just begun. You are just beginning to find out the little quirks that I have tried to help you to identify before buying a system. It will still take time to get used to performing daily operations with your system. The chances of making mistakes, especially at these times, are high. Therefore, I strongly urge you to continue to utilize the old system. This way you will not immediately become totally dependent on the new computer, and any errors made in those first few weeks will not be disastrous. You will still be able to get all of the bills and insurance forms out under the old system. At the end of the first month you should be able to compare your totals on items like accounts receivable, producer reports, and day sheets to make sure you've entered the data correctly in the first month.

Now you are ready to begin Month Number Two. This is the month you think you can totally rely on your new toy, the computer. Wrong. I again caution you to play it safe and continue the old system, just in case something unexpected happens. And, as you are checking the computer work with the backup system, you should be able to prepare to do the billing from the computer for patients and insurance companies at the end of the second month.

There is another reason why a 2-month time period is essential. In designing the billing format and insurance forms, you are going to need time to complete those layouts. You are also going to need time to print the statements and to purchase the insurance forms to be used in the computer. You want these to be pin-fed or continuous so that once the first sheet of paper is entered into the printer, all the rest are attached and automatically come through. It will take time to get the materials, and it will probably be the end of the second month before you have these forms in your possession and can begin to use them. The standard health insurance claims (HIC) forms are available as a stock item in many different computer supply companies. It is simply a matter of ordering them; a 12-month supply would be a sufficient order. I would suggest a more cautious approach in ordering the statements for the patients, however. You may decide to change the format after using it for several months. It is certainly cheaper to order a large quantity, but for the first order, I would recommend a supply no greater than 3 months'. You're also going to need some blank paper for the computer. This is available by the carton, usually for around $25.00. Two cartons should last several months. This paper is used for in-house reports. There are some other supplies you probably will want to have printed. While entering information into the computer on a daily basis, a method of checking to determine if something was entered correctly is essential. This is what I will call a *paper backup system*.

Charge Tickets. We have several forms that we utilize. One is called a *charge ticket*. The charge ticket has the patient's name, account number, and diagnosis number. It also lists all of the standard procedure codes. After a patient is seen, the doctor checks off what procedure was used and what the charge is. These forms also have the doctor's license numbers and tax identification numbers and come in two copies, so it can be used by the patients as a "superbill" to send to their insurance companies if they are to be reimbursed. This saves the difficult and costly procedure of having to provide additional information for patients for their insurance companies.

Each of the charge tickets should be numbered consecutively when they are being printed. The appointment book should list the charge ticket number alongside the patient's name. It then becomes possible to look in the appointment book and see that for August 1st, charge tickets numbered 001 to 025 are being utilized. Then, either at the end of the day or at the beginning of the next day, while preparing to enter the charges into the computer, make sure all of the charge tickets have been submitted. If one is missing, you will be missing that charge for the day. If the charge tickets are numbered, you can identify for which patient a charge is missing. The other purpose of the charge ticket is to allow the data-entry person to come up with a total of the charges for the day simply by totaling the amount of all the charge tickets. This should coincide with the total charges for the day, as printed out on the day sheet.

Multiple-Transaction Form. A multiple-transaction form is also helpful. On this form you can list five days' charges for one patient; this form is used for all patients who are seen outside of the office and therefore do not get charge tickets. This includes patients in the hospital as well as patients in a board-and-care home or convalescent facility. By adding all the charges on the multiple-transaction forms to the charges on the charge tickets, once again, there is a balance to compare with the total amount of charges listed on a day sheet.

A third form needed is for the day's receipts. This would list the patients' names, account numbers, source of payment, and the amount of payment. One part of this form would actually become a deposit slip for the bank. The total of receipts on this form should match the total of the receipts on the computer's day sheet. Thus, there is a paper copy to verify all of the work being done. By double-checking the system you can find out if errors have been entered into the computer, and there is a way of catching them and correcting them.

There are many, many considerations when deciding to install a computer system into your office. Yes, it can save time. Yes, it can be cost-effective. Yes, it can provide a tremendous amount of information about your practice. However, the system will do none of these things if you purchase a patient-accounting system that does not take into consideration the items we have discussed. Computers can be fun. They can also be a tremendous source of frustration, disappointment, and anger if you buy the wrong system. When reviewing a system, look at it step by step. By taking into account the items we have discussed, you should be able to purchase a system that meets your needs.

PART IV

Word Processing for the Clinician

One of the most common applications of computers in the mental health setting is word processing, a capability that permits rapid creation and easy editing of written materials. Part IV introduces word processing and some of its applications that are especially relevant to the mental health setting.

Although the preparation of reports, proposals, and correspondence can be rendered efficient to a degree that is difficult to imagine by those who have not used a word processor, the introduction of a word processor can cause some initial disruption in the office. Its use requires skills that personnel in a mental health organization may not have. Also, the ease with which changes and modifications can be made in a document is conducive to an author's making much more frequent revisions than the secretarial staff may be accustomed to. Once secretaries become familiar with its use, however, they are generally pleased with the changes it brings, since the effort of repetitiously retyping materials requiring only minor modification is minimized.

With a word processor, individualized letters or consultation reports can be quickly constructed from a series of electronically stored files, each consisting of a standard paragraph or sentence. By selecting and merging the proper files, an author can construct a document that is tailored to describe a particular patient or situation. With minor revision, editing, and polishing, a letter or consultation report can be written that might have taken many hours more to write without the use of a word processor. This capability is described in more detail in Part VI, "Psychological Reports."

Part IV starts off with a short lesson in word-processor terminology. Frank Gallo then presents a comprehensive review of word processing, discussing the factors you should consider in evaluating various systems you might use in your practice or organization. Finally,

105

Peter Keller gives an introduction to the use of word processing in the clinical office.

It will be well worth your time to spend a few extra hours comparing various word-processing systems before buying. Their features vary. Some are easier to learn to use, but may not have the full range of functions you need. Others may be harder to learn, but may have extraordinary capabilities. Be assured there are some that are hard to learn and have few useful features. If possible, talk to friends or get the names of users from your word processor dealer and ask them about their experiences with various systems. Do not assume that the word processor made by the company that manufactured your computer is the best word processor for that computer. A number of books are available providing comparison charts. Look around. Ask around. You'll be grateful you did.

12 | What Word Processors Do: A Glossary of Terms

Kathy Chin
Tom Shea

When you first get your hands on a word processor, chances are you won't ever let go.

Before dashing off to begin your writing career, take some time to learn how the thingamajig works. Here are some basic terms, in alphabetical order, that set out the abilities of word processors.

Automatic pagination causes the program to put page numbers at the top, on the bottom, on the left, on the right—anywhere you please.

Boldface is especially useful when you want to section off a portion of an article for your readers. This feature types each character two or more times, creating a darker impression on the page.

Block move transfers sections of text into other areas of your story or even to another file. This eases the dilemma and hassle of cutting and pasting. You simply mark the beginning and ending of your material and move the cursor to the proper point of insertion. Some word-processing packages allow you to copy blocks of text. The original block remains where it is and its twin is sent elsewhere.

A buffer is a memory area for temporary text storage. More and more programs are now featuring this item on their menus. If you write a paragraph but are unsure whether or not to keep it, you can transfer the material in the buffer along with other unused portions until you decide to use it or delete it from the file. Very useful for the indecisive author.

Centering positions your titles, names, and headlines in the middle of the line. You can forget the typing formula of starting on the center of the page and backspacing one letter for every two. On a word processor, you just press a key, and the centering is done automatically. Sure saves on correction fluid.

Chain features connect multiple files together so that you can have lengthy documents printed at one time.

The cursor, a moving symbol on the display screen, tells you where you are at any given moment in the text you're working on. With some word processors, you use arrow keys to move the cursor up, down, right, or left. With others, you use two or more keystroke combinations to do the same thing.

Depending on your word processor, the cursor can move slowly from character to character, or it can jump from word to word, from page to page, or to the beginning or the end of the document. Many programs let you do it all.

File insertion permits you to incorporate additional files of text into the file you are editing. You can also duplicate your text and insert into other sections.

File length shows you how many letters are available for you to use. Two thousand bytes equal one double-spaced, typed, 8½ × 11-inch page; some of the lowest-priced programs allot you two pages of text at a time. Others can handle anywhere from 70,000 to 400,000 characters—or between 35 and 200 pages of text.

Footing and heading means the program can display titles or page numbers on the top or bottom of every page automatically. Some pages come with a one-line heading feature only. The newer ones will have multiline headings at the top for your convenience.

Global search is search through the entire file. See *Search*.

Horizontal scroll moves the text on the screen from left to right. On some systems the scroll feature jumps; on others the scroll glides smoothly. It's great for making monster charts.

Justification lines up your margins, left and right, according to your tab setting. It makes your copy look professional when you are compiling newsletters or other types of printed material.

Kerning tightens the text horizontally, for a cleaner appearance. It reduces the amount of space between your letters.

Mail merge is loved by secretaries who are plagued with typing innumerable form letters. In mail merge, one file contains the text and the other file has the address and name list. You use this feature to insert the name and address into the text.

Overprinting prints one character over another. This is useful when you are writing foreign words and need an accent mark or some other type of symbol.

Page display shows where the page ends so you can avoid beginning another page in the middle of a paragraph.

Pitch determines how many characters are printed per inch. Most wordsmiths already know the meaning of pitch if they have ever wrestled with a typewriter. A few programs allow you to alter the pitch without interrupting the printing process.

Proportional spacing allots more space to, say, a *W* than to an *I*. Typeset copy is proportionally spaced.

Screen-oriented editors allow moving the cursor up and down through the text, as opposed to line-oriented editors, which operate on one line at a time.

Search and replace allows you to locate all instances of a specified word or phrase in your text and replace each with another word or phrase, if you wish.

Spell check prevents you from misspelling words such as *hypercholesterolemia*. If you're unsure about the spelling of certain words, you can move the cursor throughout the file to check against an existing list of 1,000 to 45,000 words. If the word is misspelled, an asterisk or some other symbol appears before the word when you use the global-search feature. You can add to the dictionary as well.

Subscript and superscript, in case you haven't heard, would be perfect for mathematicians and scientists. When you write H_2O or 10^4, the little number really looks like it belongs there.

Typeover is a mode of text entry in which typed text replaces any text already entered. The alternative is the *insert mode*, in which old text is pushed ahead as the new text is entered.

Word wrap refers to the program's automatic justification of lines and moving of words to the next line, as necessary. The words "wrap" around from one line to the text, without your having to type a carriage return.

Wild card is the general computer term for a symbol that represents a don't-care or an all-of-the-above option. In word processing, wild cards are used in search and replace operations to, for example, replace all instances of *father* with *dad*.

Windowing allows you to display several files on the screen simultaneously. You can even edit by moving the cursor from one file to the next.

13 | Word Processing on a Small Computer

Frank Gallo, PhD

One of the difficulties clinicians face in selecting a computer for their practice is finding one that can perform as many tasks as possible. Mental health practitioners should look for more than just a business computer designed to do billings and financial statements. They should have a computer that also can help with record storage, with testing and diagnosis and, as will be discussed here, with all writing tasks.

Just as data processing involves a computer to manipulate figures, word processing is the computerized manipulation of words. The purpose of this article is to describe word processing and its applications for people who practice psychotherapy.

BACKGROUND

A few years ago, some companies—Wang Laboratories and Digital Equipment Corporation, for example—developed computers specifically for the purpose of word processing. These so-called *dedicated word processors* represented the state of the art in word processing and subsequent manufacturers did everything possible to replicate them. There were two major limitations to these machines, however, which made them a rarity in small businesses or professional offices. First, they were expensive (over $10,000) and second, they could only do word processing. A clinician who wanted a computer to perform billing and other non-word-processing functions could not do so with a dedicated word processor without making costly hardware and software additions.

With the onslaught of microcomputers in 1980 and 1981, efforts were rapidly made to provide these less-expensive machines with word-processing capabilities. Apple and Radio Shack were the most popular, although the most sophisticated word-processing package, Wordstar, was designed for slightly more powerful computers, which used an operating system called CP/M. (An operating system is the

111

computer's own built-in program that "tells" it what to do, how fast to do it, and when to do it.)

Although these systems were much less expensive (computer, software, and letter-quality printer for about $5,000–$6,000) and the computers were able to do many of the other things people wanted, the word-processing programs left much to be desired. Word-processing software for these early microcomputers could perform a wide range of word-related tasks. However, in order to accomplish them, operators had to learn complex commands, and were required to swap diskettes often and perform other tasks that sometimes made word processing more of a nuisance than typing. The original Wordstar program is so complicated that several guides have been published, independent of the manufacturer's, to help users understand the program.

The inconveniences of these word-processing programs were never much of a bother to people who were "bitten" by the computer bug. But for those who had a computer thrust upon them by a boss who believed that production would magically improve with a word processor instead of a typewriter, the experience was quite intimidating.

To the rescue comes the latest stage in the development of microcomputers and accompanying software. Due to advances in the manufacturing of computer chips, the fingernail-sized electronic components that control the computer's "brain," computer companies are now able to make microcomputers powerful enough to perform word processing in a way formerly reserved for much larger, more powerful, and more costly machines. Examples of computers that typify this generation are the IBM Personal Computer, the Apple III, the Decmate II, and the Wang Personal Computer.

A concurrent advance in the manufacturing of lower-cost letter-quality printers means that one can purchase a rather powerful computer system with excellent word-processing ability for as little as $5,000. Other systems in this category cost as much as $10,000, although the modal price in 1982 is somewhere between $6,000 and $7,000. All further discussion of word processing in this article will refer to this latest generation of systems.

APPLICATIONS FOR CLINICIANS

Most forms of written communication can be performed more quickly and accurately with a word processor than with a typewriter. In my own work, the only times I opt for a typewriter are with one-time brief notes and in addressing individual envelopes. (When several envelopes are to be addressed, it usually pays to use the word processor to produce mailing labels.)

Correspondence

There are several specific applications of a word processor that are important to most clinicians. The first is correspondence. Besides the obvious speed factor, word processing offers the user the ability to store letters in files. Letters can be recalled easily for reference or reprinting. They can be modified and printed in the new form with the options of either saving or deleting the old letter.

For clinicians who send letters to other professionals thanking them for referrals, the process can be simplified by preparing a basic "boiler-plate" letter. This would include the basic layout of the letter with a place for date, addressee, salutation, and a reference (for the particular client). Then there could be an introductory sentence or two such as, "Thank you for referring————. ————was first seen in my office on————1983 with a presenting problem of————." This could be followed by more "boiler-plate" sentences, such as one regarding diagnosis, prognosis, or the treatment plan. You could end the letter with a final sentence or two and your usual closing and signature lines.

Each time you wish to send one of these letters, all that is required is to call up the "file" in which your "boiler-plate" is stored, edit it for date, addressee, client name, etc., and insert whatever you wish into the body. You need not worry about tabs, spacing, margin or any other of the concerns you would have each time you type a letter, because those mechanical functions were already accounted for in your "boiler-plate." After printing the new letter, you only need to proofread the additions. If you find an error in the new letter, it is a simpler, quicker, and neater process to correct it in the computer and reprint it than to use a correcting ribbon or other such manual method on a typewriter.

Another feature applicable to correspondence and other word processing is the ability to program your computer to "remember" certain commonly used words or phrases and print them without your having to retype them each time. For example, "adjustment reaction to adolescence," could be reduced to "a r a" or "schizophrenia—paranoid type" could be printed by typing "sp." This task is performed by using a word-processing function sometimes referred to as a glossary or a library. The usual procedure is to "store" commonly used phrases in the glossary or library and assign them codes such as those above. The listing with codes can be printed out so that the codes need not be memorized and can be kept next to the keyboard for easy reference.

A few words about electronic typewriters are in order. If your primary writing requirements are for correspondence and you are not interested in other features of a computer such as finances or data storage, then perhaps an electronic typewriter is for you. They have the "boiler-plate" and "library" capabilities described above and are much faster than electric typewriters. Their price is approximately one-third that of a computer system. However, their functionality is very limited. They are sophisticated typewriters, nothing more. Unless you are only interested in upgrading the clinical function of your practice, do not invest in an electronic typewriter.

Reports and Publications

For clinicians whose careers involve more extensive writing than just correspondence, the benefits of word processing will be quickly noticed. The ease of editing, storage function, and glossary abilities noted above become more valuable as time-savers when preparing long reports.

A feature of word processing called *block moving* allows a user to perform the cut-and-paste function. In a manually prepared document, the writer often decides to move a paragraph from one section to another. This is sometimes accomplished with the help of scissors and paste. With word processing, the cut-and-paste process is more easily accomplished. Sentences, paragraphs, or larger sections can be moved to other positions with little effort. If, after reviewing the new format, it is decided that it looked better the first way, it can just as easily be revised again. Some writers extol the block move function as a boon to their creativity. It allows them to see their writing in different formats and choose which looks and sounds best.

A second valuable feature applicable to the preparation of lengthy documents is the *search and replace* function. With this feature, the computer is programmed to search a document for a particular word or phrase and replace it with another. For example, suppose you have prepared an article for publication and have used the pronoun "he" in several places. After review, you decide to substitute the term "he/she." If you did not have your draft entered on a word processor, you would have to locate each case of the word "he," determine if it should be changed, and then manually change it to "he/she." With word processing, you have the computer locate each case of the word "he." You then decide if it is appropriate as is, or should be changed to "he/she." Then, with one or two keystrokes, the change is made. Because it is done electronically, you are sure that the computer did not miss any cases of the original word in its search.

The search and replace function can be used globally as well. If you are certain that you wish to change all cases of a word to something else, you simply program your computer to do this. An example could be a change from *Anderson* to *Andersen*. This otherwise tedious process is accomplished quite rapidly and accurately with a word processor.

Statistical tables are prepared more simply with a word processor than with a typewriter. If you can prepare a format for a table, you need only fill in the numbers each time you wish to print it. Then, if you are writing a paper describing the findings of a research experiment and you wish to show results in tabular form, you can prepare a basic table to portray results of the experimental group. To present the data for the control group, it will only be necessary to change the figures. It will not be necessary to retype the entire table. Your printer will print each version of the table separately. This function is also applicable for forms, lists, bibliographies, tables of contents, and cover pages.

Another point to consider when writing articles for publication is that draft revisions can be made quite simply and quickly on a word processor. Furthermore, each new draft does not have to be proofread entirely if it was already proofread at an earlier draft. Printing revised letter-perfect drafts then becomes a matter of pushing a few buttons.

Proposal Writing

Word processing provides an efficient method of writing grant proposals. All of the features described above are applicable. Anyone who writes proposals knows that certain information is almost always required. For example, it is usually the case that funding sources require background information, resumés, and prior accomplishments. These can be written and stored in the computer for use each time a new proposal is generated. Furthermore, the format for title pages and budget pages can also be stored. All that would be needed to type out a new budget, for example, would be to enter the new numbers in the appropriate places on the form you had programmed for an earlier proposal.

Proposal writers know that a key to success is the ability to respond promptly. It is not uncommon to hear about a funding opportunity only a few days before a deadline. With the help of a word processor, you will be better able to meet a funding deadline than if the proposal is done manually. Furthermore, your proposal will look like an original, even though you may have used much of it before. The alternative of having photocopies of certain sections on hand is often a clue to a potential funder that your proposal was not prepared solely for the current project. With a word-processed proposal however, there is no indication that any section of the proposal was not written expressly for that proposal.

Other Uses of Word Processing

The application of word processing to clinical practice is limited only by the creativity of the clinician. Several of my colleagues have used a word processor to write their doctoral dissertations. Not only is this the most efficient way to handle the numerous revisions required by reviewers, but it also provides the basis for subsequent related publications. After the initial document is entered in the computer, it then requires only minimal typing to revise it for an article.

A psychiatric social worker I know uses a word processor to market his services to potential referral sources. He sends a letter to local industries describing his skills and experience. Each letter is modified to fit the particular needs of the company. His letter might mention something about executive stress, alcoholism, or family problems affecting work performance. In this way, each letter is designed specifically for each potential referral source. This clinician also sends letters occasionally to mental health centers and social service agencies, reminding them of his availability to receive referrals. He does so with a letter that specifically addresses one of the needs of the particular agency. He has a basic letter stored in his word processor and revises it slightly for each agency.

Another use of a word processor for a clinician is in the compilation and storage of mailing lists. There are special mailing-list programs, which are designed to work with word processors and can be purchased separately. These allow you to merge names from the list with letters composed on the word processor. However, if the need is simply to record and perhaps print copies of any list, a word processor is a good tool to handle the job. Names can be edited, inserted, deleted, or moved, using standard word-processing functions.

There are also spelling programs that can be added to your word processor to check on the accuracy of your spelling. These are programs with common words stored in them. If the spelling check program does not recognize a word, it will notify you in some fashion, and you can decide if the word is spelled correctly or not. The limitation of such programs is that they cannot tell you if you have used "their" when you should have used "there." Both are recognizable, correctly spelled words. It will tell you, however, if you typed "beleive" instead of "believe." This type of error often goes unnoticed when copy is proofread manually.

Finally, there are word-processing programs that interact with other programs and, in combination with these, will permit you to alphabetically or numerically sort lists or numbers; do mathematical computations; and produce graphic displays.

CONFIDENTIALITY

We have all heard horror stories of client-related correspondence being inadvertently left behind at the copy machine. Word processors can help reduce the necessary number of hard copies of confidential data. When preparing a report or other correspondence of a confidential nature, your own copy can be stored electronically rather than in a file cabinet. Although the information is still accessible to one versed in the use of computers, it is much less likely to be located by an unauthorized person and therefore less likely to be misused. In order to avoid losing an important piece of confidential correspondence, the recommended approach is to make a backup copy on a computer diskette and to store it in a different location from the original.

A SUMMARY OF WORD-PROCESSING FUNCTIONS

All word-processing programs allow the user to generate text on a screen, edit it, and print it. Copy can be stored and maintained for as long as you wish. It can be revised, and you can either save or delete the original. While editing, you can delete or add characters, words, or lines with simple keyboard commands. The program allows you to scroll through your document, backwards or forwards. Most permit you to underline, add subscripts and superscripts, set tabs and margins automatically, set the number of spaces between printed lines, and then change these within the same document. You can line up (justify) both the left or right margins or leave a ragged margin, the kind you get with a typewriter.

The *block move-and-search* and *replace* functions were described earlier. These functions are not available on all programs. Some programs let you view on the screen exactly what you will see on the printed page. Other less costly programs will show the text, but without the margins, tabs, and other commands indicated. Thus, you will have to print your document before knowing exactly how it will look on paper.

Depending on the word-processing program and the versatility of your printer, you should be able to produce printed text with several options. You can print your draft triple-spaced and then simply reprint it in single-space after you review and edit it. You can program some printers to stop printing at the end of each page or to continue until the end of a document. You can link files together and have them printed consecutively. You can also print multiple copies. Better-quality printers allow for different typefaces, including foreign alphabets. You can also print with 10-pitch or 12-pitch type and can alter this with each printing. Finally, you can "instruct" the printer to only print certain portions of a document.

In general, there are few functions you can perform on a typewriter that cannot be done more quickly and accurately on a word processor.

GETTING STARTED

Hardware

The basic hardware for a word-processing system includes a computer or central processing unit (CPU), a keyboard, a screen, at least one disk drive, and a printer. Most basic systems include all of the above in a package. Some, such as the Radio Shack models, include all but the printer in one compact unit.

Choosing the right components, however, is not a simple task. For example, if you are using your computer for business functions and record-keeping, and you also wish to do word processing, a basic 48K (the amount of memory) system might not suffice. Wordstar, the word-processing system referred to earlier, requires more than 48K as well as a particular operating system (known as CP/M), which must be part of your computer's abilities. More memory and/or CP/M can be added to your system, but not without additional cost.

The keyboard you choose is also important. Some keyboards are identical to typewriters, while others offer numeric keys similar to adding machines. Others include special keys appropriate for word processing, such as "insert" and "delete" keys. For one who does frequent word processing, these latter features are important. A keyboard that is detached from the computer and allows you to move it around to your most comfortable position is best. Some prefer a keyboard to rest on a table, while others like to lay it on their lap. The National Institute of Occupational Safety and Health (NIOSH) recommends that the keyboard be placed 29–31 inches above the floor with the keys at or below elbow height. This allows for adequate blood flow to the fingers and results in the least possible amount of hand and arm tension.

The computer screen is one of the most important features in terms of health. Specifically, computer screen viewing has been shown to be the cause of eyestrain, pain or stiffness in the neck or shoulders, headaches, fatigue, vision blurring, and other symptoms connected with occupational stress. Although these symptoms are usually associated with long-term continuous use, they still should not be taken lightly. NIOSH recommends that the screen be of high resolution and be placed 17–25 inches from the viewer with the center located on a plane 10–20 degrees below the plane of the user's eye height. It is also recommended that you take a 10- to 15-minute break after every hour of word processing.

Some people substitute a TV set rather than purchase a computer screen. Although this will serve some purposes, it usually does not have adequate resolution and will lead to eyestrain if used excessively. Green phosphor or amber-colored screens are usually recommended.

Printers also deserve major consideration when you pick your system. The major factor for word processing is whether you require letter-quality documents. The most versatile printers for microcomputers are letter-quality printers. They can perform all of the functions referred to earlier. Their disadvantages are their high cost and their slowness. If your needs can be met by a printer that will prepare draft-quality documents, then by all means purchase one. They are much less costly, have fewer potential mechanical problems, and operate many times more quickly than letter-quality printers.

Some people have avoided the cost of a letter-quality printer by preparing all of their documents on a draft printer and then renting the use of a letter-quality printer. They simply bring the diskette to someone with a similar computer and a better printer and run their document on the letter-quality system when they need it. As mentioned earlier, however, the cost of letter-quality printers has decreased considerably. For a person who needs a smooth professional copy, the investment in such a printer is probably worth the cost.

A disk drive is the part of the system that runs the program. It is analogous to the record turntable on a stereo system. Some systems have disk drives built into the CPU, while others are connected by external cables. Most word-processing systems require one disk drive, although the work is often easier if there are at least two drives. The software usually consists of one program diskette that is loaded into the disk drive to "inform" the computer that you are about to do word processing. If you only have one disk drive, your next step would be to remove the program diskette and insert another one, upon which you will write and store your document. Having two disk drives alleviates the necessity to do this switching. You can simply load your second disk drive with the document diskette and begin typing as soon as you have started the word-processing program. These diskettes are fragile and so the other advantage of having a second drive is that there will be less handling of diskettes.

Most microcomputers use 5¼ inch floppy diskettes. These are named floppy because of their malleability. The newest phenomenon in disk drives, however, is to add a hard-disk drive to a microcomputer. These drives use hard diskettes, which are less fragile than the floppies and have a considerably greater storage capacity. Few word-processing software packages for micros require hard-disk drives, however, and their cost (about $2,000) make them an unnecessary luxury for most clinicians' word-processing needs.

Other hardware applicable to word processors are those items used to upgrade an existing system. These can provide such functions as extra memory, adding a CP/M (operating system), and the ability to expand the number of columns you can read across your screen. All of the above are usually added by inserting a small circuit board in the computer. They rarely require any soldering or sophisticated electronics knowledge.

Another feature of value to word processing is a buffer. This allows for a function known as *multi-tasking*, the ability to have the printer printing out one document while the user is writing or editing another. Some systems have this feature built in. However, most basic systems do not.

Software

The heart of word processing is in the software. In fact, experts suggest that the first job in selecting a computer for word processing is to choose the software and then simply find a computer that will run it. There have been numerous software reviews in lay magazines covering specific word-processing programs, as well as broader articles reviewing all of the popular programs and comparing them in terms of function, price, and hardware compatability.

If a clinician already owns a computer and is interested in adding word processing, then the recommended approach is to review the literature and select those programs that will work on the existing computer and are suited to the needs of the practice. Then, if possible, see the programs demonstrated at a computer store or consult with members of a local computer club who are familiar with the programs.

If you do not yet own a computer and consider word processing one of your more important tasks, you should probably choose your overall system based on which word-processing software is compatible with it. Just determine your most important computer applications, including word processing. Select the most appropriate software and then choose your computer.

Supplies

Not to be neglected in your decision to use word processing is the cost of supplies. Among these are paper, diskettes, print ribbons, and print wheels or print thimbles.

Some printers require special paper while others will use just about anything. If you wish to use your own letterhead, it can be prepared on continuous form paper so that you can print several letters in a row without having to insert new paper each time. Computer paper comes in assorted grades and sizes. It should be noted that spreadsheet paper used in accounting will not fit on all printers. Also, some printers will not handle thick envelopes with the same ease as others.

Diskettes come in different grades and are usually purchased in boxes of ten. Some can hold text on both sides of the diskette, while others are single-sided. Another feature of diskettes is their density. This also has to do with how much text the diskette will hold. Thus, a double-sided double-density diskette will generally cost more than a single-sided or single-density diskette, but will store more text. Before choosing them, it is first necessary, however, to know which types of diskettes your disk drive will handle.

Printer ribbons come in two types: a nylon ribbon that is reusable and a film ribbon that can only be used once. The film ribbon provides cleaner and more distinct letter quality. It is advisable, however, to have both types of ribbons on hand. You then can use the nylon ribbon for drafts and personal notes and the film ribbon for final correspondence and reports.

Finally, there are the print wheels or thimbles that provide the typeface. These can be purchased in metal or plastic. The metal product lasts longer than the plastic but costs eight to ten times as much. Both types are available in various type styles and pitches. Most people begin word processing with a few common-style plastic print wheels or thimbles. Then, after selecting the one or two types best suited to the needs of the practice, they consider investing in the metal version.

SUMMARY

Word processing can save time and effort in accomplishing the writing tasks of a mental health practice. In addition, it offers the clinician a chance to be more productive, and, perhaps, creative, in the development of articles, reports, and books. Some clinicians purchase computers solely for the purpose of word processing.

Hardware costs have decreased to the point where word-processing systems are now within the means of any clinical practice. When word processing is combined with other computer functions such as bookkeeping, billing, and record-keeping, the purchase of a computer becomes an attractive investment.

Clinicians use word processors for correspondence, publications, grant proposals, marketing letters, and mailing lists. Even the most simple and least expensive systems are adequate for performing these applications and are considerably more efficient than typewriters.

Some of the more common functions of word processors are the ability to insert or delete characters or words from a document, scrolling the document rapidly to get to a desired location, moving blocks of text from one point to another, searching for particular words or phrases and replacing them with others, and printing portions of text. All systems store text or lists for future reference, editing, or reprinting.

When selecting a word-processing system, it is often recommended that you select the software you require first and then locate hardware to accommodate it. This is contrary to the popular belief that the most important item is the computer itself. Also, in selecting a system, a person should be aware of the various options available in peripheral equipment such as computer screens and printers, and in the various grades of paper and other supplies required to print documents.

As a final note, it should be mentioned that although there will always be better word processors, there will never be a better time than the present to begin using one. The sooner one learns their applications and operation firsthand, the sooner one can reap their benefits. The key to a successful mental health practice is the freedom to deliver mental health service. A word processor is one tool designed to hasten that freedom by reducing the time required for clerical tasks. Whether the word processor is used directly by the clinician or by a staff member, the time saving and improved accuracy should quickly justify the investment.

Word Processing for the Clinical Office

Peter A. Keller, PhD

If you have not noticed, something called *word processing* has been taking the modern office world by storm. A product of the computer revolution, word processing was something that until recently only large offices could afford because of the high initial outlay involved in the purchase of equipment. Therefore, this technology did not affect the many professionals working in small clinics, the independent practitioner who often operated without a full-time secretary, or the clinician sharing accommodations and secretarial services with colleagues.

Just a few years ago, I was baffled when a colleague at a large university told me he had a paper we were discussing "up on cards." In response to my puzzlement, he explained how text could be entered into a sophisticated typewriter, stored on magnetic cards, and saved for revisions so that a lengthy paper would not have to be retyped in its entirety if corrections were required. At the time, it seemed pretty impressive, but today most would consider such a primitive word-processing system in the same vein as the Model T. Computer technology is moving so fast that all word-processing equipment and other computer systems seem to be, in the words of one consultant, either obsolete or not yet on the market (Veit, 1981). It may very well be true that by the time this introduction to word processing reaches print, my explanations will be out of date.

By now some of you may be asking yourself if this article has any relevance to you. You may get your paperwork, reports, and record-keeping done without too much difficulty. If you have a secretary, she may have access to a modern electric typewriter, which produces good quality copy. Just a few years ago, you probably would have been quite right, but no more. Now, many experts would say the real question is no longer, "Why should I be interested?" but, "Which system can meet my needs and when will be the best time to purchase it?"

Adapted from *Innovations In Clinical Practice: A Source Book*, vol. I, eds. P. A. Keller and L. G. Ritt (Sarasota, FL: Professional Resource Exchange, 1982), 194–198, by permission.

Advances in small microcomputers and the software (or programs) that make them function have brought word processing within reach of even the smallest professional office. It may be especially suited to your needs if you are a clinician in part-time private practice who might not even consider the cost of a secretary. A small microcomputer with word-processing capabilities has the potential to increase your output and, at the same time, improve the quality of your written work for a reasonable cost. In short, there remains little question that within the present decade, these machines will revolutionize the way most of us work.

WHAT IS WORD PROCESSING?

Word processing as it applies to most small offices refers to a computer system that allows one to type and edit almost any written document on a television-type monitor (CRT), save the document for corrections or later modifications, and have it reproduced by a printer. This approach has a number of distinct advantages over the traditional methods of dictating or writing rough drafts and then typing final copy. First, word processing allows you to examine what you have written on the CRT and make as many adjustments as necessary before you arrive at a satisfactory draft. This means that the necessity for multiple drafts of important documents is virtually eliminated after one becomes used to working on the screen.

Second, once a document is completed it can be handled in any number of ways. It can be stored, usually on a small *floppy disk* (similar in appearance to a thin 45 rpm record in an envelope) for future retrieval or modification. Or it can be printed, using a variety of printers, as a *hard copy*. This would be what happens to most correspondence or reports. Alternately, it may be a report or paper on which you wish someone else to comment. If he has suggestions that you want to include in the original document, you simply have your computer read off the disk to place the document on the CRT where you can modify it before printing a final copy.

Third, with appropriate equipment, you may be able to use your computer to transmit the document to someone else's computer via the telephone lines. With the necessary device (*modem*), your microcomputer/word processor has the capacity to open up a new world of communication through various information services, which facilitate communication among subscribers with similar interests. In addition, these services provide access to a variety of information, ranging from current stock quotations to a customized search of the psychological literature.

The available systems are of two basic types. The first type is known as the *dedicated word processor*. This system is designed primarily for word processing and may seem limited for the user who would like to adapt it to other functions such as bookkeeping, test scoring, or statistical analyses. Dedicated word processors also frequently have a high price tag, especially when their limitations are considered. The other type of system used for word processing is essentially a micro- or minicomputer with software packages that enable the computer to accomplish the desired functions. The advantage of such a system is that software can be purchased for a wide range of functions, or the user can write programs for specific needs. In short, the computer is generally felt to be far more versatile than the dedicated word processor.

CREATING AND EDITING DOCUMENTS

Virtually any type of document or report that you would want to prepare can be entered on a typewriter-type keyboard. As letters are entered, they appear on the CRT at a position marked by the *cursor*, a line or square that moves across the screen to mark the position at which you are working. In essence, you are creating a page of text on the screen. CRTs vary in size and are defined in terms of the number of lines and columns* they contain. Typical screens for small business computers contain 24 lines. Widths generally vary from 40 to 80 columns, with the wider screen being more desirable because typed pages are typically 70 to 75 characters in width.

Basic typing skills are important for efficient entry of information into the word-processing system and make it easy for secretaries to adapt to the new approach with relatively little training. However, even if you are a relatively poor typist, you may find some distinct advantages to word processing. If you make an error, corrections on the screen are easy since the text is not committed to paper until you are ready to tell the computer to print. As you work, the page on the screen scrolls to make more space as a function of where your cursor is moved. No more carriage returns either—most word-processing software contains a function called *word wrap*, which places a word on the next line when the margin you have defined is reached. If you omitted something and would like to insert a few words or even a sentence to clarify an important point in a report, it is no problem for most word-processing programs. They will allow you to insert or delete portions of text by giving a few simple commands. The experience in my office

---

*The term *column* refers to the number of letters or characters that can fit across a page of text.

where several people, both the professionals and secretaries, have learned to use word processing, is that efficient use of a system can be made regardless of your ability to type.

What I have outlined is just a small sample of common word-processing features. Most software allows the operator to automatically center headings or to underline or print portions of text in boldface. If you would like your reports to appear dressy, some programs allow you to have the text printed with both margins justified. Many programs will automatically print page numbers or page headings as you instruct. Some will search the file to find a key phrase or word. This is especially handy if you discover you accidentally misspelled a word or name and would like to check other occurrences of it in a lengthy report. There are programs that will allow you to insert key portions of text that you have stored elsewhere on your disk (e.g., a closing to a letter, a name and address, or a key statement about confidentiality that you like to include in all reports). Some programs also have optional features to check your spelling.

A word of warning: not all word-processing software is the same. Prices for a package designed to run on a microcomputer can range from less than $100 to more than $500. Obviously there will be some substantial differences between software at different price ranges, and professional use will probably require software toward the upper end of the price range. Many of the computer magazines feature frequent articles on word processing. An article by McWilliams (1982), which offers an excellent comparison of many popular word-processing programs, is listed in the "Resources" section of this chapter.

PRINTERS

An important component of any word-processing system is the printer. The quality of your print will determine the applications with which you feel comfortable in word processing. Many people initially attempt to keep costs down by choosing a relatively inexpensive dot-matrix printer. While the prices of such printers (starting at about $300) and the relatively high printing speeds make them attractive, there are also many limitations. The primary drawback is print quality. Small dots are used to form the characters and give the copy a "computerized" look. Recently, several printers on the market have attempted to improve the dot-matrix quality, but the results typically do not approach the quality of modern office typewriters. Many users of word-processing systems feel that dot-matrix printers provide an excellent means of obtaining a fast rough draft of their work, but not a satisfactory final draft.

Most small office systems have settled for a so-called *daisy wheel printer*. While considerably more expensive and also slower than the dot-matrix printers, the typical daisy wheel printer provides outstanding print quality. A metal or plastic wheel with spokes that have characters at the end spins rapidly and is hit by a hammer to enter the character on the paper. An advantage of this type of printer is that the wheel can be changed to permit a variety of type styles. Even the slower daisy wheel printers, at about 25 characters per second, are considerably faster than the common Selectric office typewriter. The slower daisy wheel printers may be purchased for less than $2,000, while the more sophisticated ones may cost in excess of $3,000. If you decide to purchase one, it will be important to learn first if it has all of the features you desire for your office. Again, there are some important distinctions associated with the price differentials. We have a Diablo 630, which has given very satisfactory and reliable performance.

Computer magazines also contain advertisements for devices costing $400–$800 that convert standard electric typewriters for use as computer printers. We have never seen these devices in use and cannot evaluate their effectiveness or reliability.

PROFESSIONAL APPLICATIONS

The most obvious professional application is correspondence. The word processor is suited to correspondence because it allows error-free typing. The correction features on the CRT and fast printing time make it easy to send letters and reports that are neatly typed and without errors, even if you do not have a secretary. Many clinicians have discovered that it is both efficient and reinforcing to prepare some of their more complex correspondence on the CRT and avoid the rough-draft stages that dictation involves.

But that is just the beginning. Psychological evaluations and other forms of reports lend themselves exceptionally well to word processing. I use a relatively standard format for reports at one agency where I consult. With word processing, I automatically direct the format to appear on the CRT, where I can fill in identifying information. Next, the headings are already in place and cue me for the organization of the report. If a certain heading seems inappropriate or another seems indicated, the adjustments are simple. Also, a statement on confidentiality is available for automatic insertion at an appropriate point. These are all time-savers that have improved the quality of my reports.

Vincent (1981) has gone further in the automation of psychological reports. Various sections of his reports are based on stored descriptions, which can be integrated into reports. For example, descriptions of certain types of test results are codified for insertion into the report. The advantage of the word-processing approach is that clinicians who use it have the option of developing formats and standard statements in their own style. As much or as little as the user desires can be automated.

RESOURCES

Interface Age. A monthly magazine for small computer users. The May 1981 issue contains several useful articles on word processing. McPheters, Wolfe & Jones, 16704 Marquardt Ave., Cerritos, CA 90701.

McWilliams, P. An introduction to word processing. *Popular Computing*, February 1982, *1*, 17–30. This article presents an excellent comparison of various word-processing programs. It appears in a magazine which is perhaps the most basic of the computer publications. Thus, it represents a good place to begin. *Popular Computing*, Subscription Department, P. O. Box 307, Martinsville, N.J. 08836.

Microcomputing. A monthly magazine for small computer users. The May 1981 issue contains several articles on word processing. Wayne Green, Inc., 80 Pine Street, Peterborough, N.H. 03458. It may also be available at your local computer store.

Poynter, D. *Word Processors and Information Processing*. Santa Barbara, CA: Para Publishing, 1982. This paperback provides a nontechnical introduction to word processing and equipment.

Veit, S. S. *Using Microcomputers in Business: A Guide for the Perplexed*. Rochelle Park, N.J.: Hayden, 1981. If you want to learn the basics about microcomputers, including word processing, this book provides a helpful beginning.

Vincent, K. R. Using a word processor to expedite psychological testing. *Computers in Psychiatry/Psychology*, October–November 1981, *3*, 8–9. This article appears in a newsletter for mental health professionals who use computers.

PART V

Psychological Testing

A unique application of the computer in mental health is for psychological testing. Part V presents the views of seasoned clinicians who have developed and used psychological tests over many years. Practical, clinical, and important ethical issues are examined.

In the first chapter in Part V, Jim Johnson gives an overview of computerized testing, a field with which he has been involved for decades. He is unusual in his ability to bring clinical, academic, and commercial experience to the task of examining the current role of the computer in testing. In his chapter he discusses adaptive testing, the construction of new test items, copyright issues, presentation techniques, and the dangers posed by mental health hobbyists. Jim believes the real contribution of the computer will come with the development of new psychological tests specifically designed for this new medium.

Bruce Duthie then raises important questions about the validity and professional practice issues associated with computer administration and analysis of psychological tests. Does the administration of a test using paper and pencil give results that are different from the same test given at a computer console? Do these two modes of administration tap into different cognitive functions? How does screen formatting affect test results? What are some of the practical problems attendant on the introduction of computerized testing into a clinical practice setting? Bruce has some interesting answers.

Gale Roid and Richard Gorsuch discuss the typology of computer-based psychological assessment and evaluate the usefulness of various test-administration and testing aids. How, they ask, can users determine on what a program's scoring schema is based? Should tests be routinely accompanied by research references? How much poetic license should the author of a testing program be given in writing canned narratives? With examples from programs that have actually been developed, they put forward some ideas on possible standards for psychological tests.

129

Part V ends with a chapter by Robert Zachary and Kenneth Pope on legal, professional, and ethical issues related to computerized testing. They point up the responsibility that test developers and test users must share in the ethical evolution of computer-generated reports. In a stimulating essay, they raise important issues, including: how test results should be communicated to clients; client access to test results; the maintenance of test security, privacy, and confidentiality; admissibility of test results as court evidence; and a number of other thought-provoking issues.

15 | An Overview of Computerized Testing

James H. Johnson, PhD

T o those of us who were early researchers on the application of computers to problems in psychology and psychiatry, it has seemed a long and tedious process. There have been many frustrations and few rewards—other than the excitement associated with small breakthroughs and the large prospects for the future. Often it has seemed as though the really important developments in the area would not come in our lifetime.

Now, however, there are developments occurring that will radically alter the practice of psychology and psychiatry. These developments are mainly in the area of psychological testing and involve commerce almost as much as they involve theory and practice.

The most radical development at the theoretical level is adaptive testing. Adaptive testing, at its simplest, involves branching to determine which questions should be asked to which persons. For example, questions about marriage would not be asked to a single person. At a more complex level, sophisticated mathematical approaches are used to determine item presentation based on previous responses. For example, in a test of mathematical ability a simple addition problem would not be presented to a person who had already correctly solved a complex algebraic equation. Computerization is obviously required for this approach.

Another development at the theoretical level involves item construction. Radically different kinds of items are possible using the computer medium. Examples include testing responses to the presentation of television like situations, complex cognitive tasks such as "flashing" stimulus presentations, and learning tasks. When these new types of items are combined with the developments in adaptive testing, it is easy to understand why most future psychological assessment will require computerization.

At the applied level, computerized testing has already had a major impact on the practice of psychology and psychiatry. More than 300,000 computerized test interpretations are processed annually by various scoring services. In addition, there are now approximately 500 clinicians who either have terminals connected to or own prepackaged computerized assessment systems. Finally, there are probably as many individuals who have programmed their own personal computer to administer and score psychological tests.

The impact of computers in the applied testing area is perhaps most dramatic at the institutional level. For example, the joint armed services have recently announced that all abilities assessment for recruitment will be computerized and will involve the adaptive methodology. In addition, companies such as Continental Bank in Chicago have begun implementation of computerized adaptive testing procedures for employment screening. Examples such as these illustrate how widespread the use of computers for psychological assessment has become during the last few years.

These changes have had a major impact on the commercial aspect of test publishing. Test publishers who once dedicated their efforts to the paper and pencil medium of assessment are now pushing hard to enter the computer market. This fact has gone hand in hand with one further change in the field: publishers are becoming more proprietary about the usage of their tests.

When I began work in this area, it was relatively easy for a qualified professional to write test publishers and obtain copyright permission to use test questions and norms on a computer. The only requirements involved the recording of usage and paying appropriate royalties. Now all that is changed. Few, if any, test publishers will respond to the individual professional. Test publishers are treating their tests as assets that are proprietary. Hence, the age of the individual computer-researcher/clinician is well nigh over insofar as standard published tests are concerned.

This change in posture by the publishers has been harshly attacked by many in the field for numerous reasons, many of which are just and correct. However, it should be pointed out that there are positive aspects to this change as well.

Consider, for example, the case with the MMPI. Many psychologists and computer programmers have begun their work automating assessment devices using this test. The MMPI has had several good "cookbooks" developed for its interpretation and, hence, was a natural for automation. However, the apparent ease of automating these cookbooks is somewhat deceptive.

People such as Jim Butcher, Alex Caldwell, Joe Finney, Ray Fowler, David Lachar, and myself have spent years of our lives learning to interpret MMPIs, reading a large portion of the literature, doing research with the test, using it in practice, and teaching its use. Still, we have found its automation to take years, with updates and changes continuing on and on as new findings from research and practice are presented.

It seems to me that mixing a little knowledge of computer programming with only a little knowledge about the interpretation of a test such as the MMPI, as many hobbyists are wont to do, and developing an automated interpretation in a matter of days or weeks cannot possibly be an ethical and responsible position for any professional in the field. The amount of knowledge and practice required to do this task right is more than most hobbyists are likely to possess in undertaking such a task. Without this knowledge base and years of work, it seems highly unlikely that a valid computerized interpretation will be developed. As I forever remind my students, psychology and psychiatry are scientific disciplines that involve years of study for certification. Either there is something in this process of gaining knowledge based on research and practice, or we should open the doors to everyone. Adding a computer to the process does not change this fact.

Thus, when the University of Minnesota Press began "tightening up" on who could develop and offer computerized MMPI interpretations, it seems to me that they were acting in a manner consonant with the ethics of the field. In most cases the same can be said for other publishers who have restricted computerized interpretations of their tests.

This aspect of the changes that are going on in the field of computerized assessment need not dampen our enthusiasm for future research in the area. As I have already indicated, the major theoretical advances of the future are going to come in item construction and presentation techniques. Why not begin work in these areas? It is here that all of us can make contributions to the field.

Hobbyists are going to do themselves and the field a disservice if they continue to do a poor job of attempting to automate tests previously developed for the paper and pencil medium. The real fun and real contributions will come by developing testing procedures specifically designed for the computer medium. It is in this area where I believe we should begin to concentrate our efforts.

16 A Critical Examination of Computer-Administered Psychological Tests

Bruce Duthie, PhD

With the advent of microcomputer technology, the potential for computer administration of psychological tests on a large-scale basis has become a reality. Many firms now offer microcomputer systems that administer, score, and interpret psychological tests. While the computer administration of psychological tests offers some advantages, there are several disadvantages and professional issues associated with the computerization of psychological test administration. The purpose of this chapter is to examine the professional issues associated with the microcomputer administration of psychological tests and to examine some alternative ways to use microcomputers in testing, which may be more cost-effective than computer administration.

Does the Response Set to Computers Contaminate Test Results?

The computer administration of a psychological test is not a standardized administration. Most psychological tests are printed on white paper and the client writes an answer on the booklet or on a standard answer sheet. It may seem, at first thought, that a computer-administered test on a CRT (TV screen) differs little from the more common paper-and-pencil administration, but there are in fact some important differences between these two kinds of test administrations. One important difference is the mystique associated with computers in general. Some individuals project awe and power on to the computer. The computer HAL in *2001 — Space Odyssey*, R2D2 in *Star Wars* and TWIKKI in *Flash Gordon* are examples of an emerging cultural computer archetype. Many individuals have had bad experiences with computers. They have been billed for products that they did not receive or have been displaced from the job market by computer technology. To some people a computer is an impersonal powerful, inhuman beast. John P. Mello, Jr., in "Deep in Your Heart It Will Creep" (Mello, 1982), estimates that 30% of this nation's office workers dread computers. He calls these people *cyberphobes*. He goes on to state that 5% of these people have phobic symptoms of clinical severity.

One study (Angle, Ellinwood & Carroll, 1979) compared the responses of patients interviewed by psychiatrists and a computer. The study reported that the patients reported a significantly larger amount of alcohol consumed to the computer than to the psychiatrists. This suggests that some individuals may respond more honestly to computers. The above-mentioned two articles suggest that there might be a computer response set that could affect the test-taking attitude of computer test respondents. The author knows of no published studies that have investigated computer response sets, yet many companies are marketing computer-administered psychological tests, the validity and reliability of which are based on conventional paper-and-pencil test administration. At least five companies now sell computer-administered versions of the MMPI.

Are There Cognitive Differences?

Two differences between computer-administered tests and conventional administrations suggest that they are separate cognitive tasks. The response time from first reading a test item to responding is much longer on a conventional test. When answering a conventional test, the client usually reads the question, decides upon the answer, and then transfers the answer to a separate answer sheet, where he marks in a dot or fills in between the lines. The time it takes to transfer his answer gives the client some reflection time. When answering a question on a computer-administered test, there is virtually no time between reading the question and pressing the chosen response key on the computer. Taking a test by computer is a much less complex task, which resembles a reflex. From our experience with the Rorschach, we know that respondents think of several responses before they decide upon which one they will articulate. Given this fact, it is possible that answers given to a computer will be less thought out and may not represent the client's best answer. Given that responding to a computer is a reflex, it is also possible that different parts of the brain are involved in responding to and processing questions presented on a CRT.

Another cognitive factor influencing computerized testing is mental fatigue. It takes much less time to take a test by computer. The average MMPI administration takes about 30 minutes when administered by computer. A client will experience much less mental fatigue while taking the test by computer. This may affect the test results.

Screen Format

Another problem with computer-administered tests is the lack of a standard presentation format. Some computers print only 40 characters across the CRT screen. Others print 80, and some print 64. Computers that feature color can have one or more colors in the background and another color for the printing on the CRT. Other computers only print in black-and-white, while some only come with a green-and-black CRT. Some computers are "streamlined and sexy," others look strictly businesslike. Most have 12-inch screens, but one popular computer has a 5-inch screen. Computers are as varied as their designers and the specific market to which these designers are appealing. This lack of standardization is confusing and may further compromise the validity of a computer-administered psychological test.

Computerized testing materials may become difficult to control. Most computer-administered psychological tests employ a metered disk that allows the administration of a certain number of tests (the number of test administrations paid for). This is a form of copy protection that is intended to insure that the test copyright holder gets a royalty just as if an answer sheet were paid for and used up, as happens in conventional test administration. Manufacturers of computerized testing systems charge from $2 to $10 per administration of the MMPI. Higher priced systems administer and also interpret the test. At this price, unscrupulous individuals will likely break the copy protection and enjoy unlimited use of the software. Once the copy protection is broken, the disk can be reproduced for about $2, the cost of a diskette. Copy protection is relatively easy to break, and programs are commercially available that are specifically designed to break copy-protected Apple and TRS-80 programs. Broken programs could find their way into lay user groups, which would place them totally out of the control of the psychology profession.

Are Computer-Administered Psychological Tests Practical?

For the high-volume clinic or the clinician on a time-sharing computer system with a remote dedicated psychological assessment computer, computer-administered psychological tests may be practical. In this setting, where several computer terminals are used to give several tests at once, the cost of test administration and computer hardware may be justified by the savings in administration time. For the clinician in private practice or the small clinic using a multi-purpose microcomputer, the cost and inconvenience of computer-administered tests may make this approach to psychological testing impractical. Another practical problem for the private-practice clinician or small clinic is the use of computer time. If the office microcomputer is tied up administering tests, there may not be time for the computer to do office record-keeping, interpret tests, do financial projections, or do research and statistics.

Approaches to Computerized Testing

There are several alternatives to computer-administered tests that take advantage of the microcomputer's speed, memory, and fast turn-around time and are practical, cost-effective, and do not violate instrument standardization. With all of the alternatives, the test is administered in the conventional, paper-and-pencil way.

Several microcomputer programs are available that score and interpret psychological tests. Some of these programs can be bought outright; others must be leased. The leased programs charge a small fee per use of the program. This fee is usually substantially less than the charge for administering, scoring, and interpreting the tests. Software that is purchased can be used as many times as the purchaser desires, without any usage fees. The user should be aware of the differences between leasing software and purchasing it before he or she actually gets the software.

Employing this alternative, an office assistant must type the individual test responses or standard scores into the computer, and the software converts the responses or standard scores and produces an interpretation. Several programs are available for the Wechsler scales, 16 PF (Personality Factor Questionnaire), Rorschach, and the MMPI that operate this way. This method does take some typing time. Entering the 566 T's and F's needed to interpret an MMPI takes about 10 minutes. The advantage of this alternative is a lower cost per test administration than a computer-administered test.

Another alternative is to employ an optical scanner to read mark-sense answer cards. This alternative uses an optical card reader, costing about $1,000, to enter client responses into the computer. The software then analyzes the responses to yield standard scores and creates an interpretation. This system is currently available for the Bi-Polar Psychological Inventory. This is a fast but more expensive alternative than the above one. Unfortunately, this type of system is not available for other psychological tests.

Canned test interpretations can be entered into a computer functioning as a word processor. The word-processing software then can enter canned statements into a psychological report, thereby saving typing time and test interpretation time. Canned statements are available for several psychological tests, including the Wechsler scales, Holtzman, and MMPI. The *MMPI Semi-Automated Interpretative Statements*, and *Semi-Automated Full Battery*, two books written by Ken Vincent, contain well-written canned statements for word-processing systems. (Vincent, 1980a & 1980b).

Psychologists can take advantage of the power and speed of microcomputers without compromising the standardized testing conditions. This chapter has examined several cost-effective, practical options for doing so.

REFERENCES

Mello, J. P., Jr. Deep in your heart it creeps. *80 Micro, 33,* 1982, 373–374.

Schwartz, Marc D. Review of assessment of psychiatric patients' problems by computer interview. *Computers in Psychiatry/Psychology, 2* (2), 1979, 8–10. (This article also appears as chapter 24 in this book.)

Vincent, K. R. *Semi-automated full battery.* Houston, TX: Psychometric Press, 1980(a).

Vincent, K. R. *MMPI semi-automated interpretive statements.* Houston, TX: Psychometric Press, 1980(b).

17

Development and Clinical Use of Test-Interpretive Programs on Microcomputers

Gale H. Roid, PhD
Richard L. Gorsuch, PhD

The availability of low-cost microcomputers for home and office opens new possibilities for psychological assessment and computerized test interpretation. At the same time, the proliferation of microcomputers and software raises issues such as cost, feasibility, and standards for quality control of software. This chapter discusses each of these issues under three interrelated headings: (1) the usefulness of various aids to test-administration and scoring, (2) a typology of computer software for psychological assessment, and (3) some thoughts on standards for the development of computer software for psychological assessment, with examples from actual developed programs.

USEFULNESS OF COMPUTER AIDS TO TEST-ADMINISTRATION AND SCORING

Microcomputers can be an aid to testing in a number of ways, including the actual administration of test questions on the computer screen. Conventional types of multiple-choice achievement tests, parent rating forms, self-report inventories, and questionnaires of many kinds can easily be programmed for display to either the examiner or the examinee.

An earlier version of this chapter was presented as part of the symposium, "Issues in the Clinical Use of Computerized Test Interpretation" at the meeting of the American Psychological Association, Washington, D. C., August 1982. Requests for further information should be sent to Dr. Gale Roid, Director of Research, Western Psychological Services, 12031 Wilshire Blvd., Los Angeles, California, 90025.

A criterion-referenced approach to the diagnosis of psychopathology can be computerized as an aid to forming diagnostic conclusions from test results and other patient information. Several DSM-III programs are available, but it is yet to be established whether these are cost-effective improvements over the simple turning of pages in a printed DSM-III handbook. Soon to be available for microcomputer administration and diagnosis is the Psychiatric Diagnostic Interview or PDI (Othmer, Penick, & Powell, 1981), which is a branching-style series of structured interview questions with established validity for identifying psychiatric syndromes. The PDI is based on the Feighner criteria (Feighner, Robins, Guze, Woodruff, Winokur, & Munoz, 1972), a forerunner of the DSM-III diagnostic criteria. Fifteen syndromes, such as alcoholism, depression, and anorexia nervosa, are assessed by preliminary criterion questions, followed by more in-depth questioning if a syndrome appears positive.

Another way in which micros may aid test-interpretation is by the indirect effect of having new types of psychological tests available that can test abilities that might be difficult to assess with paper-and-pencil methods. Cory, Rimland, and Bryson (1977), for example, have shown that computerized assessments of abilities such as visual tracking, short-term memory, and resistance to distraction are feasible. Response latency and distractibility are increasingly mentioned as important factors in interpreting borderline performance on ability measures such as the WISC-R (Kaufman, 1979) and in forms of learning disabilities such as dyslexia (Rudel, Denckla, & Broman, 1981). Whether the computer is more cost-effective than the widely used traditional methods of using a stopwatch with unique test batteries, such as those of Santostefano (1978), remains to be seen.

As a more futuristic aid to test interpretation, one can imagine commercially available programs that allow for tailored testing (e.g., Lord, 1980; Urry, 1977; Weiss, 1979), which might employ item banks or scale banks. Applications of these methods are nearly all in the research laboratory at this time and require a great deal of statistical sophistication for proper implementation. However, the promise is in having available numerous psychological and educational measures virtually at the tip of the finger. This would allow branching from one test to another, or from item to item, to probe the reasons behind test performance. For example, quick and accurate estimates of reading ability or verbal intelligence could be used to determine the acceptability of certain self-report inventories, if reading ability was suspected to be interfering with accurate reporting. Also, research has shown that tailored testing, particularly in the achievement domain, can decrease error of measurement by matching the item difficulty to the ability level of the examinee (Haladyna & Roid, 1983).

Future applications of microcomputers will depend to some extent on whether or not it is concluded that patients can directly interact with the computer keyboard or display without affecting test performance or interpretation. Fortunately, there is already considerable research that points to the feasibility of subjects' direct interaction with the computer. Studies such as those of Katz and Dalby (1981) on the Eysenck Personality Inventory and Klinge and Rodziewicz (1976) on the Peabody Picture Vocabulary Test have shown nearly equivalent results for computer vs. paper-and-pencil versions. Other studies such as Scissons (1976) and Biskin and Kolotkin (1977) indicate that some differences, such as those on the Paranoia scale of the MMPI, can be expected to occur, depending on the severity of psychopathology in the subjects tested. Beaumont (1975) encountered no problems in automated administration of the Category Test to organic and psychiatric patients. O'Brien and Dugdale (1978) found some tendency for respondents to be more honest about personal habits when given a computer-administered questionnaire as compared with a field interview.

A TYPOLOGY OF COMPUTER PROGRAMS FOR PSYCHOLOGICAL TESTING

Table 17–1 shows a matrix of the input and output characteristics of computerized testing programs, which may be helpful in understanding and evaluating available software. The inputs include direct keyboard entry of responses from subjects; item responses from other sources, such as from an assistant who types in a previously completed protocol, or information from a peripheral input or storage device; and entry of scores, whether raw scores or derived scores. The outputs from a computer program can be classified into at least five types, each of which will be discussed in turn.

Types of Output

Scoring Programs. A large number of computer programs currently available for microcomputers are simply scoring routines. This may be cost-effective for large inventories or batteries with multiple scales, indexes, and profiles, but simple scoring is often a clerical task that can be done without the overhead of the computer. Some would claim that even the saving of a half-hour is important for a clinician, if scoring must be done personally, and, also, that increased accuracy is obtained by using a computer. Although not frequently done, scoring by computer would make feasible the computation of precise factor scores (if factor scales are used), rather than unit-weight factor scales, such as are typical with standard scoring keys.

TABLE 17–1. A Typology of Computer Programs in Psychological Testing

Types of Input	Types of Output
1. Item Responses from Subjects	1. Scoring Only
2. Item Responses from Other Sources	2. Test-Administration and Scoring
3. Scores Only	3. Descriptive Interpretation
	4. Clinician-Modeled Interpretation (Exemplary or Statistical)
	5. Clinical-Actuarial Interpretation

Test-Administration and Scoring Programs. To use the full potential of microcomputers, test-administration programs ideally would go beyond a simple page-turning function and programs would present new assessment functions in a manner that would not be possible with paper-and-pencil methods—for example, complex memory or pattern-recognition tasks, tailored testing of items or scales, and criterion-referenced diagnostic tests that rely on complex calculations. For conventional inventories, it would seem preferable to have patients respond on optical-scan answer sheets for later input to the micro.

Descriptive Interpretations. A descriptive type of program would generate descriptive sentences, such as "A very high score on . . .", or "Scale 1 is significantly higher than Scale 2 . . .", along with a printed profile or list of scores. Some commercially available programs we reviewed have such sentences, but use a redundantly similar format to report multiple-scale scores. To avoid this redundancy, the computer program to interpret the Barclay Classroom Assessment System (Barclay, 1983) was designed as a highly sophisticated generator of descriptive sentences that read as if they were individually written for each student. An example is provided below:

> This student is seen as having an outstanding thrust for achievement and is viewed as superior in persistence. She demonstrates impulsive, unpredictable and inconsistent behavior. She appears to be generally open and verbally expressive. In physical activities or working with her hands, she is seen as having an above average level of effort and perseverance.

This descriptive paragraph is composed by scanning the score levels of three separate factor scores, determining a sentence that describes each score level, and adding appropriate pronouns of "she" or "he." Separate sentences are then pieced together to form a narrative paragraph. The computer routines required to generate a three-page report of this nature are complex indeed, but are necessary to make the report truly readable by the school psychologist or other user.

Clinician-Modeled Programs. These interpretive programs could take two forms: (1) the process used by a renowned clinician is simulated by the program; and (2) a statistical model of the process used by expert clinicians is validated and programmed for computer (e.g., Goldberg, 1970; Wiggins, 1973).

An example of the first type of program is the forthcoming one for the Louisville Behavior Checklist (Miller, 1981), which will include a sequential, mostly descriptive report involving the same kind of profile analysis used by the test-developer, Dr. Lovick Miller. These include interpretations that are indirectly backed by much empirical research, such as the identification of "externalizers" vs. "internalizers" (e.g., acting-out vs. withdrawn), a distinction drawn by numerous researchers using factor-analysis of childhood rating scales.

The second type of clinician-modeled program would be based on statistical analyses of the judgment of one or more expert clinicians, using the methods suggested by Goldberg (1970). Wiggins (1973) noted that a statistical model of an expert clinician functions as well as, and often better than, the clinician can, since the program is more consistent. To develop such a model, an external criterion, such as confirmed psychiatric diagnosis, is established for each patient in a sample who has been given a psychological test or battery. A relatively large number of clinical judgments is needed (e.g., a sample of 200 patients), and these judgments can be regressed on the external criterion. One accurate clinician may be chosen or the composite judgment of a set of clinicians may be used. If an external criterion is not available, a potentially less valid method would involve using the composite judgment of clinicians as the criterion and an additional exemplary clinician as the predictor. The statistical model derived from these analyses is usually a simple linear model, which weights each of several psychological scales or other data, using a regression equation (Goldberg, 1968).

Clinical Actuarial Program. An actuarial type of program is represented by the widely used MMPI test-scoring and interpretive services. These include extensive narrative descriptions and clinical hypotheses based on the clinical research findings for particular score patterns. Other examples include the 16 PF programs of the Institute for Personality and Ability Testing (IPAT), the Strong-Campbell Interest Inventory scoring program, Behaviordyne's narrative programs for the California Psychological Inventory, the Western Psychological Services' (WPS) program for the Personality Inventory for Children (PIC), and others. These represent the most complex and sophisticated interpretive programs (those that have integrated the research on test interpretation), and it is probably just a matter of time before they are implemented on microcomputers (such as the Apple II version of the PIC program by WPS). These programs show great promise, but increasingly they are the focus of scrutiny over the empirical basis of their conclusions. Thus, it is a natural evolution that the APA/AERA/NCME Committee on Test Standards is now considering a section of the new revised standards to be devoted to computerized interpretive programs.

RECOMMENDATIONS FOR THE STANDARDS FOR INTERPRETIVE PROGRAMS

The consideration of standards for interpretive programs is complex; a brief, tentative list of suggestions is presented below.

1. Given that a flood of new microcomputer software is being released, it is imperative that some method of labeling or standard description be provided to distinguish between elemental scoring programs (those which calculate scores only—without interpretative or narrative discussion of results) and others. Perhaps the typology in Table 1 will be helpful in this regard, as it further distinguishes between descriptive, clinical, and fully actuarial programs. The authors have recently reviewed a large number of programs and have found a surprising number that include only scoring and profiling, with very primitive narrative reporting or none at all. Others that appear to be fully actuarial are actually modeling an expert clinician at best, or the subjective, unvalidated opinions of one clinician at worst, and the program's descriptive literature may not acquaint one with facts.

2. Although it is a detailed and tedious undertaking, a quality interpretive program must provide extensive references to the empirical basis for the decision rules used. In the case of the PIC, for example, this documentation required a separate hardbound monograph (Lachar & Gdowski, 1979). The requirement for references or documentation is particularly challenging for well-researched instruments such as the MMPI, because it is easy for the developer to assume that the user is familiar with the extensive literature on the instrument. However, in the experience of the present authors, all too often a computerized interpretive service is approached by otherwise qualified users who are not intimately familiar with the research on an instrument. They may need research references to be able to determine if unusual circumstances not taken into account by the program could temper the results.

3. It is tempting to refer to the computer-generated interpretation as "the IBM Computer Report" or "the APPLE-85 Program." But the quality of the report is totally unrelated to the type of computer that

generated it. The quality of the report is a function of its authors: those who specified the decision-making rules (they may often be different people from the ones who programmed it). Someone must take responsibility for the suggestions made by the report. Just as the quality of a book is suggested by its author and publisher, and not by its color, so the quality of a computer interpretation is suggested by its author and publisher, and is independent of the type of computer.

4. One of the areas where it is tempting for developers to depart from an empirical base is in the narrative portions of a computerized report. Lachar and Gdowski (1979) developed a technique for validating descriptive words and phrases that is a good example of the clinical actuarial method. They obtained independent clinicians' ratings and checklist data for families and children who were subsequently subjects of completed PIC protocols. Profile scales for the resulting PICs were scored, and each scale was divided into levels or "elevations," such as 80T +, 70–79T, 60–69T, 41–59T, 40T–. The frequency of clinicians' descriptive ratings for subjects whose scores fell in each level were then obtained. High-frequency descriptors were called "correlates," and were subsequently cross-validated on new samples. The correlates of profile elevations then provided the basis for narrative sentences and descriptors used in the computerized interpretive program. This procedure adds an element of external validity to the narrative portions of the test reports.

SUMMARY

The proliferation of low-cost microcomputers has made possible some new aids for psychological test interpretation. With the increasing availability of new software for microcomputer-based testing, some system of labeling or definition for programs seems required to prevent confusion over scoring vs. interpretive programs and to highlight those programs that include research-based actuarial interpretive systems.

We presented in this chapter a proposed typology that distinguishes between programs that can be labeled Test Administration and Scoring, Descriptive Interpretation, Clinician-Modeled Interpretation, and Clinical-Actuarial Interpretation. In cases where a test or test battery has an extensive array of scores or scores that are difficult to compute by hand (e.g., factor scores), the Test Administration and Scoring programs can save the practitioner many hours of scoring time. Although the clinical-actuarial programs have the advantage of being based on extensive validation research, the user should investigate the empirical research behind the original test, its scores, and their interpretation, regardless of the level of the program in the typology presented in this chapter. Presentation of research references and findings in the marketing of such programs would aid the users in determining the applicability of each program to their clinical needs.

REFERENCES

Barclay, J. R. *Barclay Classroom Assessment System (BCAS) Manual.* Los Angeles: Western Psychological Services, 1983.

Beaumont, J. G. The validity of the category test administered by on-line computer. *Journal of Clinical Psychology,* 1975, *31,* 458–462.

Biskin, B. H., & Kolotkin, R. L. Effects of computerized administration on scores on the Minnesota Multiphasic Personality Inventory. *Applied Psychological Measurement,* 1977, *1,* 543–549.

Cory, C. H., Rimland, B., & Bryson, R. A. Using computerized tests to measure new dimensions of abilities: An exploratory study. *Applied Psychological Measurement,* 1977, *1,* 101–110.

Feighner, J. P., Robins, E., Guze, S. B., Woodruff, R. A., Winokur, G., & Munoz, R. Diagnostic criteria for use in psychiatric research. *Archives of General Psychiatry,* 1972, *26,* 57–63.

Goldberg, L. R. Simple models or simple processes? Some research on clinical judgments. *American Psychologist,* 1968, *23,* 483–496.

Goldberg, L. R. Man vs. model of man: A rationale, plus some evidence for a method of improving on clinical inferences. *Psychological Bulletin,* 1970, *73,* 422–432.

Haladyna, T. M., & Roid, G. H. A comparison of two item-selection procedures for building criterion-referenced tests. *Journal of Educational Measurement,* 1983, *20*(3).

Katz, L., & Dalby, J. T. Computer and manual administration of the Eysenck Personality Inventory. *Journal of Clinical Psychology,* 1981, *37,* 586–588.

Kaufman, A. S. *Intelligent testing with the WISC-R.* New York: Wiley, 1979.

Klinge, V., & Rodziewicz, T. Automated and manual intelligence testing of the Peabody Picture Vocabulary Test on a psychiatric adolescent population. *International Journal of Man-Machine Studies,* 1976, *8,* 243–246.

Lachar, D., & Gdowski, C. L. *Actuarial assessment of child and adolescent personality: An interpretive guide for the Personality Inventory for Children Profile.* Los Angeles: Western Psychological Services, 1979.

Lord, F. M. *Applications of item response theory to practical testing problems.* Hillsdale, N.J.: Lawrence Erlbaum, 1980.

Miller, L. C. *Louisville Behavior Checklist Manual.* Los Angeles: Western Psychological Services, 1981.

O'Brien, T., & Dugdale, V. Questionnaire administration by computer. *Journal of the Market Research Society,* 1978, *20,* 228–237.

Othmer, E., Penick, E. C., & Powell, B. J. *Psychiatric Diagnostic Interview (PDI) Manual.* Los Angeles: Western Psychological Services, 1981.

Rudel, R. G., Denckla, M. B., & Broman, M. The effect of varying stimulus context on word-finding ability: Dyslexia further differentiated from other learning disabilities. *Brain and Language*, 1981, *13*, 130–144.

Santostefano, S. *A biodevelopmental approach to clinical child psychology: Cognitive controls and cognitive control therapy.* New York: Wiley, 1978.

Scissons, E. H. Computer administration of the California Psychological Inventory. *Measurement and Evaluation in Guidance*, 1976, *91*, 22–25.

Urry, V. W. Tailored testing: A successful application of latent trait theory. *Journal of Educational Measurement*, 1977, *14*, 181–186.

Vincent, K. R. Using a word processor to expedite psychological testing. *Computers in Psychiatry/Psychology*, 1981, *3*(6), 8–9.

Weiss, D. J. Computerized adaptive achievement testing. In H. F. O'Neil, Jr. (Ed.), *Procedures for instructional systems development.* New York: Academic Press, 1979.

Wiggins, J. S. *Personality and prediction: Principles of personality assessment.* Reading, Mass.: Addison-Wesley, 1973.

Legal and Ethical Issues in the Clinical Use of Computerized Testing

Robert A. Zachary, PhD
Kenneth S. Pope, PhD

The proliferation of programs for administering, scoring, and interpreting psychological tests by computer offers many advantages to test-users but also raises novel legal, ethical, and professional issues. In this chapter we discuss several major issues confronting both developers and users of computerized test reports. These include maintenance of professional standards, user qualifications, client welfare, communicating test results, test security, privacy and confidentiality, admissibility of computer-generated reports in court, copyright violations, client access to computerized test information, and vulnerability of computerized test data and client information to subpoena.

Test-developers and test-users bear a joint responsibility for the ethical and professional use of computerized tests (American Psychological Association, 1974; see also Novick, 1982). In sorting out these responsibilities it is useful to define some essential roles. *Test-developers* are individuals who create, publish, or market tests and test-related materials, including software. *Test-users* are individuals who use tests for some decision-making purpose. *Test-takers* are those who take the test, whether by choice or necessity. While test-developers and test-users have traditionally had the greatest influence over policies governing the use of tests, the growth of consumerism and concern about discrimination has made the test-taker a more prominent force. The

An earlier version of this chapter was presented as part of a symposium, "Issues in the Clinical Use of Computerized Test Interpretation," at the annual meeting of the American Psychological Association, Washington, DC, August 1982.

right of the test-taker to examine his or her scores on individual tests, and the interpretation of these scores is an issue which we shall take up later.

RESPONSIBILITIES OF TEST-DEVELOPERS

Maintenance of Professional Standards

An issue of major importance to test-developers concerns the maintenance of appropriate professional standards in the development, documentation, and promotion of computerized test reports. There are several problems to consider. Computerized interpretive reports vary tremendously in comprehensiveness, flexibility, and in the methods used to develop them (Roid, 1982). The use of a computer to interpret psychological test data may create an aura of objectivity. However, the sophistication, appropriateness, and clinical utility of the conclusions drawn from computerized interpretive reports are limited by the skills and sophistication of the individuals who formulate the decision rules on which the programs are based, and by the clinician who has to decide how to integrate the interpretive report with information from other sources.

A concern for professional standards affects test-developers in several ways. First, organizations or individuals who produce interpretive programs must be competently staffed. For individuals, this means having technical expertise in several areas: computer programming, measurement theory, and the interpretation and clinical use of specific tests. For organizations, this means having a mix of qualified individuals on staff who can blend their separate areas of expertise to produce high-quality programs. Second, the development of programs should be empirically based and must be backed up by sufficient documentation of the program—the rationale and specific decision rules—so that the procedures used to produce test reports can be examined and independently evaluated. Third, automated assessment systems should not be distributed prematurely (see Farrell, 1984, for specific criteria on when a program is ready for distribution).* Fourth, programs should be periodically revised and updated so that they remain current with the professional literature and with changes in normative data. Fifth, debugging and technical assistance should be available. Finally, test developers and publishers should avoid making inflated claims, which are not independently verifiable.

How can an individual clinician, who does not have specialized knowledge in computer programming, responsibly evaluate alternative

---

*[Farrell, 1984 appears in Part VII of this book.—Ed.]

programs or computerized testing services? A direct approach is to score and interpret the same test protocol using different programs, and then compare the output. Technical manuals and users' guides, when available, may offer more detailed information about the programs' rationale, empirical basis, and specific procedures for determining decision rules and classification statistics. In addition, independent reviews of some automated scoring and interpretive programs are available (e.g., Buros, 1978, pg. 938–962), along with comparative studies of user satisfaction or judged accuracy of reports (Lachar, 1974; Green, 1982). Other useful sources of information include journals such as *Computers in Psychiatry/Psychology*, which provide a network for sharing information, and other, less specialized journals, which discuss computer-related issues.

To facilitate such comparisons, we need a uniform method for describing and classifying computerized reports, along with a clear set of standards detailing the essential and desirable characteristics of an acceptable program and prescribing ethical guidelines. At a time when the *Standards for Educational and Psychological Tests* (American Psychological Association, 1974) is being expanded and revised, it is important to confront directly the unique technical and professional issues posed by the development of computer-based interpretive programs. The chapter in this book by Roid and Gorsuch, "Development and Clinical Use of Test-Interpretive Programs on Microcomputers" represents a heuristic step in this direction.

User Qualifications

There are two different types of individuals who are at risk to misuse computerized test information: unqualified users and unsophisticated users. Unqualified users are those who lack the appropriate professional training and background to use and interpret psychological tests appropriately. Unsophisticated users are those individuals who, while they may have a general background in measurement theory and testing, are unsophisticated or inadequately informed about a particular test. This frequently occurs in the use of more complex tests such as the Minnesota Multiphasic Personality Inventory (Hathaway & McKinley, 1967) or the Luria-Nebraska Neuropsychological Battery (Golden, Hemmeke, & Purish, 1980). Users of such tests often lack specific knowledge of the test rationale and psychometric properties, or lack familiarity with the literature in specialized content areas.

The availability of automated interpretive reports increases the likelihood that they may become available to individuals who lack the professional qualifications to use and interpret them appropriately. Because of the ease with which they produce a readable, seemingly "objective" report, computerized reports will be especially attractive to organizations such as small businesses, who employ psychological test data but do not always make appropriate use of outside consultants. This is a particular concern because small- to medium-size corporations are especially likely to purchase microcomputers.

A second area of ethical concern involves the use of computerized interpretive reports by unsophisticated users. These are individuals who, while they may have a general background in psychodiagnostics, are not sufficiently familiar with a particular test to use and interpret it appropriately. There is a risk that these individuals will use the test results for purposes other than those for which they were specifically validated. In particular, they may be unaware of the limitations of the test and/or the interpretive program; they may try to use tests for individuals, settings, and assessment purposes for which there is no documented empirical evidence; they may not be sensitive to situational variables, such as unusual distractions or sensory or physical handicaps, which may lead to invalid inferences; or they may not be able to integrate actuarial and clinical data appropriately.

At present, the major method for dealing with this problem involves routine screening by test publishers and distributors to prevent use by unqualified individuals. However, the effectiveness of such procedures is questionable. Usually publishers rely on user-supplied information to determine their eligibility to purchase particular kinds of tests. Unless publishers define their eligibility in a very restrictive fashion (e.g., only members of APA or only licensed psychologists can purchase tests), there is no readily available means of verifying user qualifications. In addition, a degree per se—or even a state license or diplomate status—is no guarantee that an individual will administer and interpret a particular test appropriately. Concern that computerized test materials may be distributed without sufficient screening of potential users is especially great because of the attraction of individual entrepreneurs into this area. Although some independent producers of computer software may adhere to very high professional and ethical standards, there is nothing to bind these individuals to these standards.

Concern for Client Welfare

A concern for the welfare of the individual client is central in all clinical endeavors, but is especially important in testing. Those who develop interpretive programs and/or market them should be concerned with the typical uses and potential misuses of these programs, what Messick (1981) calls the "value consequences of a test." The potential for misuse is high in all areas of testing, but the use of computer-generated reports places an added burden on the developer because of its potential use by unqualified or unsophisticated users. In creating narrative statements, program developers must be sensitive to the damaging consequences that may result from their statements, especially because computerized reports may have an added aura of authenticity. They should make appropriate use of confidence intervals or equivalent verbal descriptors (e.g., "90% sure") in interpreting test data. They should also be careful to represent accurately the empirical basis for any clinical decisions obtained from the program, and build into the program appropriate cautionary statements about the limitations of the test and/or the computer-generated report.

Communicating Test Results

Developers of computerized reports should insure that the content and style of their reports are appropriate for the assessment purposes for which the test is intended and that they take into account the level of sophistication of the person who will actually make use of the report. Particular caution should be exercised in writing programs that will be given directly to clients, as for example in providing feedback on a vocational guidance inventory. The probabilistic nature of the conclusions derived from the tests should be emphasized and the results explained in language that the average client will find useful. The use of individually tailored reports written for different audiences (Krug, 1982) is desirable when the same test can be used appropriately in a wide variety of assessment contexts (e.g., the MMPI, 16-PF, and CPI).

Test Security

Another professional issue confronting users of test-related software concerns the maintenance of test security. Developers of computer programs to interpret tests are concerned with two types of security. First, they are concerned with security of the test itself, including actual items or stimulus materials, test rationale, and scoring and interpretive procedures. The major focus of these concerns is to limit the public dissemination of information about tests, which would tend to invalidate their future usefulness. A second type of security concerns the actual program that is used to administer, score, and/or interpret the tests. Again, the concern is to restrict the program to its intended professional use and avoid any practices that would contaminate the future use of the test. The issue of safeguarding programs against possible copyright infringement is somewhat separate, and is discussed along with other important legal issues below.

As more interpretive programs become available, the risk to test security is greater. The problem is certainly not unique to computer-ized reports. However, computer programs provide more detailed in-formation that could potentially harm test security, such as flagging of critical items and clear identification of validity scales. In addressing this issue, test publishers and users bear a joint responsibility for insur-ing test security. From this perspective, the maintenance of test secu-rity (e.g., preventing unauthorized copying of disks for microcom-puters) is important to insure the appropriate use of the test, not just to protect the publishers' financial investment.

Privacy

Another area of concern is the threat to individual privacy posed by computerized test reports (Hoffman, 1980). Privacy involves three re-lated issues: justification for testing, avoiding unwarranted intrusions, and informed consent.

Professionals who make use of programs to interpret tests should be able to provide a reasonable explanation for their choice of tests. The intent is to use tests for a specific assessment purpose, not because they are readily available or because the clinician can charge more for his or her services.

The increased availability of interpretive reports makes it more likely that they will be used routinely or indiscriminately. Casual ad-ministration of tests for which there is no bona fide purpose poses the threat of unwarranted intrusions into an individual's privacy and may even cause personal harm. Professionals should avoid the indiscrimi-nate use of tests, especially in employment batteries where irrelevant but potentially harmful information could readily be obtained.

As with other types of testing, the use of computerized tests as-sumes that the individual clinician has adequately informed the client about the purpose of the test, what he or she can reasonably expect to gain from the test, and any limitations or potential harm associated with the test procedures or eventual computerized report. Having been appraised of these issues, the client must give his or her informed con-sent prior to being tested.

While the primary responsibility for insuring individual privacy in the use of computerized tests rests with the test-user, test-developers should be sensitive to these issues and should restrict the sale of com-puterized reports to individuals who agree to use them in a manner that insures individual privacy.

Confidentiality

An area of particular ethical concern involves the use of archival re-cords, which are routinely stored and accessible by computer. The maintenance of archival records by institutions or individual clinicians is highly desirable for specific purposes, such as the development of local norms. Moreover, the maintenance of research files in settings that act as clearinghouses for scoring and providing computerized test reports facilitates research and updating of norms. However, the routine storing of raw test data also poses a potential threat to confidentiality of individual clients and opens the way for possible misuses, such as use of obsolete data to make decisions about individuals and unauthorized access to data. A related issue concerns the legal status of such archival data. Are such records privileged and, if so, under what circumstances?

Many test-report services do not use client names when processing or archiving test data. To protect confidentiality, unique identification numbers are assigned not only to individual clients, but also to the clinician who bears the professional responsibility for interpreting and using the test data. A separate coding system for linking up test data with individual client records can be created so that, if questions are raised about the accuracy of a particular individual's report, it is possible to go back to the files and check for errors in scoring or interpretation. In this respect, automated procedures may be more efficient than relying on clinicians or technical and clerical staff to maintain confidentiality (see also Anastasi, 1976, pg. 54–55).

RESPONSIBILITIES OF TEST-USERS

Maintenance of Professional Standards

Test-users, as well as test-developers, need to be concerned with maintaining professional standards. Test-users should be able to justify their use of specific tests. They should be able to state precisely what it is they hope to gain by the use of a specific test and how the test will be used along with confirmatory or disconfirmatory information from other sources to make clinical decisions. It is unethical for test-users to "pad" test batteries with unnecessary tests in order to charge more for testing.

Automated reports are useful tools but can't replace skilled clinical judgment. Users have a professional responsibility to recognize the limits of their knowledge and areas of competency, and to avoid misrepresenting their qualifications to others. If necessary, users should supplement their present knowledge with continuing education courses and other sources of information on content areas and tests that are unfamiliar to them. In addition, it is essential that they have available and use the technical manuals and other documentation for programs. Finally, users should show reasonable judgment in consulting experts in areas outside their field of specialization. The ultimate responsibility for the appropriate use of tests, whether or not computerized interpretations are used, resides with the individual user.

Communicating Test Results

Test results should be communicated in a form that takes into account the ability of the individual client to use the results and his or her current emotional state and attitudes. Unless the reports are specifically designed to be read by unsophisticated test-takers, clients (like unsophisticated clinicians) may misunderstand the technical language of reports and may be harmed by their misconceptions. Even if reports are specifically designed to be read directly by clients, as is the case with some vocational guidance instruments, the responsible professional should insure that each individual who receives the reports fully understands the results and the professional should be available to answer any questions. Leaving it up to the client to initiate contact is not enough.

Privacy

As was the case with test-developers and publishers, test-users are responsible for insuring the privacy of the test-taker. This entails guarding against unwarranted intrusions and obtaining informed consent. If anything, the test-user should be more responsible for this function because he or she will have the most direct contact with the test-taker and is the one who decides which tests to give.

Confidentiality

Test-users can help to protect the confidentiality of their clients by replacing clients' names with unique identifying codes. In general, computer-generated materials should be afforded the same safeguards as any other clinical material. The storing of data either to collect local norms or to develop research files should include specific procedures to protect confidentiality. However, care should be taken so that the clinician can go back and link up existing client files with new data, if desired. For a more detailed discussion of issues concerning privacy and confidentiality in mental health practices, see Siegel (1979).

Test Security

Test-users also share a responsibility for maintaining test security. Users should not make available the test or test-related materials, including computerized reports, to the general public. Similarly, they should not allow unqualified users to use tests or test software. This is a particular problem because purchasers of specialized hardware may wish to recover some of their initial expenses by leasing time to other professionals in their area. Once they do this they become, in effect, test-distributors and should be bound by the ethical and professional guidelines discussed above.

LEGAL ISSUES

Wide-scale use of computers to score and interpret psychological tests also raises a number of legal issues. These issues include the admissibility of computer-generated reports as evidence in court proceedings, copyright violations involving computer software, client access to computerized test information, and vulnerability of computerized test data and client information to subpoena.

Admissibility of Computerized Test Reports as Court Evidence

The issue of admissibility of computerized test reports as evidence in criminal or civil court proceedings is difficult to address in the abstract. Although there are some cases where a computerized report may be introduced directly as evidence—for example, if the validity of the report itself is at issue—for the most part psychological test data is introduced indirectly as part of the testimony of expert witnesses. The 1962 decision of the District of Columbia Court of Appeals in *Jenkins* v. *United States* set a precedent for accepting the testimony of psychologists on a multitude of legal issues (Perlin, 1980). However, the impact of psychological testimony on courtroom decisions is highly variable. The general criticism leveled at psychological testimony is that it is too subjective and inexact to satisfy legal standards for evidence (Szasz, 1963, 1970).

From a legal perspective, computerized reports may be better than those generated by an individual clinician because the rules for making particular decisions and for classifying individuals are explicit and readily accessible. Thus, a computerized interpretive report is potentially less subjective, more impartial, and more directly tied to empirical data, which are explicit and testable. At the very least, computer interpretation makes explicit and public what it is that is "inexact" in making inferences from psychological tests. In addition, interpretive reports can be programmed to make systematic use of qualifiers such as setting confidence intervals around obtained scores or stating the degree of certainty for various clinical decisions—procedures that are especially important in giving expert testimony (Delman, 1981), but which are generally not systematically reported in most standard test reports. The legal status of computerized reports is still unclear. However, informal feedback from some psychologists who have been called to testify in court cases involving computerized test reports indicate that the initial response from the legal community has been generally positive.*

As a practical matter, clinicians must be able to document fully any statements made from test data and address more general questions concerning the appropriateness of the test for particular individuals and clinical/legal decisions. In other words, the existence of a computerized report does not eliminate the need to be thoroughly informed about the research basis for particular tests and to be able to articulate this information clearly in court. If an individual is using the computerized report as a substitute for a thorough understanding of a test, this will probably become abundantly clear in court. For a more detailed discussion of the courtroom use of psychological testimony and some pragmatic suggestions on how to prepare, see Caldwell (1960) and Ziskin (1975).

Copyright Violations

With the proliferation of computer programs, a major problem confronting those who develop and market tests is that of providing adequate security for their products. Although programs, like published test materials, may be protected by copyright, specific provisions have not yet been made to deal with the added complexities of computerized testing. The Copyright Revision Act of 1976 affirms that:

> . . . In the area of computer uses of copyrighted works—the use of a work in conjunction with automatic systems capable of storing, processing, retrieving, or transferring information—the problems (are) not sufficiently developed for a definitive legislative solution. . . . In view of this, the purpose of the Sec. 117 of the revised law is to preserve the status quo. This provision is not intended to cut off any rights that now exist or to create any new rights, but merely to maintain existing conditions. Also, the provision deals only with the exclusive rights of a copyright owner with respect to computer uses. The revised law will apply with respect to the copyrightability of computer programs, the ownership of copyright, the term of protection and the formal requirements, etc.
>
> Sec. 117 provides that . . . the owner of a copyright is not afforded any greater or lesser rights with respect to use of the work in conjunction with automatic systems capable of storing, pro-

---

*Personal communications from A. Caldwell to authors, August 23, 1982, and from S. Krug to authors, August 23, 1982.

cessing, retrieving, or transferring information, or in conjunction with any similar device, machine, or process, than those rights afforded to works under the law in effect on December 31, 1977. [Copyright Revision Act of 1976, pg. 36, paragraph 292]

In other words, the committee charged with revising the copyright law in 1976 deferred acting on specific issues relating to the copyright protection of computerized versions of previously copyrighted materials. The committee felt it was necessary to allow case law (precedents in individual cases) to develop before enacting specific laws in this area.

The vagueness of the present law confronts test-developers with a difficult choice. From a professional standpoint, it is important to fully inform professional users of tests about their psychometric properties and to make available normative data and scoring procedures to promote further research on an instrument. However, this makes it possible for others to take the normative data and develop their own computer programs to score and interpret tests. Since these individuals bear none of the responsibility or expense for developing and refining these instruments, they can undercut the original publisher by offering programs at seemingly bargain prices. In response to this situation, some publishers have been forced to withhold normative data or restrict use of test items to prevent others from marketing their products.

Client Access to Computerized Test Material

Traditionally, client access to test protocols has been strictly limited for clinical reasons and to protect test security. However, the enactment of a series of consumer-disclosure laws at both the state and federal levels has made test materials more accessible to individual consumers. The Family Education Rights and Privacy Act, *Detroit Edison* v. *NLRB* (1979), and the "truth-in-testing" laws of New York and California are examples of a trend in state and federal legislation and case law making test materials more accessible to individual consumers (Bersoff, 1981). They reflect a movement toward greater involvement of clients, subjects, examinees, and other consumers of psychological services in their own evaluation and treatment (Fischer & Brodsky, 1978). But this is an area in constant flux and, for the most part, we are operating without a comprehensive set of clear guidelines.

Access of Others to Computerized Client Information

The rights of others to gain access to confidential client files, whether or not they involve computerized reports or information stored on a computer, depend on several factors: the nature of the client-professional relationship; the client's attitude toward the release of the documents; and the specific circumstances of individual court cases in which the release of confidential client information becomes an issue. In the case of practitioners who use computerized devices in their own offices to interpret or store client information, such information would probably be regarded as "privileged." Originally designed to protect information between professionals (doctors, lawyers, and ministry) and their clients, the notion of client privilege has also been affirmed for psychotherapists. However, a major point of confusion is who "owns the privilege"—who decides whether or not certain confidential information can be released under particular circumstances. Clinicians do not "own the privilege"—only their clients do. Thus, clinicians do not have any legal recourse if their clients waive their privilege to restrict the access of others to confidential test material. Clinicians, of course, can refuse to turn over confidential information but, if they do so, they may be held in contempt.

Whether this privileged relationship extends to organizations who score and interpret tests for clinicians has not yet found its way into judicial opinion. Because of the uncertain legal status of such organizations, there is a particular need for caution in maintaining archival files. It is important to note that in California, for example, the Evidence Code is quite specific about which therapy clients enjoy privilege: only those whose therapist is a *licensed* psychiatrist (or other physician), psychologist, social worker, or marriage, family, and child counselor.

CONCLUSION

Test-developers and test-users share a joint responsibility for using computer-generated reports in a professional and ethical manner and for being aware of the associated legal issues. To avoid ethical and legal pitfalls, the users of computerized materials and services need to be aware of these issues and take them into consideration in their professional practices. In addition, the proliferation of computerized testing materials makes it important that test-developers also pay more attention to these issues and institute appropriate procedures and safeguards. While it is too early to delineate any hard-and-fast rules to govern the use of computerized tests, the present chapter has sought to raise a number of the more important issues.

REFERENCES

American Psychological Association. *Standards for educational and psychological tests* (Rev.). Washington, D. C.: Author, 1974.

Anastasi, A. *Psychological testing* (4th ed.). New York: Macmillan, 1976.

Bersoff, D. N. Testing and the law. *American Psychologist*, 1981, 36(10), 1047–1056.

Buros, O. K. (Ed.). *The eighth mental measurement yearbook*, Vol. I. Highland Park, N. J.: The Gryphon Press, 1978.

Caldwell, A., Jr. Courtroom use of psychological testing. *Trauma*, 1960, 111–164.

Copyright Revision Act of 1976 (P. L. 94–553). Chicago, Illinois: Commerce Clearing House, Inc., 1976, pg. 36, paragraph 292 (Computer Uses of Copyrighted Works).

Delman, R. P. Participation by psychologists in insanity defense proceedings: An advocacy. *The Journal of Psychiatry and the Law*, 1981, 9(3), 247–262.

Detroit Edison v. NLRB, 440 U.S. 301 (1979).

Farrell, A. D. When is a computerized assessment system ready for distribution? Some standards for evaluation. In M. Schwartz (Ed.) *Using Computers in Clinical Practice: A Guide for Psychotherapy and Mental Health Applications.* New York: The Haworth Press, 1984, 185–189.

Fischer, C., and Brodsky, S. *The Prometheus principle: Informed participation by clients in human services.* New Brunswick, N. J.: Transaction, 1978.

Golden, C. J., Hemmeke, T. A., and Purisch, A. D. *The Luria-Nebraska Neuropsychological Battery.* Los Angeles: Western Psychological Services, 1980.

Green, C. J. The diagnostic accuracy and utility of MMPI and MCMI computer interpretive reports. *Journal of Personality Assessment*, 1982, 46(4), 359–365.

Hathaway, S. R., and McKinley, J. C. *The Minnesota Multiphasic Personality Inventory: Manual.* New York: Psychological Corporation, 1967.

Hoffman, L. J. (Ed.). *Computers and privacy in the next decade.* New York: Academic Press, 1980.

Krug, S. E. Tailoring interpretive programs to specific users. In J. Butcher (Chm.), Issues in the clinical use of computerized test interpretations. Symposium presented at the 90th Annual Convention of the American Psychological Association in Washington, D. C., August 1982.

Lachar, D. Accuracy and generalizability of an automated MMPI interpretation system. *Journal of Consulting and Clinical Psychology*, 1974, 42(2), 267–273.

Messick, S. Evidence and ethics in the evaluation of tests. *Educational Researcher*, 1981, 10(9), 9–20.

Novick, M. R. (Chm.) *Draft Joint Technical Standard for Educational and Psychological Tests.* Washington, D.C.: American Psychological Association, 1983.

Perlin, M. The legal status of the psychologist in the courtroom. *Mental Disability Law Reporter*, 1980, 194(4), 41–54.

Roid, G. H. Clinical uses of microcomputers. In J. Butcher (Chm.) Issues in the clinical use of computerized test interpretations. Symposium presented at the 90th Annual Convention of the American Psychological Association in Washington, D. C., August 1982.

Roid, G. H., & Gorsuch, R. L. Development and clinical use of test-interpretive programs on microcomputers. In M. Schwartz (Ed.) *Using Computers in*

Clinical Practice: A Guide for Psychotherapy and Mental Health Applications.
New York: The Haworth Press, 1984, 141–149.

Siegel, M. Privacy, ethics, and confidentiality. *Professional Psychology*, 1979,
10(2), 249–258.

Szasz, T. *Ideology and Insanity.* New York: Doubleday, 1970.

Szasz, T. *Law, liberty, and psychiatry: An inquiry into the social uses of mental health
practices.* New York: Macmillan, 1963.

Ziskin, J. *Coping with psychiatric and psychological testimony* (2nd ed.). Beverly
Hills, California: Law and Psychology Press, 1975.

## PART VI

Psychological Reports

O ne of the advantages of the computer is that it-can help us do things that are repetitive and mindless, thereby freeing our time and energy for more productive and creative endeavors. Ken Vincent has found a novel way to use the computer to help write parts of the narrative psychological report. He has found a way to use the filing system of the word processor to store certain sentences and paragraphs that are commonly used in a test report. He carefully selects those files that are descriptive of the client, integrates them with information that identifies the client, and then incorporates this information into a structured report, producing a polished test report in a fraction of the time formerly required. Ken describes the development of his system and tells how other clinicians can develop similar systems of their own.

19 | The Full Psychological Report via a Word Processor

Ken R. Vincent, EdD

A word processor can be a major time-saver for the psychologist writing psychological test reports. At the most basic level, typing time is reduced. This is no small matter. Anyone who is familiar with the field is all too well aware that the lag time between psychological testing and the receipt of the psychological report by the user is the most frequently cited complaint regarding psychological testing. Using the word processor for typing alone, the psychological examiner's time can be significantly reduced. Our system, which uses the Xerox 850 display typewriter, has cut the typing time on an average full psychological battery from an hour to 30 minutes and has reduced the time of psychological analysis and writing from an hour to an average of 25 minutes.

Selecting from a worksheet of preformatted statements and creating a report constructed in part of those statements, the tester can speed the process of report writing. Furthermore, the statements utilized by the word processor are more apt to be carefully compiled and well worded, thus facilitating readability and understanding by the user of psychological testing.

Psychological-test reports written on a word processor have the advantage over computer-generated reports in that they are indistinguishable from the traditional report. In other words, the "canned" aspects are invisible.

In its present form, our system automates the writing of identifying information; notation of psychological test instruments used; impression and comments section; a structured social history (the Vincent Biographical Inventory); the entire section of intellectual assessment, including neuropsychological and psychoeducational screening; the personality-assessment section; the diagnostic impression section (DSM-III diagnoses); and a summary and comments section.

Interpretive statements are codified into call numbers, which are written by the psychologist on a worksheet (see example below). All typing instructions are codified into a series of numbers. Also included on this worksheet are those statements about low-frequency behavior, which are written out by the examiner. The patient-identifying information, two dozen or so call numbers, three or four written sentences to cover low-frequency or unusual behavior, and the diagnosis is easily converted by a secretary with a word processor into a 3- to 3½-page psychological report.

Our system is outlined in a journal article (Vincent, 1980a). The entire collection of interpretive statements is covered in a recent monograph (Vincent, 1982). The Semi-Automated Full Battery (Vincent, 1980b) covers 16 tests relating to intellectual, neuropsychological, and psychoeducational assessment, as well as projective tests and rating scales. The *MMPI Semi-Automated Interpretive Statements* (Vincent, 1980c) is a handbook that analyzes over 300 research articles, and specifies 201 automated statements covering virtually all MMPI validity scale configurations and, in addition, one- and two-point clinical scale codes, as well as a considerable number of three- and four-point code types for the MMPI. All in all, 326 validity and clinical scale configurations are covered in the *MMPI Semi-Automated Interpretive Statement*. These books can also serve as guidelines for those wishing to build their own systems. A detailed description of how to go about devising one's own interpretive statements has been spelled out in "Psychological Test Analysis and Report Writing via a Word Processor" (Vincent, 1983). However, the following examples from the author's previously cited work can give the individual psychologist an idea of how to devise his or her own system if he/she does not wish to modify or add to the system described above.

The following examples are statements from Vincent 1982. This example is in the section used in differential diagnosis:

DIFFERENTIAL DIAGNOSTIC STATEMENTS

60. While a case could be made from the test data that the patient is suffering from————
61. the data generally favor the above impression.
62. the data favor the above impression.
63. the data strongly favor the above impression.
64. the data slightly favor the above impression.

One will note that after statement 60 one can insert a differential diagnosis and then, on the amount of certainty for the differential, add any one of statements 61 through 64. For example, if the differential for whatever diagnosis as given in the report was that of a major affective disorder, then on the worksheet the psychologist would write *60, a ma-*

jor affective disorder, and (if the psychologist was fairly certain about the diagnosis that had been given) he/she might write 63. When this is picked up from the worksheet by the secretary, the statement entered into the word processor would read, "While a case could be made from the test data that the individual is suffering from a major affective disorder, the data strongly favor the above impression." Another example from Vincent 1982 covers medical psychiatric recommendations:

MEDICAL PSYCHIATRIC RECOMMENDATIONS

106. Medical psychiatric intervention is definitely indicated, and in all probability the patient will need outpatient monitoring and follow-up for the indefinite future.
107. Medical psychiatric intervention is indicated, as is supportive therapy.
108. Medical psychiatric intervention should be considered.

When one is fairly certain that the individual has either schizophrenia or manic depressive illness, statement 106 may be used; 107 typifies things that are not forever (such as major depressions); and 108 is for when the psychologist is uncertain as to whether psychoactive medication might be a helpful recommendation.

As can be seen, there is a certain amount of constraint in utilizing such a system. After the individual psychologist becomes familiar with it and accepts the constraint, the relief gained from the tedium of repetition in psychological report-writing and the fact that the reports are generally of an overall superior quality because they have been thought out in advance should more than compensate for adapting to the structure.

REFERENCES

Vincent, K. R. Semi-Automated Full Battery. *Journal of Clinical Psychology*, 1980(a) (9), 36 (2), 437–446.

Vincent, K. R. *Semi-Automated Full Battery*. Houston, Texas: Psychometric Press, 1980(b).

Vincent, K. R. *MMPI semi-automated interpretive statements*. Houston, Texas: Psychometric Press, 1980(c).

Vincent, K. R. *Automated interpretive statements for the impression, Vincent Biographical Inventory, and summary and comments section of a psychological assessment battery*. Richland, Washington: Psychological Software Specialists, 1982, 4–7.

Vincent, K. R. Psychological test analysis and report writing via a word processor. In *Innovations in clinical practice: A source book*. Vol. 2. Mansfield, Pennsylvania: Professional Resource Exchange, 1983.

PART VII

Clinical Assessment and Interviewing by Computer

One of the uses of computers in mental health that has not achieved the kind of widespread use and success that it deserves is clinical interviewing. On first glance, it would seem apparent that it would save much clinician time if the client or patient could sit down at a terminal and answer questions about his or her clinical history. Pertinent results would be summarized and given to the clinician. Completely thorough and tireless, the computer would miss nothing. Responding to its nonjudgmental qualities, the patient would tell all. Part VII explores what has been accomplished in the area of clinical interviewing and what we might expect of the field in the future.

In the first chapter, Leigh McCullough and her colleagues take a refreshingly open and informative look at what goes into the development of a computer-based assessment system. Step by step, they chronicle the development of their own assessment program from conception to implementation. Anyone planning to develop or use any kind of clinical program can benefit immeasurably from their revelations.

Albert Farrell, who was involved in the same project as Leigh, raises the question in the next chapter, "When Is a Computerized Assessment System Ready for Distribution?" Many share his concern that the answer too often seems like "never." Just as disturbing are the programs that he fears may be distributed before they have been found to be clinically valid or reliable. Is there a way, Farrell wonders, to establish some standards?

John Greist, one of the fathers of the use of computers in psychiatry, shares with us his views about clinical interviewing programs. He

171

believes the quality and power of existing hardware and software far exceed our capacity to use them at anything approaching their capacity. He has a very interesting and somewhat disturbing explanation for this phenomenon.

As an example of how the computer can be used in interviewing and assessment, David Comings describes how he got involved in writing a 27,000-step piece of software. He finds the overwhelming advantage of the computer system is its standardization and replicability, issues of critical importance for anyone using the results of the interview for research purposes. His programs can be obtained from him upon request, as can the programs written by many of the authors in this book.

In the next chapter, the work of Hugh Angle and his associates, who interviewed almost 700 patients in a variety of mental health settings, is reviewed. Would you believe that no patient refused to complete the interview, even though some remained at the console for up to eight hours? This study concludes with the interesting results of a survey of the reaction of clinicians at the facility where the computer-interviewing system was used.

Part VII contains a chapter that provides a specific example of the use of computerized assessment. Victor Krynicki and Charles Gould present their use of the computer in assessment in their chapter on computerizing the SCL-90 (Symptom Check List 90).

A review of the classic work of Doug Gustafson and his colleagues, who used a computer program to identify probable suicide-attempters, concludes part VII.

The Making of a Computerized Assessment System: Problems, Pitfalls, and Pleasures

Leigh McCullough, PhD
Albert D. Farrell, PhD
Richard Longabaugh, EdD

This chapter will describe a behind-the scenes view of how the idea for a computerized psychotherapy assessment system was first conceived. It will also describe how we wove the skills of three psychologists, each with different areas of experience, to transform an idea into a functioning reality. The result of this effort has been a computer-based design to provide the profession with a fast and comprehensive system of evaluation.

There are many systems on the market that have "computerized" standard psychological tests and offered them to the consumer, often at high prices. We hoped that the system we developed would provide a great deal more by offering a complete clinical research package that could be used in private practice. (By *clinical research* we are referring to features such as pretesting and posttesting; session-by-session ratings of the problems focused on in treatment; ratings of client-therapist interaction; diagnoses; treatments provided; and so on.) In addition, our goal was to accomplish this task with an economy of time and cost, with the aid of a microcomputer. Not only would this assist the clinician in case management, but it would also provide a broad, readily accessed, and ever-increasing data base for psychotherapy research.

Our goal here is to describe the form of the creative process—not the content. That is, in this chapter we will discuss how this task was accomplished rather than issues such as what specific questions are asked in the computerized interviews. We felt that the best way to focus on how this system was developed was to descend into anecdote. Leigh McCullough, the first author of this paper, will guide the descent.

PROJECT HISTORY

I came to work with Dick Longabaugh in 1979 as Project Director of NIMH grant 26012, a major outcome study of problem-oriented systems and treatment.* We call this grant the *POST Study*. I had been trained as a clinical psychologist and wanted further research experience because my long-range goal was to have a private practice that incorporated the evaluation of therapy process and outcomes.

An NIMH report had described Dick and his team as "an excellent group of researchers." Therefore, this setting promised exactly what I was looking for, a chance to see patient evaluation close up and to draw from the research methodologies used on this grant for use in my own private practice in the future.

The task of the POST Study was to interview a total of 500 psychiatric patients, their families, and treatment staff. A battery of assessment instruments was used, which included several paper-and-pencil measures and a computerized interview. Each day, interviewers had to be matched with incoming patients. There never seemed to be enough time or research staff to administer the paper-and-pencil measures, but the computer interview took very little staff time and was well-received by the patients. Just in terms of economy, I began wishing that all our data could be put directly into a computer, including patient self-reports, interviewer's rating, and treatment staff ratings. If all the data-collection were done by computer, there would be a tremendous savings both in the number of staff required and in the errors of transferring data from paper into the computer. Also, data directly entered into the computer could be manipulated and synthesized immediately, whereas we were waiting months at times for keypunching and cleanup of our massive paper-and-pencil-collected data sets.

Dick Longabaugh had been working on a computer system to assist clinicians for several years. The computer interview in the present grant represented one step along the way. But what he had in mind was a complex and sophisticated system that was still several years away in development. Other researchers, such as John Greist and his colleagues at the University of Michigan, had also been working on impressive and highly sophisticated computer systems to assess therapy and assist clinicians. However, both Longabaugh's and Greist's systems required expensive computers and advanced computer technology, which made them inaccessible to someone in private practice. I felt impatient and frustrated. From a practical standpoint, what good

---

*This study, (NIMH #26012) completed collection of one-year followup data in August of 1982. Data is presently being analyzed and prepared for publication. Preliminary reports may be received by writing Richard Longabaugh, Department of Evaluation, Butler Hospital, 345 Blackstone Boulevard, Providence, Rhode Island 02906.

would such systems be if they were restricted to two or three grant-funded sites? So I started musing about how these systems could be adapted for simpler and cheaper applications and could be made available to the private professionals in the front lines.

A lot of time at this point was spent entertaining ideas about my own private practice and how I could do there what was being done on our grant, i.e., collecting data before, during, and after treatment. I started looking around at what might be available. I found several companies that sold fancy computers that administered psychological tests—the MMPI and the like—but this offered little more to me than did paper-and-pencil tests, and the cost was prohibitive. On one hand, computerized tests with immediate reporting of results were intriguing, but, given their cost, they did not offer substantial advantages over their paper-and-pencil counterparts. For one thing, when would a busy practitioner find time to administer a series of psychological instruments that might take three to four hours? How many patients would sit at a computer terminal for that amount of time? Also, since research requires repeated measurement before, during, and after therapy, who would do this kind of assessment repeatedly? Surely a few zealous clinicians and a few motivated clients might undertake such a task—but it would not be applicable to a wide variety of practitioners.

Particularly important, it would not be applicable for my practice. I had tried to get clients to take a battery of psychological instruments at intake. I even had folders of tests made up and ready. I had a system to pick out "target complaints" to focus on in therapy. But I was repeatedly frustrated in my attempts to have clients fill out forms reliably and bring them back. Many clients would not have the time to fill them out in the office. Once taken home, tests would be lost, dropped in a puddle, or eaten by the client's dog. Rarely was a complete package returned, and when it was, it was difficult to score all the instruments on the spot and put them to immediate use. Weeks would pass without data being collected or tallied. The system was not working, and when it did, it was the exception, not the rule; I knew that would never do for large-scale research. So I started daydreaming about the amount of time I could reasonably afford and the amount of time most clients would reasonably give. I had had some outpatient clients try our initial version of the computer interview, which took about a half-hour. Clients found the computerized test pleasant to take and not a burdensome task. I was pleased to have the data collected and stored so easily. The particular test we used generated a problem list that I could immediately print out and go over with the patient. I decided that I would set a half-hour as a limit for every major test, and ask for only five minutes or less for quick problem ratings after each therapy session.

Since the computerized test seemed so efficient, I looked around at small computers that I could afford and discovered microcomputers. To my delight, I learned that they could be obtained for under $2,500, or for monthly payments of $200 to $250. To paraphrase McCracken (1982), I will refer to the microcomputer I chose as a *Pomegranate* so no one will think I'm referring to an apple or a lemon. I chose the Pomegranate, not due to any discernible superiority over other brands. (As I knew nothing about computers, I couldn't evaluate them.) I decided to use the Pomegranate because the hospital I worked in had just acquired one and I knew I could borrow it and test out some ideas. My fantasies continued with vigor. Now I put a fantasized Pomegranate in my fantasized office. My problem was to find out if I could do the sort of ongoing testing I wanted to do with it.

The next step was to find a programmer who could tell me if a system that combined some of our grant's research protocol and some of the systems that Dick conceptualized could be simplified and programmed on the Pomegranate. I had no programming knowledge at all, so I had no understanding of such things as memory, or storage capacity required.

The mathematical psychologist on our grant, Bob Stout, was the ideal person to consult. He is a computer whiz and, to the novice like me, he seemed to know everything there was to know about computers. I explained what I wanted to do and he said with his dry wit that theoretically it was possible to do what I wanted to do, but that it would require a "non-negligible amount of effort." He also explained to me that the Pomegranate was greatly limited in the sophistication of the systems it could provide because of storage capacity and so forth. However, all I heard was that he said that it was possible.

Being much less pragmatic, Dick was supportive and encouraging and was also very interested in seeing a prototype of his system in action. (We now refer to his system as the Cadillac model and mine as the VW Bug.) But he emphasized that time should not be taken from our major effort, the POST Study.

So the fantasies continued for several weeks—as just fantasies—and with the addition of an imaginary programmer.

Then I remembered my friend and colleague Al Farrell, who was on the faculty at Virginia Commonwealth University. Al and I interned together at Brown University, and he not only had a clinical background and research skills, but had also been using the Pomegranate for several years in his own research in behavioral assessment of social competence.

We made Al an offer he couldn't refuse: to work in his spare time for no money on an interesting project. Al's interest was immediately captivated, but his first comment was "Surely something this important has already been done?" We explained that we knew of nothing yet, so Al came aboard in an unaccustomed role of programmer. The bonus this gave the project was Al's varied background and skills in both therapy and research, qualities not found in a programming professional. Al became the link between technology, research methods, and clinical practice. The prospects took a giant forward step.

Thus, the project got underway. The three of us, in minutes snatched from our research and academic duties over several months' time, designed a research package.* By way of mail and phone calls, we tried to assist Al in translating it into a computer program. This was a slow and cumbersome process, but not impossible. His clinical and research training enabled him to weave into the fabric of the program the needs of the practitioner in treating a patient as well as the needs required for sound research methods. While designing a system that would be practical and helpful on the individual case, Al also planned for ways in which data could be pooled by phone for group analysis. We began to see our fantasy becoming a reality.

We tested the product by having Al send us a floppy disk with the programmed system on it for us to attempt to use. We had spent months (for Dick, it had been years) imagining how a system would work. So, when Al mailed us the first disk, it was a momentous occasion. Neither Dick nor I had ever seen the hospital's Pomegranate. Neither of us knew any programming. But we felt that we would be good test cases of computerphobic clinicians who would be attempting to use this system with no prior training whatsoever. Our only instructions from Al were to put the disk in the disk drive and to type "RUN INTERVIEW."

Separately, we took the floppy disk Al had sent us and, with instructions about how to run the machine, we headed to a borrowed Pomegranate on the other side of the hospital.

To our surprise, it worked the first time for both of us! That is, we successfully found the buttons to turn on the Pomegranate and managed to insert the disk into what we figured was the disk drive (and managed to set the disk in right-side up and not backwards). We were able, with a few tries, to correctly type "RUN INTERVIEW." After that, the computer did the rest for us. We just sat back and answered questions. Then, we started passing the disk around and asking other computerphobic clinicians and staff if they would attempt to run the program and take the interview. In our pilot sample of 20, every single individual was able to accomplish this task. The only trouble encountered was figuring out how to turn on the Pomegranate. (There were three buttons, including one to the printer, and people couldn't find

---

*More information on this research project may be obtained by writing to the authors.

them all!) The Computerized Assessment System was by no means perfect. There were still a lot of bugs in it, but we felt we had a product with much potential that might not only be useful to us, but to others as well.

In the spring of 1982, Dick and I noticed an APA call for papers and thought this project would make a good presentation. But even more than that, it seemed that we could present to the private-practice sector of APA (Division 42) and maybe spur some interest in a few clinicians, who would be willing to work with us in further testing and developing this model. Dick had long been aware of the pitfalls of designing computer systems in the laboratory that later proved clumsy in the clinical setting. We felt strongly that this system should be piloted in actual private-practice settings.

We sent in an abstract, and to our surprise it was accepted! This meant we had to deliver. We had 95% of the work complete and we were dauntless. But, as the convention approached, we became more and more nervous. We didn't have any idea how it would be received. Many of our colleagues told us we were crazy, that clinicians would never want to receive feedback on their work or evaluate what they do. Several friends thought we might be laughed at or, more likely, ignored. We could see that there would be resistance in some of our colleagues to evaluating their work. But since we were clinicians and *we* wanted to evaluate what we did, we suspected that there were others like us.

Whenever our confidence started slipping, we reminded ourselves that our project was relevant to the whole issue of accountability. Whether or not clinicians willingly wanted to evaluate their effectiveness, there had been much evidence that government and third-party payers would be demanding proof of effectiveness in the not too distant future.

August arrived, the APA presentation was well-attended, and we were pleasantly surprised to find that people were quite receptive. Several people in the audience commented that they were very frustrated by technological gimmickry being sold at high prices, before there was demonstrated efficacy. We emphasized that our system was in an intermediate stage of development and that we were asking people who would actually use such a system to assist in its development. Our goal was to work slowly over several years to develop a system that offered something substantive to the clinical researcher. Twelve clinical psychologists volunteered their support and gave us their names and later sent disks. Suddenly we had more support than we ever considered!

But we were not at all prepared for the later response. For months after the APA convention, there were calls and letters from all over the country. A newsletter published an article on what we were doing and generated more interest. Daily, people were sending us disks. However, we only had our system programmed for the Pomegranate and people were sending us floppy disks for a variety of microcomputers. We had to return these disks with notes expressing the regret that we did not have programming for their systems. We began receiving more disks and also offers from people who volunteered to program our system into their language, to be shared with us and others. (These offers to give up spare time for no money were greatly appreciated and their work is now underway.) This gave us the sensation of the "The Sorcerer's Apprentice" segment of the movie *Fantasia*—the more we tried to slow down the process, the more things mushroomed.

We were well-prepared for the possibility that we would meet with resistance or be ignored. We had not seriously considered favorable responses from so many practitioners. This attention generated a number of problems that we had never anticipated.

First, we could no longer develop our system with a handful of colleagues over the phone. We had two dozen disks and even more letters asking for information.

Just handling the correspondence became a full-time job. We rushed to work up a form letter that would address all the issues that were raised, but many of the letters required specific responses. We also had to quickly put together information packages to describe all the details of what we were doing and explain that we were cleaning up the programming and there would be a delay.

Furthermore, suggestions given at the conference and ideas we had come up with had to be integrated into the system, and all the bugs had to be worked out. When was it going to get done? Although 95% of this work had been completed, the last 5% seemed to be endless. (Apparently, this is a truism in computer programming.)

We remembered the warning about the non-negligible amount of effort involved in the months of nights and weekends it took to finish! But it wasn't impossible. It just required relentlessly sticking with it.

Several calls came in from people excited about the system and offering to publish a story about it in their newsletters. We begged them not to. "Keep it quiet for a while," we said, "until we are able to respond adequately to all the requests."

Another thing we were not prepared for was being contacted by people who wanted to sell our system. It seemed to make no difference that we emphatically pointed out that the system was in a developmental stage and had not been tested in actual private practice. We had initially been willing to share whatever we had done in the interests of furthering research. However, Al was concerned that someone could take our system and copyright it before us and then require us to buy it in order to use it. Suddenly, copyrighting became another job that had to be done before sharing our system with others.

Just as things were piling up over our heads, Nancy Keenan, a housewife and student interested in computers, volunteered one afternoon a week as partial fulfillment of course credit. She took over the correspondence and input test data into the program and was invaluable in completing the last 5% of the project.

When the project was small, many things could be overlooked. Now, with a larger audience, much more structure and formality became essential. Yet the benefits far outweighed the costs. The opportunity to develop an instrument in multiple settings and to share experiences with a wide variety of clinicians will provide a wealth of interchange that will greatly enrich this product. It will also continue to require a non-negligible amount of effort.

We have told this story in anecdotal form, hoping to encourage others who might be in the creative-fantasy stage with a computer-system idea and who would like to bring their fantasy into reality. Our experience has shown us that there are many mental health professionals who have microcomputers with power that they don't fully utilize. We also feel that the possibilities for computers in the mental health field are wide open and that there is much need for innovative programs and systems. The following discussion will be concerned with problems and pitfalls we encountered in the development of our system and will give some suggestions for those who might want to undertake similar projects.

SOME CONSIDERATIONS IN MAKING A COMPUTERIZED ASSESSMENT SYSTEM

Usefulness. We have found that the major consideration in developing a computer system is that the system has to meet a need and give the user something of value. Often computer systems have been developed, particularly with research in mind, that have lofty long-term goals. But clinicians have not put them to use because day-to-day incentives are lacking. Consequently, our system is not only a research protocol for collecting, storing, and analyzing data—it also provides the client and therapist with various reports or progress ratings printed out in easily readable formats immediately after each session. Feedback, presented in printed reports or on the monitor, is just one of many ways to promote short-term user satisfaction and help keep up motivation towards the longer-term aspects of the program.

Costs—Financial and Temporal. Many beautiful and sophisticated computer systems are not able to be widely used because they cost too much and take too much time. As emphasized earlier in this paper, economy of time and money is most important. Our plan was to decide how much time and money the average user (in this case both the client and the therapist) would reasonably be willing to spend. Then we absolutely did not extend those boundaries. We forced ourselves to stay within a certain number of minutes with a set type of equipment. This is one of the main reasons people have expressed interest: our system is practical.

Programming Knowledge Required. Many people in the mental health field have creative ideas but do not know computer programming. We hope that our experience is good evidence that you do not need to know programming, you just need to know a programmer. Furthermore, there are many young programmers with newly acquired skills who want to cut their teeth on an interesting project. In exchange, they often want to cite the project on a resumé and/or be given letters of recommendation. Two computer programming students have joined our project on this basis and are working on modifying Al's programs for use with other systems.

Debugging. Computer programs once written often need much testing to detect "bugs." Volunteers can be of tremendous help in this way.

Nancy Keenan not only volunteered time to help test Al's program, but also volunteered her Pomegranate at home. While supper was cooking, she went over and over the system in multiple ways, taking the role of both client and therapist, taking dozens of interviews and session "updates." She carefully recorded every error, and we sent them to Al for correction. Her volunteered time counted as course credit in college and she wrote a term paper with us. She plans to continue with us for independent-study credits for two more semesters. She has been invaluable to the completion of the project, and we feel very fortunate to be able to swap a "learning experience" for her services.

One of the biggest problems that faces the development of computer systems is the final cleaning up and debugging. This invariably takes far more time than anyone ever anticipates and should not be underrated as an obstacle. The last 5% of the project work tends to drag on for about 50% of the total project time. This is where so many potentially good programming projects bite the dust. Debugging a program takes a tremendous amount of time. We think the difficulty lies in the unpredictability of programming. It is not a linear process; therefore, problems that appear simple and straightforward are often more complicated than anticipated.

When to Stop. Another problem is that one can continue to improve upon the program ad infinitum. We found ourselves doing just that and had to be very firm with ourselves in accepting that the system is not and never would be perfect. After a certain point of relative "goodness," we just decided to quit and go with what we had. We do not feel that there is any way to avoid this unpleasant aspect of programming reality. A nose to the grindstone and sense of humor help a lot. We present this problem not to deter anyone's fervor; quite the contrary, we hope, by anticipating this difficulty, it will be more easily dealt with and overcome. This leads to the next pitfall, that of tenacity.

Tenacity. Tenacity is a crucial element in making a good computer idea work. Given the obstacles in one's path, such as "glitches" in the program and perfectionism and so on, something has to help pull one along. We found that insecurity about one's own creativity was a major obstacle. Tenacity doesn't just emerge out of nowhere. We think it is a product of the contingencies involved (real or imagined). For example, while feeling quite uncertain about our system, we reminded ourselves that it was meeting an important need. This pulled us through 95% of the project. Then, after presenting the system at APA and promising to send people disks, we were pulled along by our fear of losing credibility. People's expectations that we would do what we said pulled, or rather dragged, us through the remaining 5% of the project. Our message is this: do whatever is necessary to force your project to completion. It is often the case that your own ideas are worth more credit than you yourself give them.

Copyrighting. Once developed and completed, the fledgling program is often thrust into a dog-eat-dog world. We have found that a novel system must be copyrighted immediately. Not only could others copy the program overnight and attempt to put their names on it, but they might in fact charge large sums of money for it. Stand forewarned.

When to Market. The last concern in software packages is when and when not to market one's project. We do not pretend to have the answers. We chose not to sell our system at present because it has not been adequately tested. No reliability or validity data have been established to support its efficacy. We can only say that we have gained in credibility and volunteer support from all over the country far more than we have lost in terms of the limited sales that we might have generated for an underdeveloped project. We have also heard repeated complaints from mental health professionals about high and sometimes exorbitant prices that are being charged for computer systems that sometimes amount to nothing more than technological gimmickry. It appears that the consumers are wising up and that innovators would be prudent to meet quality standards before charging money for their product. (See Al Farrell's chapter in this book—"When Is a Computerized Assessment System Ready for Distribution?")

Our system represents only one of many possibilities for the use of computers in the mental health field. The microcomputer in the office and the home provide limitless possibilities. Evaluation is only one area, and we are just scratching the surface here. Mental status examination, memory tests, concentration exams, computer versions of "card sorts," etc., are a few examples of how much more "active" computer testing could be done. Also, the microcomputer as a treatment tool (videogames for cognitive structuring, biofeedback for self-control) offers many other possibilities.

In conclusion, it has been said that run-of-the-mill minds can do today what geniuses of the past could not do because we are lifted on the shoulders of this "giant," i.e., computer technology. It is a tremendous, exciting area for exploration and development. There is tremendous power to be harnessed and put to good use. We hope we have taken a step in this direction and that we can encourage others to do the same.

REFERENCE

McCracken, D. D. Maintaining a grapefruit. *Datamation*, April 1982, 164–168.

When Is a Computerized Assessment System Ready for Distribution? Some Standards for Evaluation

Albert D. Farrell, PhD

Recently I became involved in a collaborative effort to develop a computerized assessment system for use on a microcomputer by the private practitioner (McCullough, Farrell, & Longabaugh, 1982). As is true in any relatively new area, in the course of working on this project, my colleagues and I encountered a number of problems for which there were no established precedents. One of the critical problems was to determine when our system was sufficiently developed to be shared with others. Developing a computerized assessment system is like embarking on a road where the final destination continually seems just around the corner. Deciding if the system is ready involves far more than determining if the program will run. When the project nears completion, there always seems to be just one more revision to make.

I see this as a rapidly growing problem as more and more individuals become involved in developing computerized packages. Apparently many others share this concern. The development of user-friendly, relatively inexpensive microcomputers, and the attention focused on these developments as the wave of the future, has caused many individuals who a few years ago had never seen a computer to

"When Is a Computerized Assessment System Ready for Distribution? Some Standards for Evaluation" originally appeared in *Computers in Psychology/Psychiatry*, 1983, 5 (1), 9–11, and is reprinted by permission.

become "programmers" overnight. While I see this as a positive trend, it is not without adverse side effects. In what may be (or will become) a common scenario, the private practitioner buys a microcomputer for use with billing, record-keeping, etc., and as a result of well-designed tutorials, he or she gains some facility with writing programs over a fairly short time period. Out of a desire to facilitate the collection of client data, it may not be long before a computerized assessment system, based on the clinician's idea of what is important, emerges. Much satisfaction will likely result from developing such a system in terms of conquering the computer (i.e., getting it to do what you want) and the utility of such a system for efficient collection of client data. Who could keep such a system to him/herself? It will not be long before this system is shared with colleagues. As this network of colleagues and associates expands, it is not long before one considers packaging this system for a wider market. In a less altruistic scenario, many individuals who have computer skills but lack psychological sophistication may see the potentially lucrative market for systems to "aid" the private practitioner, and may put ill-devised but impressive-looking systems on the market. The inevitable consequence of these events is a proliferation of programs for the private practitioner. While the result of such proliferation has positive features, I fear that the unbridled growth of untested programs in this area will have very deleterious effects in the long run.

In most other areas, there are fairly clear criteria for determining when a product is ready for market. In the area of drugs, for example, the FDIC has fairly rigorous standards, which must be met before a drug can go to the market. Unfortunately, there are no equivalent standards for computerized packages, to my knowledge. The purpose of this paper is not to set such standards, but to begin a dialog that may hopefully lead to the development of such standards. This paper represents an attempt to rough out some important criteria for evaluating computerized assessment systems. Criteria will be presented that deal with the fact that these are computerized systems and assessment systems.

Evaluating the Software Aspect

In evaluating the software aspect of these systems, three criteria should be considered: (1) freedom from logic and syntax errors; (2) accuracy of storage and retrieval of data; and (3) adequate documentation.

It is a common myth among people new to computers that debugging a program simply means getting the program to run. While a program that will not run presents obvious problems, a program that runs but contains errors poses a less obvious and consequently more serious problem. As one writes increasingly complex programs, the number of runs necessary to confirm that the program works appears to increase exponentially. Programs should be thoroughly tested under many of the possible combinations of options before distribution.

In developing programs that store data for later use, one of the most important considerations is the accuracy of the input and storage system. Before any program is made available for other users, the accuracy of the data stored in the files must be assessed by verifying a number of sample data sets. Comparing the original raw input data with the data retrieved by the program is the best test of accuracy. This determines whether errors occurred during any step in the process from input to retrieval.

Finally, there is the important and often neglected area of documentation. A program is only useful to the extent that others can understand how to use it. Some very sophisticated programs are worthless as they cannot be used by the intended consumer. Based on firsthand experience, it is apparent that developers of computerized systems may become too intimately familiar with their own systems to be able to evaluate the adequacy of their documentation. Ideally, the developer should solicit the assistance of colleagues completely unfamiliar with the system and send them the program and documentation to determine if the programs "travel" well. Documentation should be self-explanatory. The critical test is whether the consumer can use the system without the developer looking intently over his/her shoulder (unless the developer intends to aid every user in this manner). Ideally, the individuals testing the program should be representative of the population of consumers for whom the program is written. For example, the test subjects should have no more or less computer expertise than the target population. In developing our own system, we have enlisted the assistance of clinicians who have volunteered to use a preliminary form of our system in their practice.

Evaluating the Assessment Aspect

In addition to criteria related to the computer aspect of computerized assessment systems, it is also important to evaluate the assessment aspect of these systems. Computerized assessment systems should be developed according to well-established principles of test construction (cf. "Standards for educational and psychological tests," 1974). Prior to bringing such a system to market, the reliability and validity of the system should be thoroughly evaluated. Reliability concerns the consistency of test scores across different conditions of measurement and can take a variety of forms depending on the purpose of the assessment procedures (cf. Cronbach, Gleser, Nanda, & Rajaratnam, 1972). For

some systems, the consistency of scores over time, or test-retest reliability, should be determined. For other tests, which employ subscales,
internal consistency should be evaluated (i.e., split-half reliability,
Kuder-Richardson reliability). For tests that involve ratings, the
interrater or interjudge reliability should be assessed. In some cases,
investigators may take a well-established assessment instrument and
"put it into the computer," for example, computerization of standard
psychological tests such as the MMPI. Before such users invoke the
psychometric properties of the original scale, the comparability of
scores obtained on the computerized and paper-and-pencil version
must be established. This obvious evaluation is seldom seen in the literature.

In addition to evaluating the reliability of the package, it is also important to evaluate its validity. (For a more extensive discussion of reliability and validity, the curious reader is referred to Anastasi, 1982.)
Validity can also take many forms, depending upon the purpose of the
test. For computerized systems such as interviews, which provide information about a variety of areas, perhaps the most important consideration is content validity. Content validity concerns the extent to
which the domain of behavior of interest to the investigator is adequately covered by the items in the interview. Developers of computerized assessment systems cannot simply sit down and write a list of
items they feel are important and assume this list adequately covers
the domain of relevance to other investigators. While brainstorming
with other investigators represents an improvement, a more systematic
approach to sampling the relevant domain of behavior is desirable. In
developing our own assessment system we attempted to collect a pool
of items representing the most frequently asked questions from over a
dozen well-established psychological tests (see McCullough et al.,
1982). Systematic approaches to developing items with content validity
will insure that the information provided by the system is relevant to
more than a small handful of users.

In addition to content validity, it may often be important to evaluate the criterion validity of a computerized assessment system. Criterion validity is the extent to which scores on an assessment system are
correlated with the criterion of interest to an investigator. While defining and measuring criteria are often a difficult problem, systems that
purport to predict various events, such as response to particular treatments, medications, or institutional release, should empirically demonstrate that they can, in fact, do so. In the absence of such data, the utility of these systems remains unclear.

In summary, the burgeoning growth of computerized assessment
systems must be checked. There is a growing need to develop guidelines for determining when a system is ready for distribution in order

to maintain quality-control in this important area. The ease of writing programs and the potentially lucrative market for such efforts puts pressure on the developer to market a system prematurely. This is made worse by the tremendous competition in this fast-growing area, coupled with the painstaking effort required to adequately evaluate these systems. Standards must be established to protect the consumer and to keep the data base provided by this technology on a solid ground.

It was my purpose in writing this paper to propose some tentative guidelines for determining when computerized assessment systems are ready for distribution. These systems are both software packages and assessment instruments. As such, it is my recommendation that both aspects of these systems be evaluated before a system is distributed. It is hoped that these preliminary recommendations will open a dialog that may eventually lead to firm guidelines and established standards in this exciting and rapidly growing field.

REFERENCES

Anastasi, A. *Psychological Testing*, Fifth Edition. MacMillan: New York, 1982.

Cronbach, L.J., Gleser, G.C., Nanda, H., & Rajaratnam, N. *The dependability of behavioral measurements: Theory of generalizability for scores and profiles.* Wiley: New York, 1972.

McCullough, L., Farrell, A.D., & Longabaugh, R. Toward a model of computerized assessment in private practice. Paper presented at the annual convention of the American Psychological Association, Washington, D.C., August, 1982.

Standards for educational and psychological tests. Washington, D.C.: American Psychological Association, 1974.

22 | Conservative Radicalism: An Approach to Computers in Mental Health

John H. Greist, MD

W e have at least two major and seemingly contradictory problems with computers in psychiatry and psychology. First, the computing tool is already so powerful and its potential applications so promising that we have difficulty recognizing and accepting the necessity of hard, persistent, and painstaking work still needed to reach our lofty goals. Second, advances in clinical computing have such radical implications that they have been slow to gain acceptance.

The steadily and rapidly increasing power of computers has, for some, become an addiction akin to that which some adolescents experience when describing how many horsepower a car has and fantasizing how fast they could go if only the car were theirs. I would argue that present hardware and driver software is more than adequate for most needs in practice, research, education, and administration. Driver programs permit comparatively unsophisticated users to define content for data bases, interviews, consultations, bibliographies, etc., which are "driven" by sophisticated, high-level programs.

I would further argue that most clinicians should not program. Learning to program is a pleasant two-year distraction—some would say *addiction*—but the major contribution clinicians can make lies in the development of applications using driver programs already available. For example, our computer/operating system (Data General Eclipse/

This work was supported in part by Dr. Greist's NIMH Research Scientist Development Award (MH70903–08) and by NIMH Grants MH16477 and 16464–02 and MH32624–02 and by a grant from The National Library of Medicine, LM03713–02. The present article originally appeared in *Computers in Psychiatry/Psychology*, 1982, 4 (3) 1–3, and is reprinted by permission.

MIIS) has been stable and highly reliable for more than eight years. Available driver programs have also met most of our needs over the last five years and promise to do so for the next five years. Similar driver programs are already available for microcomputers (e.g., PILOT, an interview driver for the Apple). Our great need is for better use of present driver programs to construct better computer interviews and consultations and to actually use existing drivers for data-base management systems, bibliographic retrieval programs, and word processors. Still better word processors will not produce deathless prose. The challenge is to make the best use of the excellent driver programs we already have.

Marvin Eidinger (1982) reports that he has had over 100 requests for a catalog of software from psychiatrists and psychologists, but only three programs to include in that catalog. Waiting for advances in computer technology to solve problems is rapidly becoming a diagnosable neurosis. I am reminded of an aphorism by an author whose identity is lost from memory: "Our duty is not to see what lies dimly at a distance but to do what lies clearly at hand."

It seems to me that the most fertile and least developed area for applying computers in psychiatry and psychology is direct patient interviewing. Even in internal medicine, over half of the useful information in diagnosis is verbal and the next largest fraction comes from physical examination. In psychiatry and psychology, patient reports are the mother lode, hard to find and mine, but yielding an enormous payoff. The problems with the patient report, as shown over the past decade with the advent of structured diagnostic interviews (SADS and DIS), lie partly in the clinician's inability to collect complete data and systematically apply standardized criteria for diagnosis. Clinician training, recent experience, immediate distractions, and foibles of memory are among the factors that may compromise our competence as diagnosticians. In virtually every instance in which computer interviews and clinicians have been compared, the computer outperforms the clinician in terms of completeness and accuracy.

The complexity of the problems that patients present is great and clinicians' training is often incomplete, outdated, or forgotten. A personal example may be instructive.

Although I work each day with mood disorders and have written books on depression and lithium, I cannot remain truly current with the literature in either field. By contrast, the Lithium Index and Lithium Consultation programs (see *Computers in Psychiatry/Psychology*, Vol. 3, No.3, p.8) are more current, knowledgeable, and never forget. I at times omit important items in assessing individuals with mood disorders and find, in honesty, that I have not yet completely mastered the complexities presented by DSM-III. Our DSM-III consultation (*Comput-*

ers in Psychiatry/Psychology, Vol.3, No.4, p.11) and Diagnostic Interview Schedule (DIS) patient diagnostic interview never skip important materials, ask questions in a polished and standardized manner, and wend their ways unerringly through their respective diagnostic logics. These computer interviews and consultation programs surpass my abilities as a data-gatherer and general diagnostician but not yet, I hope, as a well-rounded clinician, making ultimate evaluations based on a myriad of factors and helping patients reconcile sometimes divergent and often ambiguous data.

Acceptance of advances in the use of computers in psychiatry and psychology is our second and even more vexing problem. Thomas Kuhn eloquently described the problem of paradigm shifts in his book, *The Structure of Scientific Revolution* (Kuhn, 1970). William Faulkner put it another way: "What the heart loves becomes truth." There is at least one generation of mental health clinicians who have grown up to love certain paradigms and cannot face with equanimity the ordeal of change that computers represent.

Our experience with resistance to computers is not new. Max Planck concluded in his scientific autobiography that, "A new scientific truth does not triumph by convincing its opponents and making them see the light, but rather because its opponents eventually die, and a new generation grows up that is familiar with it." I think that history will rank computers with the revolutions initiated by Copernicus, Freud, and Darwin. Darwin waited a decade after arriving at his conclusions on natural selection before publishing *The Origin of Species* in 1859. At the end of that work he wrote, "Although I am fully convinced of the truth of the views given in this volume. . . , I by no means expect to convince experienced naturalists, whose minds are stocked with a multitude of facts all viewed, during a long course of years, from a point of view directly opposite to mine. . . . But I look with confidence to the future—to young and rising naturalists, who will be able to view both sides of the question with impartiality."

When I began working with computers in 1967, I felt that all the important and interesting work in computer interviewing would be completed within five years. What we still need fifteen years later is for a number of individuals to develop and carefully evaluate computer interviews for a wide variety of problem areas. The scientific method is somewhat antithetical to our more intuitive, dynamic, interpretive psychotherapeutic heritage, but there is no substitute for controlled research. If enough clinicians carefully pursue interviewing problems in single areas, we can assemble and possibly integrate a large system of computer interviews in five, ten, twenty, or more years that will do our professions proud. The short-term promise of a comprehensive, integrated mental-health information system is an alluring siren's song.

As Kierkegaard said, "to promise the system is a serious thing." And as Kenneth Kenniston said to radical undergraduates at the University of Wisconsin in 1970 as they were advocating the radical change or immediate overthrow of many of society's institutions, "You have been radical for a few months. To make the kinds of changes you talk about will require people prepared to be radicals for life!"

The potential for computer applications in psychiatry and psychology remains enormous. In my opinion, the quality and power of existing hardware and software far exceeds our capacity to use it at anything approaching its capacity. We do not need another generation of computers or even of programming languages. We need a generation of clinicians who will take the powerful tools presently available and apply them with care, ingenuity, diligence, and patience to difficult mental health problems, which will gradually yield to our steady efforts. Over time, this basically conservative approach can produce radically beneficial changes in our professions and in patient outcomes.

REFERENCES

Eidinger, M. From the librarian's desk: call for software. *Computers in Psychiatry/Psychology*, *4* (2), 1982, 11–12.

Kuhn, T. *The structure of scientific evolution* (2nd ed.). Chicago: University of Chicago Press, 1970.

Planck, M. *Scientific autobiography and other papers*. New York: Philosophical Library, 1949, 33–34.

A Computerized Diagnostic Interview Schedule (DIS) for Psychiatric Disorders

David E. Comings, MD

I would like to share with you how I, a clinician, got involved in writing a 27,000-step piece of software for making standardized and replicable DSM-III psychiatric diagnoses. My interest is in the mechanisms of neuropsychiatric disease and attempting to identify the specific genes responsible for disorders such as Huntington's disease, Alzheimer's disease, severe endogenous depression, manic depression, schizophrenia, alcoholism, Tourette syndrome, and related disorders that have a very high genetic component. Just as the whole field of the hemaglobinopathics and sickle cell disease took an exponential leap after Linus Pauling demonstrated that patients with sickle cell disease had a molecular defect in their beta-globin molecule, a similar giant increase in our understanding of various neuropsychiatric disorders will occur if we can identify the specific mutant genes involved. Following the Willie Sutton law,* we have felt that the most logical place to look for mutant proteins in neuropsychiatric diseases is in the human brain. Utilizing a highly sensitive technique called two-dimensional gel electrophoresis, we identified a mutant protein which we termed Pc1 Duarte, which was brain-specific and was present at a significantly increased frequency in individuals who had committed suicide with severe depression (Comings, 1979). Following up on this initial observation, we submitted a proposal to collect many more brains of individuals who had committed suicide; perform psychiatric autopsies on these individuals to identify those who had chronic, long-standing histories of depression; and compare those to a series of con-

---

*When Willie Sutton was asked why he robbed banks his reply was, "Because that's where the money is."

trols without mental illness to determine if this mutant protein was a susceptibility factor in depression. During the course of the review of this proposal, we were introduced to the DIS (Diagnostic Interview

---

72. In your lifetime, have you ever had two weeks or more during which you felt sad,
O   blue, depressed, or when you lost all interest and pleasure in things that you
    usually cared about or enjoyed?   DECK 03

                        No .... ①
                        Yes .... ⑤   32/

73. Have you had **two years** or more in your life when you felt **depressed** or sad almost
O   all the time, even if you felt OK sometimes?   ① ②   ⑤
                                                                                              33/

> **INTERVIEWER:** IN Q. 73, DID R TELL DOCTOR?
>
> F   NO .... ①
>   YES .... ⑤   34/
>
> **INTERVIEWER:** ASK QS. 74-89. **OMIT** WORDS IN [ ]. CODE IN COLUMN I.

		I EVER IN LIFETIME	II [WORST PERIOD]	
A P P E T I T E	74. Has there ever been a period of two weeks or longer when you lost [Did O you lose] your **appetite**? CAN BE POSITIVE EVEN IF FOOD INTAKE IS NORMAL. MD: _____ SELF: _____	① ③ ④ ⑤	① ⑤	35/ 36/
	75. Have you ever **lost** [Did you lose] **weight** without trying to—as much as O two pounds a week for several weeks [or as much as 10 pounds altogether]? MD: _____ SELF: _____	① ③ ④ ⑤	① ⑤	37/ 38/
	76. Have you ever had a period when your eating increased so much [Did O your eating increase so much] that you **gained** as much as two pounds a week for several weeks [or 10 pounds altogether]? MD: _____ SELF: _____	① ③ ④ ⑤	① ⑤	39/ 40/
S L E E P	77. Have you ever had a period of two weeks or more when you had [Did O you have] **trouble falling asleep**, staying asleep, or with waking up too early? MD: _____ SELF: _____	① ③ ④ ⑤	① ⑤	41/ 42/
	78. Have you ever had a period of two weeks or longer when you were O [Were you] **sleeping too much**? MD: _____ SELF: _____	① ③ ④ ⑤	① ⑤	43/ 44/

FIGURE 23–1. A sample page from the DIS. The numbers in circles represent potential answers after entering the probe routine (see Figure 23–3).

Source: Lee N. Robins, John Helzer, Jack Croughan, Janet Williams, and Robert Spitzer, *NIMH Diagnostic Interview Schedule (DIS), Version III*, U.S. Government Printing Office: Washington, DC, 1981, p. 15.

Schedule) as a means of producing reliable and replicable, inclusive and exclusive, diagnoses of not only depression but of 32 other DSM-III diagnostic categories. The DIS is an outgrowth of many years of involvement in the process of standardizing psychiatric diagnoses by the St. Louis group of investigators including Spitzer, Feighner, and E. Robins. Version three of the DIS is a highly structured interview consisting of a minimum of 263 questions designed to diagnose organic brain syndrome, mania, major depressive episodes, bipolar disorder, schizophrenia, alcohol- and drug-abuse, somatization, panic disorder, and many others, for a total of 32 different DSM-III diagnostic categories (Robins, Helzer, Croughan, & Ratcliff, 1981). Figure 23–1 shows a typical page of a test booklet. The interview booklets and detailed in-

```
                 DIAGNOSTIC INTERVIEW SCHEDULE

NAME = JOHN DOE
ID#  = 246-56-46

MANIA
     AGE OF FIRST MANIC EPISODE =  27
     AGE OF LAST MANIA =  37
     TOTAL NUMBER OF MANIA SYMPTOMS EVER =  7

MAJOR DEPRESSIVE EPISODE (TWO WEEKS OR MORE)
     AGE FIRST DEPRESSED =  23
     LAST EPISODE SIX MONTHS TO ONE YEAR AGO
     TOTAL # POSITIVE DEPRESSION SYMPTOMS =  9

BIPOLAR DISORDER

ALCOHOL ABUSE AND DEPENDENCE
     AGE AT FIRST ALCOHOL PROBLEM =  23
     LAST SYMPTOM WITHIN LAST THREE YEARS
     TOTAL # OF ALCOHOL SX =  14

BARBITURATE AND SEDATIVE/HYPNOTIC DEPENDENCE

OPIOID DEPENDENCE

COCAINE ABUSE

AMPHETAMINE DEPENDENCE

HALLUCINOGEN ABUSE

CANNABIS DEPENDENCE

DRUG SUMMARY = DRUG DEPENDENCE REQUIRING HELP OR INTERFERING WITH LIFE
     AGE OF FIRST DRUG DEPENDENCE =  14
     AGE OF LAST DRUG PROBLEM = 39
     TOTAL NUMBER OF DRUG ABUSE SYMPTOMS =  7

OBSESSIVE COMPULSIVE DISORDER (WITHOUT EXCLUSION CRITERIA)
     AGE FIRST HAD OBSESSION OR COMPULSION =  13
     AGE LAST HAD OBSESSION OR COMPULSION = 38
     TOTAL # OF OBSESSIVE COMPULSIVE SYMPTOMS =  3
```

Continues

FIGURE 23–2. Printout on a hypothetical patient.

```
AGORAPHOBIA (WITHOUT EXCLUSION CRITERIA)
SOCIAL PHOBIA (WITHOUT EXCLUSION CRITERIA)
SIMPLE PHOBIA
PHOBIA (SUMMARY)
AGE OF FIRST PHOBIC SYMPTOMS (DIAGNOSTIC HIERARCHIES NOT INCLUDED) =   30
    AGE OF FIRST PHOBIC SYMPTOMS =   30
AGE OF LAST PHOBIC SYMPTOMS (DIAGNOSTIC HIERARCHIES NOT INCLUDED) =   34
    AGE OF LAST PHOBIC SYMPTOMS =  34
    TOTAL NUMBER OF PHOBIC SYMPTOMS =   11


SOMATIZATION DISORDER
    AGE OF FIRST SYMPTOMS =   18
    LAST ATTACK TWO WEEKS TO ONE MONTH AGO
    TOTAL # OF SOMATIZATION SYMPTOMS =   19


PANIC DISORDER (IN THE PRESENCE OF OTHER DISORDERS)
    AGE OF FIRST PANIC ATTACK =   24
    LAST ATTACK SIX MONTHS TO ONE YEAR AGO
    TOTAL # OF PANIC SYMPTOMS =   11

AGORAPHOGIA (WITHOUT EXCLUSION CRITERIA) WITH PANIC ATTACKS


ANOREXIA NERVOSA
    AGE OF FIRST SYMPTOMS =   20

TOBACCO USE DISORDER
    AGE FIRST SMOKED DAILY =   18
    LAST SMOKED THIS MUCH ONE MONTH TO SIX MONTHS AGO

PATHOLOGICAL GAMBLING
    AGE OF FIRST TROUBLE WITH GAMBLING =   22
    LAST SYMPTOM TWO WEEKS TO ONE MONTH AGO

PSYCHOSEXUAL DYSFUNCTIONS (WITHOUT EXCLUSION CRITERIA)

TRANSSEXUALISM
    FIRST AGE MET DIAGNOSIS OF TRANSSEXUALISM =   24
    LAST SYMPTOM TWO WEEKS TO ONE MONTH AGO

EGO-DYSTONIC HOMOSEXUALITY
    AGE OF FIRST HOMOSEXUAL RELATIONS =   19
    LAST SYMPTOM WITHIN LAST TWO WEEKS



            SUMMARY

TOTAL # DSMIII POSITIVE SYMPTOMS    = 130
# OF GROUPED DSMIII   POSITIVE
    DIAGNOSES                       = 11
# OF DSMIII DIAGNOSES WITH
    SX  REPORTED TO A PHYSICIAN     = 12
# OF DSMIII DIAGNOSES
    PRESENT IN THE LAST TWO WEEKS   = 1
# DSMIII DIAGNOSES
    PRESENT IN THE LAST   MONTH     = 4
# DSMIII DIAGNOSES
    PRESENT IN THE LAST SIX MONTHS  = 5
# DSMIII DIAGNOSES
    PRESENT IN THE LAST YEAR        = 6
```

FIGURE 23–2. *Continued.*

```
TOTAL OF INDIVIDUAL SYMPTOMS

ORGANIC BRAIN SYNDROME SX              = 6
SCHIZOPHRENIC SX                       = 10
OBSESSIVE COMPULSIVE SX                = 3
PHOBIC SX                              = 11
PANIC SX                               = 11
SOMATIZATION SX                        = 19
ANTI-SOCIAL PERSONALITY SX             = 18
    + GROUPS BEFORE 15     = 9
    + GROUPS AS ADULT      = 8
ANOREXIA NERVOSA SX                    = 2
TOBACCO SX                             = 2
GAMBLING SX                            = 4
SEXUAL DYSFUNCTION SX                  = 3
DEPRESSIVE SYMPTOMS                    = 9
MANIC SYMPTOMS                         = 7
ALCOHOL SX                             = 14
DRUG SX                                = 7
TRANSSEXUAL SX                         = 4

DIAGNOSIS SUMMARY

    DIS002 =   46   AGE
    DIS001 =    1   MALE
  ORGBRAIN = ⁄  1
  DSMMANIA =    3   MANIA
    DSMDEP =    3   MAJOR DEPRESSIVE EPISODE
  DSDYSTHY =    1
  DSMBIPOL =    3   BIPOLAR DISORDER
  DSMDEPSE =    1
  DSMDEPRT =    1
  DSMBIPII =    1
    DSMALC =    3   ALCOHOL DEPENDENCE (DSM III 303.9)
   DSMBARB =    3   BARBITURATE DEPENDENCE (DSM III 304.1)
  DSMOPIOD =    3   OPIOID DEPENDENCE (DSM III 304.0)
   DSMCOKE =    2   COCAINE ABUSE (DSM III 305.6)
   DSMAMPH =    3   AMPHETAMINE DEPENDENCE (DSM III 304.4)
   DSMHALL =    2   HALLUCINOGEN ABUSE (DSM III 305.3)
    DSMTHC =    3   CANNABIS DEPENDENCE (DSM III 304.3)
  DMDRGSUM =    3   DRUG DEPENDENCE REQUIRING HELP OR INTERFERING WITH LIFE
  DSMSCHIZ =    1
  DSMSZFRM =    1
  DSMOBCOM =    5   OBSESSIVE COMPULSIVE DISORDER (WITHOUT EXCLUSION CRITERIA)
  DSMAGPHB =    5   AGORAPHOBIA (WITHOUT EXCLUSION CRITERIA)
  DSMSMPPH =    3   SIMPLE PHOBIA (DSM III 300.29)
  DSMSOCPH =    5   SOCIAL PHOBIA (WITHOUT EXCLUSION CRITERIA)
   DSMPHOB =    3   PHOBIA
    DSMSOM =    3   SOMATIZATION DISORDER (DSM III 300.81)
  DSMPANIC =    5   PANIC DISORDER (IN THE PRESENCE OF OTHER DIAGNOSES)
  DSMAGPAN =    5   AGORAPHOBIA (WITHOUT EXCLUSION CRITERIA) WITH PANIC ATTACKS
    DSMASP =    1
  DSMANORX =    3   ANOREXIA NERVOSA (DSM III 307.10)
   TOBACCO =    3   TOBACCO DEPENDENCE (DSM III 305.1)
  GAMBLING =    3   PATHOLOGICAL GAMBLING (DSM III 312.31)
   SEXDYSFN =   5   PSYCHOSEXUAL DYSFUNCTION (IN THE PRESENCE OF OTHER DIAGNOSES)
  DSMTRSEX =    3   TRANSSEXUALISM (DSM III 302.5)
   DSMHOMO =    3   EGO-DYSTONIC HOMOSEXUALITY (DSM III 302.00)
```

FIGURE 23–2. Continued.

structions on giving the interview can be obtained from Dr. Lee N. Robins, Department of Psychiatry, Washington University School of Medicine, 49040 Audubon Avenue, St. Louis, Missouri 63110.

I obtained the interview and its documentation and was excited

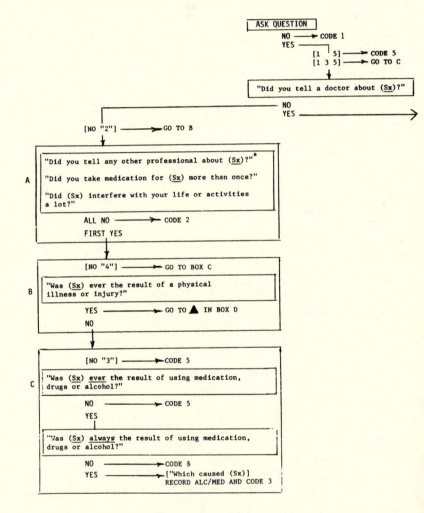

FIGURE 23–3. The probe routine required for some questions to determine whether a *yes* answer represents symptoms due to drugs, alcohol, medication, physical illness, or psychiatric symptoms.

about its capabilities, but distressed to find that computer scoring of the interview was set up for use with an expensive IBM computer and required a card punch and SAS language, all of which would come to well over $100,000 of hardware and software investment. This clearly

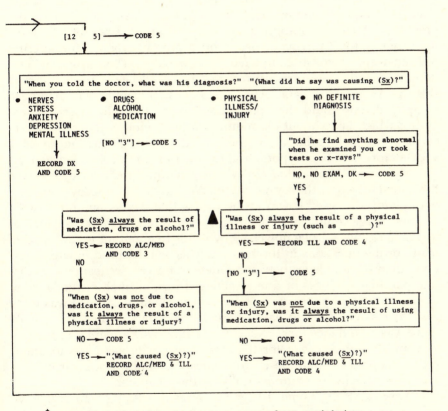

*Other professionals include social workers, nurses, clergy, psychologists, dentists, chiropractors, and podiatrists.

Source: Lee N. Robins, John Helzer, Jack Croughan, Janet Williams, and Robert Spitzer, *NIMH Diagnostic Interview Schedule (DIS), Version III*, U.S. Government Printing Office: Washington, DC, 1981, p. 79.

put it out of the realm of my resources. However, since I have long been an Apple II enthusiast and had written a number of programs in BASIC, I thought perhaps that a computer program written for SAS could be translated to BASIC. Some computer experts that I approached about this said it couldn't be done because the Apple II had too small a memory. However, I found that by purchasing a Microsoft Z80 card I could use CP/M disc operation and Microsoft BASIC. Microsoft BASIC had an extremely useful command called CHAIN, which allowed short programs to be pulled off of the disc while retaining all the variables from the previous programs. Thus, the disc could be used to effectively expand the memory of the Apple II to an almost infinite degree. Over a period of approximately four months, I rewrote the scoring program for BASIC, and also wrote a prompt program for entering the answers from a completed test booklet. This program was debugged with 32 test cases I received from Dr. Lee Robins. I termed this the *Apple DIS Program*. After a DIS questionnaire booklet had been completed, one could then go to one's own Apple II, insert the answers, which takes about ten minutes, and in another few minutes receive a complete printout of the scored results given. Figure 23–2 shows a printout of a hypothetical case with many positive answers.

My wife, who is a clinical psychologist, and I then decided to take the course given at the University of Washington to improve our skill with giving the tests. It was at the course that we became fully aware of some of the complexities of administering the test. For example, Figure 23–3 shows a probe flowchart, which is required for *yes* answers to many of the questions in the booklet. This standardized flow of questions then distinguishes between whether a given *yes* response is due to a psychiatric illness or due to taking drugs, alcohol, or medication, or if it is due to a physical illness or injury. While this probe was fairly easy to master in a few days of trial, unless one used it continually there was a tendency for it to slip away. It became apparent to me that it would be much easier for the mental-health professional to utilize this questionnaire if all these probe questions and interviewer instructions were carried out automatically by the computer.

After returning home, I began a series of 9:00 P.M. to 2:00 A.M. programming sessions, which went on for about three months, to develop the *Apple Auto-Prompt DIS*. This program presents all of the questions on the monitor, does the necessary subroutines automatically, and is then computer scored; the results are printed out as shown in Figure 23–2. In uncomplicated cases, the whole procedure takes almost one hour. After the printout is completed, the user has the opportunity of also getting a hard copy of the answers to all the questions. After this is completed, if mistakes have been made, individual answers can be corrected and rescored. It is also possible to jump from any one question to any other question on the questionnaire by either going backwards or using a jump routine. Sometimes a patient will change an answer to a question already asked, and it is necessary to go backwards. Also, if a patient has organic brain disease, it may be necessary to jump to the section on organic brain disease and complete this before returning to the main part of the questionnaire.

We are particularly interested in utilizing this questionnaire to examine psychiatric problems in patients with Tourette syndrome and their families. I have given it to several individuals whom I thought I knew very well and turned up a large amount of information that had never come out before.

The overwhelming advantage of the DIS is standardization and replicability. Thus a patient diagnosed by this means in one part of the country or world has a high probability of receiving the same diagnosis anywhere else that this instrument is used. Anyone with expertise doing interviewing techniques can give the questionnaire. The thoroughness and structured nature of the questions are apt to uncover symptomatology that might be missed in an interview directed just toward present symptoms. Further information on how to obtain these programs and the price can be obtained by writing Apple DIS, Department of Medical Genetics, City of Hope Medical Center, Duarte, California 91010.

REFERENCES

Robins, L. N., Helzer, J. E., Croughan, J., & Ratcliff, K. S. National Institute of Mental Health Diagnostic Interview Schedule. Its history, characteristics, and validity. *Archives of General Psychiatry*, 1981, *38*, 381–389.

Comings, D. E. Pcl Duarte, a common polymorphism of a human brain protein, and its relationship to depressive disease and multiple sclerosis. *Nature*, 1979, *277*, 28–32.

24 Review of "Assessment of Psychiatric Patients' Problems by Computer Interview"

Marc D. Schwartz, MD

The authors of this study [Hugh Angle, Everett Ellinwood, and Judith Carroll] believe little can be gained by automating presently available techniques of psychometric testing, such as the MMPI. They feel that the clinical utility of the tests is doubtful, that the level of training of psychometric test clinicians is declining, and that clinical outcome predictions based on the tests have not demonstrated any value.

They believe that use of the computer for clinical diagnosis is also of limited value in view of the problems inherent in psychodiagnosis even without the added complications of computerization.

What they believe to be the ideal substrate for the interviewing computer is "the idiosyncratic elements of patient problems and the situational setting in which they occur." To avoid confusion, the problems processed by this system are restricted to behaviors that demonstrate an excess or deficit of frequency, intensity, or duration. In some instances they are behaviors that occur in inappropriate settings. (Excluded are problems in the senses of symptoms, signs, diagnoses, and clinical inferences.) The major tasks of a behavioral problem-assessment are to identify problem behaviors and to detail the variables controlling these behaviors.

During the course of this study, 683 patients in a variety of settings (inpatient, outpatient, CMHC, alcohol program, and drug program)

This chapter is a review by Marc D. Schwartz of the article "Computer Interview Problem Assessment of Psychiatric Patients," by Hugh Angle, Everett Ellinwood, and Judith Carroll, which appeared in *Proceedings of the Second Annual Symposium on Computer Applications in Medical Care* (New York: Institute of Electrical and Electronics Engineers, 1978, pp. 137–148). The present review of that article originally appeared in *Computers in Psychiatry/Psychology*, 1979, 2 (2), 8–10, and is reprinted by permission.

each spent from four to eight hours completing a computer interview covering 29 life-problem areas.

The interview is carried out in two stages. The first, termed the *problem screen,* is made up of over three thousand possible questions (with branching). It obtains demographic information, information about problem behaviors related to 29 life areas (sex, job, legal, sleep, alcohol, appearance, etc.), and assesses treatment motivation. The number of computer questions about each life area varies from 21 (appearance) to 233 (alcohol). The second stage of the interview explores in depth and detail the problems identified in the first stage and obtains the characteristic situational variables that control the appearance of the behavioral problems.

Upon completion of the interview, the computer provides an immediate printout of information, including a problem data base and a Problem-Oriented Record (POR) problem list.

In a comparison of human and computer interviews, it was found that the humans covered only half the problem areas examined by the computer. Once a problem area was identified, the humans asked questions covering only 6% of the items questioned in the computer interview. In another comparison, the computer identified, on the average, 16 problem areas and 104 specific problems, compared to the human's 8 and 13, respectively. The problems identified by the computer seemed to be important ones, as judged by a panel of psychologists. In fact, three-fourths of "critical" problems elicited by the computer never appeared in the patients' clinical records.

One way both computer and human interviewers might miss important problems is if they used a branching inquiry strategy, which did not ask specific questions about a particular problem if the patient's global response to an inquiry about problems in that area was negative. Despite the negative global response, the patient might still have significant problems in that area. For example, about a quarter of the patients who denied being depressed in a global inquiry had Zung depression scores not significantly different from the depression scores of those patients who presented with depression. The authors of this program therefore opted for a nonexclusionary branching strategy. This requires the patient to take more time to complete the interview, but avoids the failure to detect problem behaviors.

The result of this decision is an interview that requires the patient to answer 60% to 80% of all questions and takes four to eight hours to complete. Somewhat surprisingly, only 13% of patients found this to be a negative overall experience. Four-fifths of patients accepted the computers' asking "personal questions," two-thirds preferred a computer interview to a human one, and more patients felt they could be more truthful with the computer than they could be with a human interviewer. Still, almost half the patients interviewed by the computer found the interview too long.

Nevertheless, no patient refused to complete the interview because of its length (or for any other reason). The authors state they were unable to determine the upper limit to the maximum size that the computer interview can reach and envision a 10,000-question survey requiring 3 to 5 days at the computer terminal.

As Stanley Milgram has demonstrated, before his work stimulated the explosive growth of human experiment committees, a person wearing the white coat can get subjects to do practically anything. Stronger evidence for the usefulness of this system will have to be marshaled before subjecting people expecting help to three to five days of computer interrogation.

A small majority of 34 clinicians who used the system rated the computer interview superior to traditional interview procedures on comprehensiveness and degree of detail. However, clinicians split 45% to 46% on whether the computer or a human would be superior in the ability to identify patients' problems. These are surprising results in view of the previous findings reported in this article. One would have expected an overwhelming majority to have found the computer superior on all counts. A closer examination of clinicians' responses showed that hospital psychiatrists found the computer much less useful in assessment, in formulating treatment goals, and in discussing treatment plans with the patient than did nonpsychiatrist mental health staff, who were generally much more positive in their evaluation of the computer's usefulness.

A testimonial to a system's usefulness, as the authors point out, "is not a suitable form of instrument validation." To explore the issue further, though, let us look at what the clinicians' evaluations of the system's utility might mean. Perhaps this kind of system actually is more useful to a less trained clinician. Or perhaps it is merely seen as more useful by one less sure of his/her skills. Or perhaps it is more threatening to one with more credentials. It may be that identification of all problems is not particularly necessary for the vast majority of patients. Working out a few major problems may have a carryover effect on many unmentioned others. Ultimately, the usefulness of this system must be evaluated in terms of certain outcome criteria related primarily to how helpful it is to patients and, if it is found to equal or be superior to the helpfulness of humans, then it should be determined how useful it is to clinicians.

## 25

A Microcomputer Program for Scoring the SCL-90

Victor Krynicki, PhD
R. Charles Gould, BA

The Symptom Check List-90 (SCL-90) is a brief screening instrument for assessing the broad range of psychopathology seen in outpatient settings. It is fully described in the *ECDEU Assessment Manual for Psychopharmacology* (Guy, 1976). It can be administered in a matter of a few minutes as a paper-and-pencil test to patients. There are 90 questions about symptoms, which are answered on a five-point scale from "Not at All" to "Extremely." These ratings are quantified by numbers ranging from 0 to 4.

The SCL-90 yields scores in 9 symptom dimensions: Somatization, Obsessive Compulsive, Interpersonal Sensitivity, Depression, Anxiety, Anger-Hostility, Phobic Anxiety, Paranoid Ideation, and Psychoticism. There are also 7 items that do not fall into any dimension, and that therefore may be defined as an "Other" cluster or symptom set.

It has been reported (Derogatis, Rickels, & Rock, 1976) that there is very high convergent validity of the SCL-90 with the set of the MMPI scales (standard clinical scales, Wiggins content scales, and Tryon cluster scales). Derogatis, Rickels, and Rock (1976) reported that peak correlations were observed with like constructs on 8 of the 9 scales. The SCL-90 by itself is not a complete intake assessment, and it should be combined with either other instruments or a clinical interview with history.

In the authors' clinical practice, the SCL-90 is used as a screening instrument. A program has been developed in BASIC to score the SCL-90 on the TRS-80 Model I, Level 2, microcomputer. The system has 32K of memory and 2 disk drives. Since the items of the 9 symptom dimensions (and the "Other" group) are intermixed, hand scoring of the results is quite laborious and slow; thus there is a need for more efficient scoring.

The microcomputer program asks for numerical input for each item and sorts and averages the ratings for each symptom dimension. If an error is made in entering a score, the item number of this error can be keyed into the next or any subsequent questions. When this is done, the program returns the user to the erroneous item for re-entry of data. Since patients occasionally skip items, there may not always be 90 responses or the expected number of responses for each dimension. Therefore, the program counts the number of responses in each dimension and the total responses. The digit "5" is entered for an item with missing data.

```
         SCL 90   RESULTS   FOR   TEST PATIENT
             TEST DATE   =   05/02/83



                            R E S U L T S
                       -----------------------------


CATEGORY #          CATEGORY              N        AVG        REMARKS
    1          SOMATIZATION              12        0.8
    2          OBSESSIVE COMPULSIVE      10        0.8
    3          INTERPERSONAL SENSITIVITY  9        1.6
    4          DEPRESSION                13        2.0
    5          ANXIETY                   10        0.8
    6          ANGER-HOSTILITY            6        2.0
    7          PHOBIC ANXIETY             7        0.6
    8          PARANOID IDEATION          6        1.7
    9          PSYCHOTICISM              10        0.3
   10          OTHER                      7        1.4


          TOTAL RESPONSES     =          90

          GENERAL SYMPTOMATIC INDEX  =              1.2

          KEY TO NUMERICAL RATINGS :
              0   =    NOT AT ALL
              1   =    MILDLY
              2   =    MODERATELY
              3   =    QUITE A BIT
              4   =    EXTREMELY

          C O M M E N T S    :


   SOMATIZATION                        MILD

       THIS PATIENT EXPERIENCES MILD DISTRESS ARISING FROM PERCEPTIONS OF
   BODILY DYSFUNCTION.   THERE ARE LIKELY TO BE COMPLAINTS FOCUSED AROUND
   THE CARDIOVASCULAR, GASTROINTESTINAL, AND/OR RESPIRATORY SYSTEM.
   OTHER POSSIBLE SYMPTOMS INCLUDE HEADACHES, BACKACHES, MUSCULAR
   TENSION, AND/OR OTHER SOMATIC EQUIVALENTS OF ANXIETY.


   OBSESSIVE COMPULSIVE                 MILD

       THIS PATIENT EXPERIENCES MILD DISTRESS RELATED TO THOUGHTS,
   IMPULSES, AND ACTIONS THAT ARE EXPERIENCED AS UNREMITTING AND
   IRRESISTABLE BUT ARE OF AN EGO-ALIEN OR UNWANTED NATURE.   PATIENT
   MAY ALSO EXPERIENCE SYMPTOMS OF COGNITIVE DIFFICULTY SUCH AS 'MIND
   GOING BLANK' OR 'TROUBLE REMEMBERING'.
```

FIGURE 25-1. Sample output of results on SCL-90.

INTERPERSONAL SENSITIVITY   MODERATE

     THIS PATIENT FEELS MODERATE INADEQUACY AND INCOMPETENCY IN
COMPARISON TO OTHERS. PATIENT HAS DIFFICULTIES WITH SELF-CONFIDENCE
AND EXPERIENCES FEELINGS OF UNEASINESS AND DISCOMFORT DURING
INTERPERSONAL INTERACTIONS. FEELINGS OF SELF-CONSCIOUSNESS AND
NEGATIVE EXPECTANCIES REGARDING INTERPERSONAL RELATIONS ARE
TYPICAL SOURCES OF DISTRESS.

DEPRESSION   MODERATE

     PATIENT EXPERIENCES MODERATE DEPRESSION. THIS PATIENT HAS GUILT
FEELINGS AND BLAMES HIMSELF/HERSELF FOR HIS/HER TROUBLES. LIKELY
SYMPTOMS INCLUDE DYSPHORIC AFFECT AND MOOD, WITHDRAWL OF INTEREST
IN LIFE EVENTS, LACK OF MOTIVATION, LOSS OF ENERGY, AND FEELINGS OF
HOPELESSNESS. IF THIS FACTOR IS RATED 'SEVERE', THERE ARE LIKELY
TO BE THOUGHTS OF DEATH AND SUICIDAL IDEATION AND/OR ATTEMPTS.

ANXIETY   MILD

     THIS PATIENT IS TROUBLED BY MILD SYMPTOMS AND EXPERIENCES
ASSOCIATED WITH MANIFEST ANXIETY. THIS MAY INCLUDE GENERAL INDICATORS
OF ANXIETY SUCH AS RESTLESSNESS, NERVOUSNESS, AND TENSION AND
SOMATIC SIGNS SUCH AS TREMBLING. IF THIS FACTOR IS RATED 'SEVERE',
THERE ARE LIKELY TO BE ACTUAL TERROR AND PANIC ATTACKS.

HOSTILITY   MODERATE

     THIS PATIENT ADMITS TO MODERATE PROBLEMS WITH ANGRY AND HOSTILE
THOUGHTS AND/OR BEHAVIORS. THERE APPEAR TO BE HOSTILE AND RETALIATORY
FEELINGS TOWARDS OTHERS, AND TENDENCIES TO BE CROSS, ANNOYED, AND
ARGUMENTATIVE. IF THIS FACTOR IS RATED 'SEVERE', THERE ARE LIKELY
TO BE UNCONTROLLABLE TEMPER OUTBURSTS.

PHOBIC ANXIETY   MILD

     PATIENT IS TROUBLED BY A MILD NUMBER OF FEARS WHICH TEND TO
RESTRICT HIS/HER LIFE AND MAKE HIM/HER UNCOMFORTABLE IN DAILY ACTIVITIES.
THIS FACTOR INCLUDES FEARS OF A PHOBIC NATURE ORIENTED TOWARDS
TRAVEL AWAY FROM HOME, OPEN SPACES, CROWDS, PUBLIC PLACES, AS WELL
AS SOCIAL PHOBIAS.

PARANOID IDEATION   MODERATE

     PATIENT ADMITS TO A MODERATE NUMBER OF THOUGHTS INDICATIVE OF A
PARANOID ORIENTATION. TYPICAL MANIFESTATIONS OF PARANOID IDEATION
INCLUDE PROJECTIVE THINKING, SUSPICIOUSNESS, GRANDIOSITY, DELUSIONS,
AND FEELINGS OF LOSS OF AUTONOMY. IF THE FACTOR IS RATED 'SEVERE',
THERE ARE LIKELY TO BE DELUSIONS OF GRANDEUR OR PERSECUTION.

PSYCHOTICISM   NOT AT ALL

OTHER   MILD

     THIS PATIENT ADMITS TO MILD PROBLEMS IN THE OTHER CATEGORY.
THE SYMPTOMS IN THIS CATEGORY TEND TO CLUSTER AROUND EATING DIFFICULTIES
(TOO LITTLE OR TOO MUCH) AND SLEEPING DIFFICULTIES.

FIGURE 25-1. *Continued.*

The output of the program includes the patient's name, date of testing, number of responses and average for each symptom dimension, total responses, and general symptomatic index (sum of all items/number of items). Comments and interpretations can either be entered into the keyboard and printed out with the above; or, alternatively, just the numbers can be printed out and the comments can be written in later. A sample output is included in this paper (See Figure 25–1).

It is possible to expand this program to actually present the test items on the microcomputer screen to the patient. Because of the practical problem of multiple offices and copyright questions, this has not been done by the present authors. The program described in this article is currently available by writing to Victor Krynicki, PhD, 28 Hollis Lane, Croton-On-Hudson, NY 10520.

REFERENCES

Derogatis, L., Rickels, K., & Rock, A. The SCL-90 and the MMPI: A step in the validation of a new self-report scale. *British Journal of Psychiatry*, 1976, *128*, 280–289.

Guy, W. *ECDEU assessment manual for psychopharmacology.* DHEW Publication No. (ADM) 76–338. Rockville, Maryland; NIMH, 1976.

26

Review of "A Probabilistic System for Identifying Suicide Attemptors"

Marc D. Schwartz, MD

C an a computer outperform experienced professionals in making clinical decisions? If it can, there are important consequences for clinical practice and teaching. If the computer processes data in a way that can predict outcome better than a clinician can, then informing the clinician about the step-by-step logic the computer used (its clinical algorithm) should enable him/her to alter accordingly the basis upon which his/her decision is made and thereby help improve it.

But *can* the computer outperform the experienced clinician? A number of studies have been carried out to answer this question and preliminary findings suggest that, under certain circumstances, it can.

John Greist, MD, of the University of Wisconsin Department of Psychiatry, and his colleagues have published a number of papers in the past few years on studies comparing the predictions made by clinicians and computers of the likelihood that a suicide attempt would subsequently be made by a patient who expressed suicidal thoughts during a clinical interview.

They first studied this question retrospectively. A group of psychiatric therapists identified 32 factors they felt were important in the evaluation of patients with thoughts of suicide (e.g., marital status, frequency of suicidal thoughts, health concerns, degree of impulsivity). They then assigned weights to each factor. For example "suicidal

"A Probabilistic System for Identifying Suicide Attemptors," by D. H. Gustafson, J. H. Greist, F. F. Stauss, J. Erdman, and T. Laughren, appeared in *Computers and Biomedical Research*, 1977, 10, 1–7. The present review by Marc Schwartz of that article originally appeared in *Computers in Psychiatry/Psychology*, 1978, 1 (2), 7, and is reprinted by permission.

thoughts all the time" was given a weight, by consensus, of 5.00; "living alone, doesn't know neighbors," a weight of 1.33.

Case histories of 20 patients, half of whom made a suicide attempt within three months of an interview, were then culled for data on the 32 factors. These data were then given to 18 psychiatrists, who were asked to estimate the probability of each patient's making a suicide attempt within the next 3 months. The same information was fed into a computer, which processed the data on the basis of the 32 weighted factors and assigned a probability from 0.00 to 1.00 to each outcome (nonattempt or attempt).

The computer accurately identified attemptors (assigned them a probability greater than 0.50) much more frequently than did the clinicians (70% vs. approximately 35%). I found that quite impressive. It was, however, a little less accurate in identifying nonattemptors (90% vs. approximately 95%). In both instances, as can be seen, the computer was more likely to predict a suicide attempt than was a clinician. (Does its unemotionality preclude its judgment's being influenced by such considerations as denial of death?) Dr. Greist's published reports do not describe the computer's clinical algorithm or present the relative weights of risk factors he has found, but I anticipate such reports will be forthcoming. In addition, a prospective study is underway.

VIII

Computer-Based Diagnosis

One application that has captured the imagination of many clinical computer specialists is the use of the computer in diagnosis. While most agree that attempts to program diagnostic thinking have been very helpful in clarifying the nature of the diagnostic process, debate rages over whether the computer as diagnostician will ever be useful in clinical practice. In Part VIII, you can get an introduction to the use of computers in diagnosis and familiarize yourself with both sides of the debate.

Part VIII begins with the description of a very simple program that aids the clinician in the diagnosis of depression. The program is straightforward and short enough to be easily implemented on any microcomputer. It is an illuminating and characteristic example of such programs in that it contains rather direct and simple questions, yet is able to generate obvious and, at the same time, very helpful conclusions from them . . . sometimes.

Marvin Miller's chapter begins with an historical overview of the use of computers in psychiatric diagnosis. He presents the various clinical and mathematical methods that have been used in this field. He concludes that the optimal diagnostic system must still include some "intuitive" information generated by the clinician.

A great deal of work has been done on the diagnostic use of computers in medical specialties other than psychiatry. In many ways, those areas lend themselves better to this endeavor, as the findings on which diagnoses are based in those specialties are more objective and measurable. So we in the mental health field perhaps can look to them for a clearer view of what can and cannot be done using computers in diagnosis. The authors of two of the chapters in this section are non-mental-health clinicians who share rather skeptical views of the computer's capabilities as a diagnostician.

27 | Review of "Direct Assessment of Depression by Microcomputer"

Marc D. Schwartz, MD

One area in which computers have demonstrated their effectiveness, yet have not been fully exploited, is in the routine collection of clinical data from patients. During diagnostic interviews, even experienced clinicians frequently fail to ask important questions or neglect to follow up on apparently obvious leads. Perhaps the clinician's attention has wandered; perhaps he has been misled by the patient's answer to a previous question; perhaps, while seeking one piece of information, he has overlooked another.

Patients' self-report of symptoms can provide a useful additional source of information that can expand the data base on which the clinician can make diagnostic decisions.

Dr. A. C. Carr and his colleagues at the Institute of Psychiatry, De Crespigny Park, London, designed a microcomputer-based assessment procedure using the Hamilton Depression Scale and compared the results of patients' self-ratings with clinicians' global clinical assessments. The study was intended not as a definitive experiment, but as an exploratory investigation of the clinical usefulness of a simple computer program designed to be used on an inexpensive microcomputer.

The computer approach offers a number of advantages, including the fact that the computer requires each patient to complete every question before handing in the questionnaire, whereas pen-and-paper questionnaires are often returned incomplete. Furthermore, the computer program can immediately encode, analyze, and report on the patient's responses.

The questions given to all subjects in this study were based on a

"Direct Assessment of Depression by Microcomputer," by A. C. Carr, R. J. Ancill, A. Ghosh, and A. Margo, appeared in *Acta Psychiatrica Scandinavica*, 1981, 64, 422–429. The present review by Marc Schwartz of that article originally appeared in *Computers in Psychiatry/Psychology*, 1982, 4 (4), 11–13 and is reprinted by permission.

modified Hamilton Depression Scale. Items on obsessionality and paranoia were omitted, as neither were easily adapted to self-rating. Assessments of agitation, retardation, and insight were also excluded,
since they rely on the judgment of a skilled observer. Extra items on
suicidal ideation were added.

Seventy-five patients who appeared at the Emergency Clinic giving evidence of depression were assessed by the computer program, as
were fifty inpatients who had been diagnosed as suffering from a depressive illness. Forty-three control subjects were obtained from the
medical and nursing staff and from relatives and friends of the patients. Each subject was briefly introduced to the microcomputer (a
Commodore PET 3052 series), usually by a nurse who had had approximately one hour's supervision in using the computer. Seated at the
computer, subjects were given instructions on the screen. In all, there
were three instruction frames followed by eighteen question frames.
All subjects understood and operated the machine without further assistance except for one particularly nearsighted patient, who could not
read the screen.

Computer interviews took less than 10 minutes for each patient.
After completion of the interview, patient response data was stored on
cassettes and analyzed later. Following a clinical interview, 99 of the
patients were rated on a 10-point global depression scale by qualified
clinicians.

The computer scores of patients and controls differed significantly
from each other. On a scale from 0 to 46, patients had a mean depression score of 25; controls had a mean score of 5. All controls scored
higher than an arbitrary (and retrospective) cutoff point of 10; only 4 of
125 patients scored lower than this. All 4 were found to be severely
and psychotically depressed, denying all depressive symptoms in clinical interviews as well as in the computer questionnaire.

Computer scores correlated highly with clinicians' global depression scores. Where there were discrepancies between information obtained from the computer and the clinician, it was found that either the
clinician had omitted asking questions due to pressure of time or the
patient had denied or minimized his symptoms.

The authors recognize that part of the difference in scores between
patients and controls may be due to the class differences between the
two groups. Generally, lower socioeconomic-class individuals tend to
score higher on depression inventories. However the authors believe
the differences are too great to ascribe to this factor. They suggest that
further research is needed to assess the reliability and sensitivity of the
method and to explore its applicability to other areas of mental illness.

The rating scale used by the program consisted of questions of
four types:

Answer type 1
    answer 0 if not at all
    answer 1 if a little
    answer 2 if a lot
    answer 3 if extremely so

Answer type 2
    answer 1 if no
    answer 2 if yes

Answer type 3
    answer 0 if no
    answer 1 if sometimes
    answer 2 if always

Answer type 4
    answer 0 if no
    answer 1 if yes but clothes still fit
    answer 2 if yes but clothes are loose

Question 1 (type 1)
How depressed are you?

Question 2 (type 1)
Do you feel guilty about things that you have done or thought?

Question 3 (type 3)
Is it taking you longer to get off to sleep?

Question 4 (type 3)
Do you sleep fitfully, often awakening?

Question 5 (type 3)
Do you waken earlier than usual and then find yourself unable to get back to sleep?

Question 6 (type 1)
Have you lost interest in your work or hobbies?

Question 7 (type 2)
Is life pointless?

Question 8 (type 2)
Have you thought of ending it all?

Question 9 (type 2)
Have you made plans to kill yourself?

Question 19 (type 2)
Have you attempted to, or do you intend to kill yourself?

Question 11 (type 1)
Do you feel that you are slower than your normal or usual self?

Question 12 (type 1)
Do you feel anxious or tense?

Question 13 (type 3)
Do you suffer from any physical symptoms?

Question 14 (type 1)
Are you worried that you might have a serious illness such as cancer or
V.D.?

Question 15 (type 2)
Have you lost interest in sex?

Question 16 (type 4)
Have you lost weight, excluding that due to dieting?

Question 17 (type 3)
Are you at your worst early in the day but improve as the day goes on?

Question 18 (type 1)
Do you feel that either you or the outside world is unreal?

The Computer and Clinical Judgment

G. Octo Barnett, MD

For a number of years it has been predicted that the use of computer technology would result in radical changes in the storage and retrieval of medical data. Only in the past five years, however, have there been major changes in the management of information in medicine. These changes have for the most part been limited to the support of such administrative functions in hospitals as admissions and discharge tracking and census activities; the communication of structured information (for example, laboratory-test orders and results); and the support of such ancillary service functions as scheduling for radiology, the preparation of pharmacy prescriptions, and the like. In general, the application of computer technology to medical care has paralleled applications in other fields, such as banking, communications, and manufacturing. The technology is most successful in the repetitive processing of explicitly defined data in well-structured tasks—activities that do not require much of what is considered "human judgment."

The optimistic expectation of 20 years ago that computer technology would also come to play an important part in clinical decisions has not been realized, and there are few if any situations in which computers are being routinely used to assist in either medical diagnosis or the choice of therapy.

There are a number of reasons why computers have had little impact on medical decisions. There is no question that many of the early attempts failed to take into account the extraordinary complexity of some elements of the diagnostic process and used greatly oversimplified mathematical models. The concept that medical judgment and the diagnostic process as practiced by medical experts can be explicitly defined and reduced to a set of rules is still the subject of lively debate. The underlying assumption that there is a well-defined, monolithic diagnostic process is almost certainly simplistic and fundamentally misleading.

Reprinted with permission of the *New England Journal of Medicine*. Vol. 307, pp. 493–494, 1982.

Nevertheless, some provocative experiments with the use of computer technology in a medical consulting role have been initiated. One of the most ambitious and comprehensive of these is represented by the INTERNIST-I model, which is described in this issue of the *Journal*.[1] Most of the experiments involving the application of computers to clinical decisions have concerned such relatively limited areas of disease as abdominal pain[2] and septicemia.[3] The INTERNIST-I program, in contrast, attempts to deal with differential diagnosis within the broad context of general internal medicine.

The size and structure of the diagnostic problem are of crucial importance in considering the possible usefulness of computers in clinical judgment.[4] Computer programs have their greatest potential use when the clinical problem is relatively well defined and well structured and when only a limited number of diseases need to be considered.

The INTERNIST-I program is correctly described as a research project and not as an imminently available consultation program. The authors employ admirable candor and insight in describing the limitations and deficiencies of the present model. Their systematic evaluation of the model's performance is virtually unique in the field of medical applications of artificial intelligence. The choice of clinicopathological conference (CPC) cases as the evaluation standard has the advantage of providing detailed clinical information on cases that are diagnostically challenging, but it also has the obvious limitation that CPC cases are not representative of the vast majority of patients seen in medical practice.

The authors describe in detail several serious limitations of the present version of INTERNIST-I. The two issues that are most troublesome are the program's inability to reason anatomically or temporally and the very limited incorporation of pathophysiologic information in the underlying statistical model. INTERNIST-I has little appreciation of disease mechanisms or of the need to formulate a differential diagnosis at different levels—e.g., at the level of the specific organ system and at the intermediate level of pathophysiologic states (low cardiac output, hypokalemia, and the like). Much of the wisdom of experienced clinicians is based on a thorough appreciation of the network of pathophysiologic causality that allows them to relate observed manifestations to underlying disease conditions.

Its lack of pathophysiologic understanding prevents the computer program from providing one of the most valuable services performed by a medical consultant. The consultant is able not only to give the differential diagnosis but also to explain why, to reason on the basis of causality, to consider whether the observed manifestations can be explained by a single disease with multiple manifestations or whether they require an explanation of multiple diseases. The experienced clinician is vastly superior to INTERNIST-I in the ability to consider the relative severity and independence of the different manifestations of disease and to understand the temporal evolution of the disease process.

The potential value of the present version of INTERNIST-I seems to lie primarily in its ability to remind the user of diagnoses that should be considered, given a specific set of signs and symptoms; to comment on the diagnostic relevance of each of the signs and symptoms; and to suggest the collection of additional data that might be of diagnostic value, given the differential diagnosis currently favored by the computer model. Perhaps the most exciting experimental evaluation of INTERNIST-I would be the demonstration that a productive collaboration is possible between man and computer—that clinical diagnosis in real situations can be improved by combining the medical judgment of the clinician with the statistical and computational power of a computer model and a large base of stored medical information.

The contribution of INTERNIST-I cannot be measured simply by its limitations or failures. Experiments like this one provide greatly needed insight into the diagnostic process and stimulate an explicit and systematic consideration of how, and in what formats and situations, a computer can be helpful as a medical consultant. The important issue is not whether the computer program uses the same strategies that a physician would use; indeed, the attempt to model such a complex phenomenon as diagnostic judgment may be far beyond the scope of any feasible experiment. The issue is whether such artificial-intelligence models can reach conclusions similar to those of a competent clinician and can then justify those conclusions in a rational and clinically acceptable fashion.

Most decisions in clinical medicine are relatively straightforward and require only that the physician be experienced in the application of a limited number of categorical rules. But when medical decisions are simple, the experienced clinician has no need to use a computer. It is in difficult problems requiring a high degree of medical knowledge and clinical judgment that a computer could potentially be most useful.[5] In such situations, however, the information immediately available is often vague, ambiguous, incomplete, or conflicting. There may be many possible diseases that could be individually or simultaneously considered, and there are frequently many possible paths of further investigation. Furthermore, the difficulties are greatly exacerbated by the fact that the diagnostic process cannot be independent of all the personal, social, family, and employment considerations of the particular patient.

In the real world it is necessary that the doctor not only understand the statistical relations of signs and symptoms to the various possible diseases but also have the wisdom and common sense that derive from the understanding and experience of everyday human existence. It is this last requirement that represents the greatest weakness (and perhaps the ultimate limitation) of computer technology in dealing in any comprehensive fashion with the problem of clinical diagnosis.

REFERENCES

1. Miller RA, Pople HE Jr, Myers JD. *INTERNIST-I*, an experimental computer-based diagnostic consultant for general internal medicine. N Engl J Med. 1982; 307:468–76.
2. De Dombal FT. Medical diagnosis from a clinician's point of view. Methods Inf Med. 1978; 16 & 17:28–35.
3. Shortliffe EH. Computer-based medical consultations: MYCIN. New York: Elsevier, 1976.
4. Blois MS. Clinical judgment and computers. N Engl J Med. 1980; 303: 192–7.
5. Szolovits P, Pauker SG. Categorical and probabilistic reasoning in medical diagnosis. Artific Intell. 1978; 11:115–44.

Computerized Models of Psychiatric Diagnosis

Marvin J. Miller, MD

The advent of numerous computerized psychiatric diagnostic systems has forced a re-examination of general diagnostic theory. The procedure of computerization requires detailed mathematical descriptions of diagnostic systems, which until now have been abstractly and globally described. We will briefly review the historical struggle between the biological and the descriptive system of diagnosis and then look at the automation of various descriptive systems. We will also review several mathematical models of decision-making, implementations of these models, and their comparative validities.

DISCUSSION OF PSYCHIATRIC DIAGNOSIS

Historically the two main approaches to psychiatric diagnosis involve descriptive diagnoses and biological diagnoses. The former utilizes historical and mental-status examination data to classify a patient, while the latter uses physical, biochemical, or genetic findings.

The biological approach dates back to the 4th century B. C., when Hippocrates postulated four body fluids to correspond to four personality types. The recent experiments with three-methoxy-four-hydroxy phenylglycol in depression and ventricle size in schizophrenics are continuing examples of attempts to delineate physiologically (and perhaps genetically) distinct classes of psychiatric patients. Persons such as Alzheimer, Nissl, Wernicke, and Korsakoff, and such contemporary individuals as Seymour Kety, have all contributed greatly to delineating the medical, biochemical, and genetic etiology of psychiatric illnesses.

An early example of the descriptive type of classification is the work of Pinel, who published in 1806 a method for dividing all types of mental illness into five categories. These were: (1) melancholia; (2) mania with delirium; (3) mania without delirium; (4) dementia; and (5) idiotism. His careful observation of the patients and his skills as a clinician allowed him to derive classifications that still have some meaning today.

The essential benefit of psychiatric diagnosis lies in the ability it gives clinicians to make *predictions* about the course of the illness, the outcome, the most efficacious treatment modality, the client's suicidal potential, his or her danger to self and others, etc. Our discussion will deal mainly with descriptive diagnosis and various methods of making predictions within this system.

MATHEMATICAL SIMULATIONS OF THE CLINICAL (OR DESCRIPTIVE) DIAGNOSTIC PROCESS

Predictions can be made by statistical and by clinical methods. Lundberg (1941) and Sarbin (1944) argue that no clinician can do better than multiple regression equations in making predictions. Meehl (1954) thinks that a clinician is at best a "second-rate accounting machine." However, the most highly predictive methods will be shown to utilize both statistical and clinical information. The only way that this can be done cheaply and rapidly on a routine basis is with computers.

Statisticians have frequently attempted to see how accurately certain clinicians could describe their own decision-making process. Hoffman (1960) devised a protocol testing clinicians' ability to predict intelligence and then tested ways to simulate the clinician's decision-making processes. Judges were asked to distribute 100 points among nine variables (e.g., length of education, study habits, etc.) in a pattern that indicated their own weighting of each of these variables in making predictions about the intelligence of the subject. A linear multiple discriminant function was devised for determining the intelligence scores of these subjects according to the weighting the judges had provided. The judges were asked to classify the intelligence of 100 individuals. These were then classified by the linear multiple-discriminant function derived earlier. The results were compared and it was discovered that for one judge, the stated method of classifying intelligence was nowhere near what he actually used in practice. For the second judge, description was close to what he used in practice.

Another study was done in 1968 by Wiggins and Hoffman, attempting to mathematically represent the decision-making model of clinicians. This was a much larger study, involving 29 clinicians and 861 psychiatric patients. Here the task given the clinicians was to classify each patient as psychotic or neurotic on the basis of 11 MMPI scales. The authors then drew inferences about the nature of the clinicians' decision-making process. They wound up with three models. The first consisted of the previously discussed linear multiple-discriminate function. The second model, which they called *the quadratic model*, included linear terms, second-degree or curvilinear terms, and interactive terms. The third was called *the sign model*, and it consisted of a combination of 70 clinical signs that clinicians had reported either privately or in the literature as being relevant to the discrimination of psychosis from neurosis using the MMPI. (An example of the sign model would be the Meehl's & Dahlstrom's (1960) sequential rules for the classification of MMPIs.) The authors then derived an equation to describe each of these models for each of the 29 clinicians and did a cross-validation study. The sign model predicted 13 of the clinical judges best, the linear model 12, the quadratic model 3. However, it was discovered that the linear multiple-discriminant function model really could do a very good job of predicting almost all of the judge's decision-making routines and the other models had only a few percentage points of increased accuracy over the linear model.

Meehl (1954) reviewed 51 studies to compare the relative accuracy of statistical versus clinical predictions. The statistical methods won in 33 cases, the statistical methods were equal to clinical methods in 17 cases, and one case was equivocally won by the clinicians. At first glance this review would indicate that statistical methods are uniformly equal to or usually superior to clinical methods in making predictions about patients, however, there are a number of problems with many of these studies. First of all, clinical methods of predictions usually focus on the individual and make a prediction for him rather than for groups of people. It is, after all, the individual, though, that is to be most immediately benefited by a good prediction. The second type of problem is that the clinician usually has the ability to sense unique patterns in patients and modify his or her predictions on the basis of these. This includes the ability to make predictions based on the observation of events that do not occur frequently enough to be included in a multiple regression equation and yet, when they do occur in certain combinations with other clinical events, assume a pivotal importance. The data base that the computer has available in any particular case is limited; the clinician often can pick up bits of data from friends, relatives, or patients that are useful in making predictions about the patient.

Sawyer (1966) reviewed 45 different studies involving the clinical-statistical debate. The mechanical composite or the mechanical synthesis methods are appreciably superior to the other methods involved. This indicates that the studies involving a mechanical or computerized combination of judgmental and mechanical data resulted in the greatest potential for prediction. Sawyer's data show that the clinician who has both judgmental and statistical data to combine can also improve his prediction ability by using this combination. In a general sense then, we can say that the combination of judgmental and systematic or statistical information can improve decision-making routines.

COMPUTERIZED APPLICATIONS

The heart of any computerized diagnostic system lies in its decision-making logic. The formal discussion of diagnostic decision-making logic rarely occurs in psychiatric education. The traditional situation in education involves a didactic presentation of syndromes (with clinical illustrations) and the assumption that the student will automatically perceive the intuitive decision-making path of the teaching clinician.

Two principle clinical models of decision-making have emerged.

The Logical-Decision Tree

The first is the *logical-decision tree* or cookbook model. The principle advocates of this model are Robert Spitzer, MD, and Jean Endicott, PhD (1975), as evidenced by the Research Diagnostic Criteria and the DSM-III, with which they are associated. An illustration of the logical-decision tree or cookbook method of diagnosis, taken from DSM-III, is given below.

Diagnostic Criteria for Panic Disorder

A. At least three panic attacks within a three-week period in circumstances other than during marked physical exertion or in a life-threatening situation. The attacks are not precipitated only by exposure to a circumscribed phobic stimulus.

B. Panic attacks are manifested by discrete periods of apprehension or fear, and at least four of the following symptoms appear during each attack:

1. dyspnea
2. palpitations
3. chest pain or discomfort
4. choking or smothering sensations
5. dizziness, vertigo, or unsteady feelings
6. feelings of unreality
7. paresthesias (tingling in hands or feet)
8. hot and cold flashes
9. sweating

10. faintness
11. trembling or shaking
12. fear of dying, going crazy, or doing something uncontrolled during an attack

C. Not due to a physical disorder or another mental disorder, such as Major Depression, Somatization Disorder, or Schizophrenia.
D. The disorder is not associated with Agoraphobia (American Psychiatric Association, 1980, pp. 231–232).

Dr. John Greist at the University of Wisconsin uses a logical-decision tree in an automated version of the Research Diagnostic Criteria (Griest, Klein, & Erdman, 1976). In his program, two approaches are possible. In the first approach, the computer asks the clinician a series of questions about a patient and then prints out an RDC diagnosis. The second approach allows the clinician to test out a specific diagnosis against the RDC. He is then told that the patient either fits or doesn't fit the Research Diagnostic Criteria for that specific diagnosis. This program is rather remarkable in that it allows for fast and smooth application of the Research Diagnostic Criteria and it has a teaching capability. The program delivers the appropriate diagnostic category, along with several other categories that were considered and that were rejected for specific reasons, which are listed. This program is not intended as a device for gathering data, but rather as an assistance in a diagnostic formulation and as a teaching tool.

Another computerized diagnostic system that also uses the logical-decision tree or cookbook approach was developed by Coddington and King (1972) at Ohio State University. This investigation attempted to determine the feasibility of using a computer as a screening device in child psychiatry. The approach is rather novel in that it gathers its information directly from the mother of the potential patient. The mother sits down at a computer terminal and answers a series of branching questions. The computer summarizes these multiple-choice questions and comes up with a decision as to whether further evaluation is indicated. The questions in the protocol attempt to elicit components of the Menninger (1963) five-stage graduated definition of mental illness. The information-gathering techniques are well-accepted by the mothers, who answer an average of 113 questions (range 77 to 181) in an average of 45 minutes. In this study, 82% of the mothers felt that they could be *as frank* or *more frank* in talking to the computer as they could be in talking to their doctors.

In the sample study, the program was able to divide patients whose pediatricians and psychiatrists could agree that they did not need referral from those felt to need referrals. This study (which had only a two-option diagnosis) used a simple cutoff point to separate the referral from nonreferral patients. More sophisticated statistical techniques might have increased the accuracy of this decision-making process. There was a good deal of overlap between the groups where referral was indicated and where it was not indicated.

A more elaborate decision-tree diagnostic system can be illustrated by the Feldman, Klein, and Honigfeld (1972) study in Glen Oaks, New York. These investigators use the Lorr Multi-Dimensional Scale for rating psychiatric patients to divide patients into one of four groups: schizophrenic, excited, character disorders, or affective disorders. Information gathered by two independent raters and diagnosis compared with the clinician show good agreement: 49% agreement for schizophrenia, 56% agreement for excited, 54% agreement for character disorders, and 87% agreement for affective disorders. (Unweighted Kappa, overall, was .508 and the weighted Kappa was .526. On a cross-validation sample, the percent of agreement ranged from 36% to 59% and the Kappa was .254, with a weighted Kappa of .272.)

This study is of note in that each fork of the logical-decision tree had a procedure in which all of the data items were used in considering the decision at that fork. The patients in this study were also randomly assigned to either a placebo, imipramine, or chlorpromazine, and the computerized diagnostic system was able to predict at a significant level how these patients would respond to chlorpromazine and imipramine. (The chlorpromazine test sample P was less than .001; the cross-validation sample P was less than .05.)

Statistical Approaches

The second general approach to modeling psychiatric diagnosis is the statistical approach. The two main subtypes of this are the Bayesian formula, and the multiple discriminant function model (or clustering). Clustering is a procedure used to divide a group of patients into their natural groupings. Purely correlational methods can be used to derive these groupings de novo, or hypothetical groupings can be postulated and then verified or disproved. The Bayesian formula is based on probability theory. Here the frequencies of various symptoms and various illnesses in a population becomes important. This method also has a "learning" capability built in as more information is collected about the symptom profile in specific illnesses.

Multiple Discriminant Analysis. Stepwise multiple discriminant analysis is felt by many to be the most mathematically sound and achievable model for computerized diagnostic procedures. The idea behind this theory is that a given patient can be described with a set of variables, which can then be used to describe his relationship to a clus-

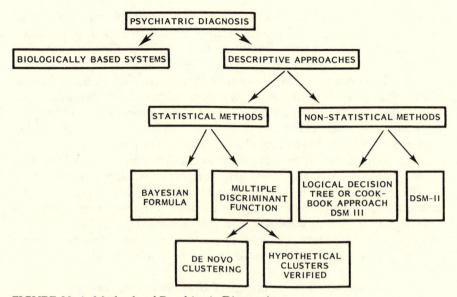

FIGURE 29–1. Methods of Psychiatric Diagnosis

ter of patients having similar features. This clustering is initially achieved by taking a group of patients and calculating a vector for each variable for each patient. These vectors are then weighted to achieve the clustering process. The weighting is done to maximize the variance between clusters and to minimize the variance within a cluster. Further analysis can then be done to see which items contribute the most powerfully and the least powerfully to this clustering and these items can then be relied upon or discarded or modified as the need may be. An excellent example of this system is demonstrated by Hautaluoma's (1971) work. He used the computerized records of 1,099 patients in the Fort Logan Mental Health Center to attempt to verify Lorr's syndromes (Lorr, Uhr, & Miller, 1960). Hautaluoma was able to identify seven of ten Lorr's syndromes.

Hautaluoma utilized both the de novo and the hypothetical methods of clustering and attempted to find if these two methods would result in similar clusters (ones corresponding with the Lorr's syndromes). He was not able to isolate "perceptual distortion" or "motor disturbances" and was only able to weakly document "paranoid projection." He attributes the failure of the latter two syndromes to be found in this clustering to the absence of certain items of information from the Fort Logan Data Base. Hautaluoma is currently repeating his clustering procedures, looking for four broader groupings: (1) schizophrenic reactive paranoid; (2) chronic undifferentiated schizophrenia;

(3) depressive neurosis; and (4) passive-agressive personality. These seem to be the largest subgroups in the Fort Logan patient population. Hautaluoma again is using methods that allow for the input of clinician hypotheses in regard to probable clusterings.

The Missouri Standard System of Psychiatry (SSOP) has a Mental Status Examination (110 items), which is gathered by a clinician and then subjected to a computerized classification procedure (Sletten, Altman, & Sundland). The method used here is a stepwise multiple discriminant analysis, which first clusters a group of patients and then assigns new patients to one of the previous clusters. It also assigns a probability of a particular case's belonging to each particular cluster.

The total of 110 items from the Mental Status Examination were factored into 27 variables. These were then combined with 29 demographic variables and were subjected to stepwise discriminant analysis to develop ten clusters. In order to perform the clustering procedure, 12 categories were hypothesized, corresponding to categories from DSM I.

The validity of this procedure shows an overall average percent agreement of 54% between the computerized diagnosis and the clinical diagnosis. This converts to an unweighted Kappa of .47.

Melrose, Stroebel, and Glueck (1970) have done a valuable study in comparing the stepwise multidiscriminant analysis with the logical-decision tree. Their data-gathering instruments were the Current and Past Psychopathology Scales (CAPPS) developed by Spitzer and Endicott (1969). In this analysis, the data from 413 psychiatric patients were first placed in 14 groups according to the clinical diagnosis and then analyzed by discriminate analysis to determine the probability that each case was in fact a member of the group to which it had been originally assigned. The 13 groups were then purified to include only those members that had an 85 percent or greater probability of membership in the group to which they were originally assigned.

This purified model was then used to test 255 new cases from the same source of the original data. The comparison between the DIAGNO II (the diagnostic system derived by the authors) and the stepwise multiple discriminant analysis was then made on the sample of 255. The discriminant analysis showed an overall agreement of 29.7% with the clinical diagnosis (K = .184), compared with an overall agreement of 40.1% (K = .305) for the DIAGNO II routine. When the first, second, or third most probable diagnosis was considered a match for the discriminant analysis routine, the overall agreement rose to 43.8%, to compare more favorably with the DIAGNO II routine. DIAGNO II had full access to the CAPPS data, while the multiple discriminant classification had access to only 70 variables because of computer limitations.

The contributions of Stroebel and Glueck (1970) also include their computer-derived global judgments, which were based on the daily nursing observations. This system is significant in that it views the standardized assessment of patients as a serial event with ongoing significance for treatment and disposition. Their program was able to diagnose no significant change versus significant improvement, or worsening, about one week earlier than the clinician was able to arrive at a similar global judgment. The hospital savings from these early judgments could be significant in terms of treatment changes or earlier discharges.

Bayes Formula. The second general type of statistical diagnostic system is the Bayesian analysis. This is a technique that is able to use clinical information in order to begin the diagnostic process and that can be updated by a *learning* process. The Bayesian formula is derived from probability theory and states that we can calculate the relative probability of an individual having a disease if we know: the probability of that disease given that symptom x_1, x_2, x_3, x_4 are present in the individual and the a priori probability of that disease in the population under study. Thus, the demand for initial clinical input is large. The clinician must make estimates of the probability that a given symptom present in a patient indicates the presence of a given disease. If a certain symptom is pathognomonic of an illness, then the assigned probability would be 1.00.

Hershfeld, Spitzer, and Miller (1974) undertook a study in which they compared the validity of the Bayesian approach with the logical-decision tree. The data-gathering instrument again was the CAPPS and the probabilities for the various symptom-disease combinations were derived from the records of 452 patients who had been rated by experienced clinicians in New York hospitals and clinics. The overall agreement between the Bayes computerized method and the clinician varied between 40% and 70%, depending upon the sample. The logical-decision tree (DIAGNO II) performed in a similar fashion, giving a range of 45% to 55% agreement with clinicians. The DIAGNO method seemed to have higher agreement with clinicians on paranoid schizophrenia, alcoholism, and drug dependency, while the Bayes method seemed to agree more with clinicians on the neuroses and the personality disorders. The overall concordance with clinicians was 69% for Bayes and 53% for DIAGNO, with a Kappa of .59 for Bayes, and .40 for DIAGNO.

A modification of Bayes is incorporated into a computerized diagnostic system designed by Brooks and Kleinmuntz (1974). Their application gathers information from a friend or relative of the patient directly, via a computer terminal. There are 113 question clusters, which are summarized to twenty diagnostic groupings. The probability of particular symptoms for specific illness is at first calculated and then after the program is in effect, each subsequent diagnosis is used to update the probabilities and thus to increase the capabilities of the system. Brooks and Kleinmuntz did not discuss any validity measures in their article, however.

Several important examples of cookbook and statistical diagnostic programs are being applied to the Present Status Examination (PSE), which is used in the World Health Organization International Pilot Study of Schizophrenia. These methods, DIAGNO (Wing & Nixon, 1974) and DIAX (Fischer, 1974), both utilize the 360 questions of the Present Status Examination to develop a smaller number of syndromes, from which an eventual diagnosis is developed. The DIAGNO program moves from 140 symptoms, which are rated 0, 1, or 2 by the clinician who conducts the standardized interview, down to 38 syndromes, and finally down to 13 classes, which correspond somewhat with categories found in DSM-II.

DIAX was developed in Denmark and generates 39 symptom groups out of the original questions in the PSE. It then separates these into 13 categories similar to the major DSM-II categories. The validity of DIAX was assessed in several ways. On a three-digit level of the International Classification of Diseases Diagnosis, the overall agreement was 90/126 or 71%. In applying the DIAX program to the data from other international pilot studies of schizophrenia centers, they reach an overall agreement of DIAX/clinical diagnosis of 74% for schizophrenia, 78% agreement for schizophrenia combined with paranoid psychosis, and a 74% agreement for the affective disorders.

Another part of the DIAX investigation included applying the Bayes formula to the 39 DIAX symptom groups. About 90% of the patients were placed by the Bayes formula into the corresponding DIAX group. The investigators also noted that in cases where the DIAX diagnosis was in conflict with the clinical diagnosis, the Bayes formula often corresponded more closely with the clinical diagnosis. The percent of agreement on two-year follow-up between DIAX and the clinical diagnosis ranged from 50% to 67% for schizophrenia.

CONCLUSIONS

In our review of current modern applications of computerized diagnosis, it has become quite clear that no particular mathematical model has yet dominated the field or proved itself clearly superior to other methods. Each method has some unique advantages (see Table 29–1). The time and expense involved in implementing various models of computer diagnosis also needs to be considered heavily in planning efforts in this area. Some have suggested that the extent to which a computerized program agrees with a clinician cannot rise above 55% to 60%, since clinicians don't agree with each other any more than that. We have also seen that clinicians show some variation in the type of approach that they use toward problem-solving. Perhaps further work should be done to attempt devising computerized programs that mimic the clinician more closely. It may be true, however, that the further research needs to occur at a more basic theoretical level. The delineation of our diagnostic categories is perhaps not yet firm because our understanding of psychodynamic and biological factors in illness is not yet complete enough to devise consistent and measurable categories. The arrival of DSM-III on the psychiatric scene should promote the science of diagnosis, since it provides for a more detailed description of syndromes and symptoms. By carefully applying these diagnostic standards, we will later be able to test the cohesiveness and validity of various syndromes.

The concomitant development of further physiologic discoveries should be used to augment our choice of drugs and other treatment recommendations. The arrival of a point in time where one illness can be postulated to arise from a specific set of molecules out of place will probably not occur, and if we continue to try to match the physiologic and descriptive diagnostic patterns too closely, we will be hampered in the respect that we will not be able to merge the two divergent dimensions of psychosis into a useful tool for the clinician.

PRACTICAL APPLICATION

The following approaches may be of use in helping the clinician to use the newer computer programs effectively in the evaluations to treatment of psychiatric patients. The current availability of a number of psychological testing packages (See Appendix I) dictates the need for some up-to-date guidelines for the clinician.

1. Computer-generated summaries or diagnoses need to be viewed as any other laboratory report. They are only preliminary reports and need to be weighed by the clinician along with all of the other clinical evidence in deciding how to treat a particular patient.
2. Computer-generated reports can improve the thoroughness and the accuracy of the clinical diagnosis, but cannot replace many complex skills of the clinician.
3. The future addition of biological and radiological information to the psychiatric diagnosis will improve on the descriptive diagnostic process, but will not likely replace it. The careful gathering and processing of clinical signs and symptoms will continue to be important and computers can improve this process.

TABLE 29–1. Summary of Recent Studies of Computerized Psychiatric Diagnosis

	Spitzer and Endicott (1969)	Greist, Klein, and Erdman (1976)	Coddington and King (1972)	Feldman, Klein, and Honigfeld (1972)	Wing and Nixon (1974)	Fischer (1974)
PERSONS	Spitzer and Endicott (1969)	Greist, Klein, and Erdman (1976)	Coddington and King (1972)	Feldman, Klein, and Honigfeld (1972)	Wing and Nixon (1974)	Fischer (1974)
PLACE	New York, New York	Madison, Wisconsin	Columbus, Ohio	Glen Oaks, New York	England	Denmark
SCOPE	Research tool	Partial patient evaluation system	Structured history	Diagnostic system only	Structured clinical interview	Structured clinical interview
COLLECTION OF DATA	Mark sense forms	Clinician is on-line and interactive	Parent enters data into computer terminal	Mark sense forms	Mark sense forms	Mark sense forms
DATA INSTRUMENTS	Research Diagnostic Criteria	Research Diagnostic Criteria	181-question, branching, multiple choice program	Lorr Multidimensional Scale for rating psychiatric patients	Present State Exam, Social History, Psychiatric History	Present State Examination
DIAGNOSTIC APPROACH	Logical-decision tree	Logical-decision tree	"Cookbook"	Logical-decision tree	Logical-decision tree	Logical-decision tree
DIAGNOSTIC CLASSES	DSM II	DSM II	"Needs further evaluation" or nonreferral	Schizophrenic, excited, character disorder, affective disorder	38 "syndromes" 13 "classes"	39 "symptom groups" 13 "classes"
VALIDITY				41%–87% agreement with clinicians		

TABLE 29–1. *Continued.*

	Hautaluoma (1971)	Sletten, Altman, and Sundland (1970)	Melrose, Stroebel, and Glueck (1970)	Brooks and Kleinmuntz (1974)	Hirschfeld, Spitzer, and Miller (1974)
PERSONS	Hautaluoma (1971)	Sletten, Altman, and Sundland (1970)	Melrose, Stroebel, and Glueck (1970)	Brooks and Kleinmuntz (1974)	Hirschfeld, Spitzer, and Miller (1974)
PLACE	Colorado State University	Missouri	Institute of Living, Hartford, Connecticut	Chicago	New York
SCOPE	Broad computerized patient info. system of Fort Logan MHC	Structured Mental Status Examination	Structured patient interview	Psychiatric history gathered from friends and relatives	Structured clinical interview
COLLECTION OF DATA	Mark sense forms	Mark sense forms or card sort	Mark sense forms	On-line, interactive	Mark sense forms
DATA INSTRUMENTS	Admission form, Social hist. form, Ment. stat. exam (Menninger)	Mental status checklist	Current and Past Psychopathology Scales (CAPPS)	113 groups of 4 questions showing degrees of psychopathology	Current and Past Psychopathology Scales (CAPPS)
DIAGNOSTIC APPROACH	3-stage cluster analysis	Multiple discriminant function	Multiple discriminant function	"Cookbook"	Bayes
DIAGNOSTIC CLASSES	7 out of 10 Lorr syndromes were found	12 classes from DSM II	13 from DSM I	20 classes from DSM II	8 categories from DSM II
VALIDITY		50% agreement with clinicians			40%-70% agreement with clinicians

4. Computers can reduce the cost of patient care through rapid gathering and processing of patient data.
5. Computer-generated reports need to be used only by professionals otherwise skilled in the diagnosis and treatment of patients.
6. The clinician should have the right to know the nature and the accuracy of the diagnostic model used in any system in which he or she participates. The clinician should assume any system has a margin of error.
7. The judicious use of computer-generated summaries can improve patient care if used along with other data or can mislead if used without adequate corroboration.

REFERENCES

American Psychiatric Association, *Diagnostic and statistical manual of mental disorders* (3rd ed.), Washington, D.C.: American Psychiatric Association, 1980.

Brooks, R. & Kleinmuntz, B. Design of an intelligent psychodiagnostician. *Behavioral Science*, 1974, *19*, 16–20.

Coddington, R. D. & King, T. L. Automated history taking in child psychiatry. *American Journal of Psychiatry*, 1972, *129*, 52–58.

Feldman, S., Klein, D. F. & Honigfeld, G. The reliability of a decision tree technique applied to psychiatric diagnosis. *Biometrics*, 1972, *28*, 831–840.

Fischer, M. Development and validity of a computerized method for diagnosis of functional psychosis. *Acta Psychiatrica Scandinavica*, 1974, *50*, 243–288.

Greist, J. H., Klein, M. H. & Erdman, H. P. Routine on-line psychiatric diagnosis by computer. *American Journal of Psychiatry*, 1976, *133*, 1405–1408.

Hautaluoma, J. Syndromes, antecedents, and outcome of psychoses. *Journal of Consulting and Clinical Psychology*, 1971, *37*, 332–344.

Hirschfeld , R., Spitzer, R. L., & Miller, R. G. Computer diagnosis in psychiatry: A Bayes approach. *Journal of Nervous and Mental Disease*, 1974, *158*, 399–407.

Hoffman, P. J. The paramorphic representation of clinical judgment. *Psychological Bulletin*, 1960, *57*, 116–131.

Lorr, M., Uhr, L. M., & Miller, J. G. (Eds). Rating scales, behavior inventories, and drugs. In *Drugs and Behavior*. New York: Wiley, 1960.

Lundberg, G. A. Case studies vs statistical methods: An issue based on misunderstanding. *Sociometry*, 1941, *4*, 379–381.

Meehl, P. E. *Clinical vs. statistical prediction: A theoretical analysis and a review of the evidence*. Minneapolis: University of Minnesota Press, 1954.

Meehl, P. E., & Dahlstrom, W. G. Objective configural rules for discriminating psychotic from neurotic MMPI profiles. *Journal of Consulting Psychology*, 1960, *24*, 375–381.

Melrose, J. P., Stroebel, C. F., & Glueck, B. Diagnosis of psychopathology using stepwise multiple discriminant analysis. *Comprehensive Psychiatry*, 1970, *11*, 43–50.

Menninger, K. *The Vital Balance.* New York: Viking Press, 1963.

Sawyer, J. Measurement and prediction, clinical and statistical. *Psychological Bulletin,* 1966, *66,* 178–200.

Sarbin, T. R. The logic of prediction in psychology. *Psychological Reviews,* 1944, *51,* 210–228.

Sletten, I. W., Altman, H., & Sundland, D. The Missouri Standard System of Psychiatry. *Archives of General Psychiatry,* 1970, *23,* 73–79.

Spitzer, R. L. & Endicott, J. Further developments in a computer program for psychiatric diagnosis. *American Journal of Psychiatry,* 1969, *125,* 12–27.

Spitzer, R. L., Endicott, J. & Robins, E. Clinical criteria for psychiatric diagnosis and DSM-III. *American Journal of Psychiatry,* 1975, *132,* 1187–1192.

Stroebel, C. & Glueck, B. Computer-derived global judgments in psychiatry. *American Journal of Psychiatry,* 1970, *126,* 1057–1066.

Wiggins, N. & Hoffman, P. J. Three models of clinical judgment. *Journal of Abnormal Psychology,* 1968, *73,* 70–77.

Wing, J. & Nixon, J. Discriminating symptoms in schizophrenia. *Archives of General Psychiatry,* 1974, *32,* 853–859.

APPENDIX

Below is a partial list of computerized testing packages and the addresses of the companies involved:

1. Psychsystems, Inc.
   600 Reistertown Rd.
   Baltimore, Maryland   21208
   1–800–368–2252

   Tests included: Minnesota Multiphasic Personality Inventory, Personality Inventory for Children, Social History, Intellectual Screening Battery, Visual Searching Task, Symptom Checklist, Rorschach Interpreter, Career Assessment System, Beck Depression and Hopelessness Scale, Index of Somatic Problems, Dissimulation Index, Minnesota Child Development Inventory, Jenkins Activity Survey, Integrated Report Writer, Medical History Survey, California Psychological Inventory, Self Directed Search, Vocational Preference Inventory, Behavioral Observations Checklist.

2. Behaviordyne
   599 College Ave., Suite One
   Palo Alto, California 94308
   (415) 857–0111

   Tests included: MMPI, California Psychological Inventory.

3. Psychological Software Specialists
   1776 Fowler, Suite 7
   Columbia Center North
   Richland, Washington   99352
   (509) 735–3427

   Tests included: Rorschach, MMPI, Wechsler, Peabody Individual Achievement Test, Detroit Test of Learning and Automated Psychiatric Diagnosis.

30 A Skeptic's View of the Computer as Diagnostician

Sydney Spiesel, MD

My prejudice has always been that any halfway competent second-year medical student is likely to be a better diagnostician than the most sophisticated program jammed into the maxiest computer. The problem is simple. Any decent diagnostician makes use of enormous numbers of variables (many of which he or she may not even consciously appreciate) in thinking about a patient. Even assuming that one could find a physician able to self-critically and objectively observe his/her own process and then reduce it to a diagnostic algorithm, there would still remain two problems:

1. How do you code the more subtle variables? (How do I enter a baby whose diaper smells like—well, like that other little kid who turned out to have the weird metabolic problem?)
2. How do I enter enough variables before I die of senility at the keyboard? ("The patient's hair began graying at 33, she has a macular reddish-brown rash with a faintly grainy surface on her trunk, the rash doesn't itch, she has a small papilloma in an inguinal skin-fold, when she sits up and leans to the left I think I hear an S4, she has a rather fetching yellow and red and blue butterfly tattooed on her left hip—nothing gaudy—her nasal mucosa is boggy, today is May 6th and the trees are in bloom, she thinks her father died of kidney something . . ." and on and on. No fair selecting—if you can do that you don't need the computer.)

Psychiatric programs have been written to establish mental status, diagnose thought disorders, and assess suicide potential. I am not persuaded that they can equal a sensitive (perhaps only competent) psychiatrist just walking into the room and sniffing the air.

*The above article originally appeared in *Computers in Psychiatry/Psychology*, 1978, 1 (2), 10, and is reprinted by permission.

Besides, their memory and speed requirements exceed most or all micros.

A more important question has to do with the moral propriety of asking a frightened, alienated patient to interact with a mechanical marvel of unfeeling, uncaring, stupid rigidity.

IX

Computers in Neuropsychology

In few clinical fields do computers offer the immediate value that they provide in the assessment and treatment of the brain-injured. The retraining of individuals with impairments of higher cognitive abilities can be enhanced by the computer in extraordinary ways. Computers, by virtue of their ability to respond immediately and to provide individualized feedback, can be programmed to address each particular patient's deficits, level of abilities, and attention span. Their tireless presentation of therapeutic and test materials frees the practitioner from the repetitious task of drill and practice often required in work with the brain-damaged. Visual perception and memory functions are especially well-handled by computer-based rehabilitative systems.

In the following chapters Bob Kurlychek, Anne Glang, and Odie Bracie discuss the use of computers, specifically microcomputers, in the assessment and treatment of the brain-injured. They look at available software, the selection of patients that can be treated, the use of video games in rehabilitation, the real hazards and problems they have found in the use of computer systems in working with the brain-injured, and new programs being developed.

31 | The Use of Microcomputers in the Cognitive Rehabilitation of Brain-Injured Persons

Robert T. Kurlychek, PhD
Ann E. Glang

Cognitive rehabilitation is the systematic application of remedial training techniques specifically intended to reverse deficits in functional areas such as memory, perception, concept formation, and problem-solving resulting from a brain impairment. This emerging area of rehabilitation is designed to supplement physical, occupational, and speech therapies in advancing a truly comprehensive rehabilitation approach for survivors of head injuries, strokes, and other brain traumas.

The philosophy of the current cognitive retraining movement challenges a long-standing pessimistic view regarding the recovery potential of higher cognitive functions following brain injury. Several authors have described successful training programs, which have improved the lives of a significant number of severely impaired individuals (Gianutsos, 1980; Miller, 1980; Diller, 1976).

Rehabilitation professionals are becoming more aware of the possibilities and potentials for the use of microcomputers in the treatment of brain-related deficits. Just as computers have been found to be effective instructional aids in higher education (Hartley, Panzer, & Harris, 1982), career guidance (Super, 1970), and special education (Taber, 1981), the instructional and interactive abilities of microcomputers are being used to address issues in the area of cognitive rehabilitation.

There are a number of advantages and desirable features that contemporary small computers can bring to the field of cognitive rehabilitation. With advances in technology and production methods, comes an increase in affordability. The feasibility of more clinicians being able to serve the brain-injured population in this fashion will surely advance the state of the art.

The self-containment of microcomputers is a great advancement. No longer does a remote terminal need to be interfaced with a main computer. This facilitates the private practitioner's use of computer-assisted treatment approaches. Previously, computers were generally limited to large hospitals or universities. With the need for continued follow-up after discharge from hospital rehabilitation units, private practitioners can better assist in the outpatient delivery of services in the patient's own community.

The high levels of interest that a computer can generate are distinct advantages when working with brain-injured individuals, many of whom have attention deficits and low arousal levels. Related to this are the interactive capabilities of a microcomputer. Immediate feedback and corrective messages, both important factors in remedial education, can be programmed into an instructional system.

A microcomputer offers precision of presentation. Factors such as time duration, response time, and display consistency can be controlled more effectively using a computer presentation. With this precision and control also comes flexibility. Computer programs can be modified or written to address a given patient's particular deficits, level of abilities, and attention span.

The remediation of cognitive losses requires numerous repetitions and presentations. A computer can provide efficiency and cost-effectiveness for both the clinician and patient. The microcomputer can, at appropriate times, relieve the therapist to focus on other duties.

A microcomputer offers assessment capabilities as well as instructional delivery. Individual skills can be measured and broken down into specific subskills. Because a computer can interface with a printer, data collection capabilities are greatly enhanced. A patient's progress can be followed over time so that both the patient's performance and the efficacy of the program can be evaluated.

AVAILABLE SOFTWARE

The application of computer technology to the area of cognitive remediation is a recent direction and the available software is very limited. This is especially the case for commercially available systems and programs.

COGREHAB is a commercially available software system developed by Rosamond Gianutsos, PhD and Carol Klitzer (available from Life Science Associates, One Fenimore Road, Bayport, New York,

11705). This material was designed specifically for the assessment and treatment of brain-impaired individuals. The system's nine programs are intended to provide cognitive rehabilitation technologies to assist patients in recovering visual perception and memory abilities. The authors believe that these two areas of mental functioning are the most likely to be affected by brain injury. Versions that will run on a 16K Radio Shack TRS-80 Model I or III, cassette or disk system, or on an Apple II disk system are now available; a version for IBM home computers is now being programmed. The listings for COGREHAB in BASIC are also available from Life Science Associates for half the cost of the available commercial systems.

The programs designed to measure and improve perceptual abilities include a Speeded Reading of Word Lists (SRWL), a Reaction Time Measure of Visual Field (REACT), and a Searching for Shapes (SEARCH).

The Speeded Reading of Word Lists is designed to diagnose and address four basic functions of visual information processing: anchoring at the margin, scanning horizontally, identification of words within the perceptual span, and monitoring the periphery. In this program, word lists are presented in three different formats. Initially, lists of nine words across are presented and the patient is required to read the lists from left to right and then from right to left. The second format asks the patient to read the words as they appear one at a time in the center of the screen. In the third presentation, the patient is again required to read words one at a time, but some of the stimulus words are unexpectedly placed to the left or right side of the screen.

The Reaction Time Measure of Visual Field procedure is designed to detect slowed response to visual stimuli. The patient is required to press any key on the keyboard to "stop the runaway numbers" on the screen. These numbers are presented in one spot and count up rapidly until the key is pressed. Two warm-up trials and five trials appear in the center of the screen. The next sixteen trials appear in spots anywhere on the screen and it is up to the patient to respond quickly. This program monitors response times and displays them on the screen.

The Searching for Shapes (SEARCH) Program is designed to detect and treat differences in attention and responsiveness on two sides of the visual field. In this program the patient is presented with an array of abstract shapes on the screen. After a shape appears in a center box on the screen, the patient is required to search for a matching shape elsewhere on the display.

Four memory-assessment and retraining programs are available as part of this system. The Free Recall (FREEREC) Program presents words, one at a time, after which the patient tries to recall entire lists of words. Twelve words are presented on each list. The interval between completion of the list and the command to recall is always of equal duration.

The Memory Span (SPAN) Program is intended to help rehabilitate short-term memory storage capacity. A list of words is displayed on the screen, one at a time. After reading this list, the patient is asked to recall a certain number of words. On the first five trials the patient is asked to recall the last two words. The requirements then get progressively harder, with the patient being required to recall one additional word for every five trials after that.

The Triplet Recall (TRIPEC) is primarily intended for patients for whom the free recall program is too complex. In this program three words are presented one at a time. A varying number of distracter words follow, which are not to be recalled. The patient is then asked to recall the initial three words.

In the Sequence Recall (SEQREC) the patient views several lists of shapes, nonsense words, or pictures presented one at a time. The patient then views a "menu" of items that may have appeared on the display and is asked to point to the items in the order in which they were shown. The computer then numbers the items in the correct order so that the patient and therapist can see whether the patient correctly recalled the items and their order of presentation. The authors feel that this particular program is helpful in addressing frontal lobe difficulties.

The COGREHAB program also includes two administrative packages. One of these programs is a cumulative record of patient activity, which keeps track of patient performance on the programs used each session. This part of the program is only available in a disk version and is most effective when used with a printer.

The Institute of Rehabilitation Medicine of the New York University Medical Center developed a comprehensive approach to the rehabilitation of head-injury victims. One of the program components is an approach to cognitive remediation, which consists of five training modules administered in the following order:

1. An orientation remedial module (ORM);
2. An eye-hand integration with a finger dexterity task hierarchy (DEX);
3. A perceptual-cognitive integration constructional task hierarchy (CON);
4. A visual-information-processing task hierarchy (VIP);
5. A verbal, logical reasoning task hierarchy (LOG) (Institute of Rehabilitation Medicine, 1981).

Recently, staff-member Jack Rattok has developed programs for microcomputers based on these modules for commercial distribution.

(Write to: Mr. Jack Rattock, Institute of Rehabilitation Medicine, 400 East 34th Street, New York, N. Y., 10016.)

These programs are based on a remediation philosophy that basic skills or "pre-training" readiness abilities must be mastered first before more specific tasks (e.g., language usage, memory training) can be addressed. These programs heavily emphasize attentional and orientation training.

For example, the Orientation Remedial Module (ORM) includes a program entitled Attention Reaction Conditioner (ARC). Following a warning tone, a signal light appears on the screen. The patient must respond by pushing a button as quickly as possible. The faster the response, the more reinforcer lights appear on the screen, providing feedback to the patient. A Time Estimate (TE) task is also part of this module.

The Visual Information Processing (VIP) module is made up of tasks that are designed to improve visual sequencing skills and visual-spatial abilities. For example, the Visual Succession task requires a patient to repeat a sequence of presented stimuli. This module, as well as others, consists of tasks of increasing difficulty.

Several computer-based cognitive remediation programs have been described in the literature, but are not now available commercially. Their descriptions can be useful leads for the computer-knowledgeable clinician who intends to take an active role in the programming of computer systems for brain-impaired individuals.

Dr. Francisco Perez and associates from the Department of Physical Medicine at Baylor College of Medicine in Houston, Texas, developed a microprocessor-based system designed to assess and rehabilitate memory deficits in stroke patients (Perez, Brown, Cooke, Pickett, Rivera, & Grabois, 1980). This program is intended to provide baseline data for the assessment of the recovery of memory function and to develop compensatory retraining procedures.

This assessment and training package consists of two recognition tasks; one program addresses problems most often found with left-hemisphere impairments while the other program addresses difficulties felt to be related to right-hemisphere functioning. Task A presents a verbal stimulus in the upper left-hand window of a display screen for one second and the patient is required to select the proper response from three choices, which appear in the other display windows after a variable time delay. Task B involves the same procedure, except that random shapes designed to measure spatial memory are employed.

The automated system is able to adjust the level of difficulty based on the patient's responses. Following a correct answer, the delay between a stimulus presentation and a display of response choices is increased by seven seconds. If the patient errs, the interval is decreased

by seven seconds. A distractor task is also displayed during the stimu-
lus-response choice interval.

In certain brain disorders, the ability to effectively use normal language skills is impaired. Difficulties with articulation (dysarthria) and
word-finding abilities (anomia), for example, are often seen with in-
sults to the left cerebral hemisphere. Researchers at the University of
California School of Medicine at Los Angeles have developed a program for a microcomputer that assists anomic patients in retrieving
words by presenting cues about the desired target word (Colby,
Christinaz, Parkison, Graham, & Karpf, 1981). The lexical-semantic
memory store is reorganized automatically, based on the patient's frequency of word usage. The memory store can also be modified to fit idiosyncratic aspects of a patient's vocabulary.

VIDEO GAMES THERAPY

Dr. William J. Lynch, Psychologist and Director of the Brain Injury Rehabilitation Unit at the Palo Alto Veterans Administration Medical
Center, has reported the successful use of Atari Home Video Games
in the cognitive retraining of traumatically brain-injured individuals
(Lynch, 1981). Lynch categorized 43 Atari Video Games into four categories that addressed various deficits often found in a head-injured
population: (a) verbal/mathematic, including games such as *Hang Man*,
which require the player to guess the letters that comprise a word; (b)
memory, composed of games such as *Touch Me*, requiring visual and
auditory sequential memory; (c) spatial/perceptual motor games such
as *Pong*, *Break Out*, and *Asteriods* (games requiring vigilance, visual
tracking, and quick reaction time); (d) table games, for example, *Video
Checkers*, a video game that requires comprehension of rules, strategies, and spatial concepts. Lynch also believes that some of the many
games that involve driving, navigation, or pursuit may be useful in
prescreening patients who are being considered for driver's training.

Dr. Lynch sees a number of positive factors related to the use of
video games with this special patient population. He points to the fun
and enjoyment aspect of most of these games and adds that a TV
screen display appears to be less threatening to the average patient
than a paper-and-pencil task, which often has strong associations with
negative schoolroom experiences.

Perhaps the most desirable aspect of using home video games is
their affordability. For under $200.00, one can purchase a video game
component and several cartridges.

At the Brain Injury Rehabilitation Unit, games are matched to a
particular patient's needs and abilities. Lynch and his associates have
developed a data recording form, "Record Form for Video Games Ther-

apy," which further allows for monitoring skill levels and patient progress. Profiles can be developed from collected data and used as feedback to the patient during training.

Controlled research examining the effectiveness of video game training is very limited. Malec, Jones, Rao, Stubbs, Flynn, and Questad (1982) at the University of Wisconsin Medical School and Rehabilitation Center reported the investigation of the effects of a simple video game (*Target Fun*) on sustained attention with head-injured patients. In an attempt to identify treatment effects independent of individual differences, nonspecific effects, and spontaneous recovery, these investigators employed a counterbalanced, double-reversal design with a nonparametric analysis of repeated measures. Individual gains in sustained attention were variable and the authors conclude that the results provide little support for the use of video games in this treatment context.

While the use of these video games is attractive, there are a number of disadvantages. These include the limited ability to select tasks at an appropriate level and the virtual inability to reprogram these games for specific patient requirements. Even individuals with presumably intact brains can become terribly frustrated and made to feel inferior when playing some of these popular video games. In learning situations, it is imperative that an individual be started at a level where success can be achieved. Tasks should be sequenced so that they become progressively more demanding. If video games are to be utilized, it is important that rehabilitation professionals supervise patients and that appropriate patient-to-game pairings are made.

Wong, Campbell, and Becker (1983) raise another cautionary consideration in their recently reported case study. These authors describe the case of a seriously head-injured male who, approximately one week following discharge from an inpatient rehabilitation unit, suffered a grand mal seizure after playing a video game for two hours without interruption. No seizures were observed during this patient's hospitalization and his phenobarbital was discontinued prior to discharge. Because of the risk potential for visually evoked seizures with patients sustaining severe head trauma, it is important to fully evaluate the patient before undertaking a cognitive retraining program with a video game component. It also becomes appropriate to caution such patients on the possible consequences of extended use.

PATIENT-COMPUTER COMPATIBILITY CONSIDERATIONS

Research from the field of human factors engineering must be applied when developing systems for cognitive rehabilitation. This existing body of knowledge regarding human-computer interactions must also be expanded to include the examination of particular concerns for brain-injured users. A number of ergonomic findings described in the literature will be seen as obvious when planning and implementing a system for brain-injured persons, while other factors are still open to empirical investigation.

An assessment and/or instructive computer system should be designed in accordance with the user's level and abilities. This is especially the case with brain-impaired patients. What may be an appropriate and stimulating video display for a normal student may be close to unintelligible to a head injury victim with shortened attention span and difficulties with visual processing.

Johnson, Godin, and Bloomquist (1981) examine human factors research and suggest applications for these findings in addressing some problems often found when employing computer technology in mental health settings. Their review also has implications for the clinician implementing a computer delivery system for remediating brain-related deficits.

These authors emphasize the need for an acceptable system to strike a balance among three important engineering factors; power, flexibility, and low complexity. Systems need to be developed that use few commands to activate a relatively complex operation. It is imperative that individuals suffering the sequelae of brain impairments not be faced with complex computer command requirements.

Information overload is a potential problem that must be avoided. The amount of information to be learned by patients to enable them to interact with the microcomputer should be kept at a manageable level. Techniques such as the programming of mnemonic variable command names can also keep interactional demands at a minimum.

Instructional programs should be progressive and allow success for patients at various levels before progressing to a more difficult task requirement. Repetition and regular feedback are other instructional strategies important in a remedial computer system.

The use of delayed vs. immediate presentation of feedback in computer-assisted instruction is an issue that must be investigated when designing software for this special population. While one study conducted with normal students found that delayed feedback was superior for retention (Rankin & Trepper, 1978), another study suggested that immediate feedback is more beneficial when the learner demonstrates a low level of mastery of the subject material (Gaynor, 1981).

Input modes are also an important consideration when planning a computer system for brain-impaired individuals. Research exists regarding error rates for various keyboard designs (Hirsch, 1976), and alternative keyboards have been proposed for special groups of users (Schneiderman, 1980). This is an important factor that merits direct investigation with brain-impaired and emotionally distressed subjects. A patient faced with a panel of keys can become easily distracted and frustrated. Alternatives to keyboards, e.g., joysticks, peripheral button boards, etc., may be appropriate (Lawrence & Horne, 1979).

CURRENT AND FUTURE CONSIDERATIONS

Practitioners intending to develop cognitive remediation systems for a brain-impaired population would do well to review developments in other professional areas that have utilized microcomputers on a fairly wide basis for a number of years. The field of special education, for example, has addressed a number of instructional issues that have implications for the remediation of brain-related cognitive deficits. Studies with this special population have examined general instructional procedures as well as the application of computer-assisted instruction.

Remedial computer programs designed for retarded and learning-disabled children have been developed addressing language-related problem areas (e.g., Hasselbring, 1982; Sevcik & Sevcik, 1980), which can be adapted or modified for application with aphasic adults.

Generalization of learned skills is an issue that has received considerable attention in education (Hammill & Larsen, 1974; Haring & Bateman, 1977), and one that must also be addressed in cognitive rehabilitation. Should the emphasis be placed on teaching readiness skills or on the instruction of specific, practical functions? The concerns here are both professional and ethical. Is the clinician teaching skills that will enable the patient to function more independently and satisfactorily in meeting demands of daily living?

Generalization of learned skills has concerned many professionals in the field of special education. Certain theorists have advocated an ability-training model, wherein the practitioner diagnoses and retrains underlying cognitive processes before beginning academic instruction. Mann (1971a, 1971b) and Ysseldyke (1973, 1975) maintain that little empirical evidence supports the effectiveness of this theory. Practitioners developing cognitive remediation programs should be cautioned by these findings. Clinicians must address the issue of generalization in selecting program components. Does successful performance on instructional tasks generalize to areas outside the clinical setting? Programming for generalization is a challenging and necessary step in the remediation process.

Rehabilitation professionals new to remedial technology must decide whether to purchase already existing software or to learn to develop their own programs. In selecting commercially available programs, the practitioner can again find assistance from prior work done with handicapped learners. Interpretive Education, Inc., Kalamazoo,

Michigan, has organized a comprehensive evaluation form, which can be used to evaluate all types of educational software (Taber, 1981). This checklist helps a perspective user rate factors related to instructional content and feasibility of the program for the intended audience.

There are many advantages for both the therapist, and ultimately the patient, when programming skills are learned. This can enable the therapist to tailor-make a flexible, interactive program for an individual patient. Often times it is inappropriate to rely on a program formulated for another special group or for normal users. A relatively new system has been developed, which allows special education teachers easier access to technology that can manage comprehensive, individualized instruction programs. This system, designed specifically for individualized instruction by Control Data Corporation, is referred to as PLATO and uses a computer language (TUTOR) developed for ease of use after only several hours of programming instruction (Carman & Kosberg, 1982).

Remedial education requires repetition and, ideally, daily practice. This can be difficult to provide on an outpatient basis. Advances in technology have led to microunits that are versatile, fairly sophisticated, portable, and inexpensive (e.g., VIC 20, Atari 400). These microprocessors can be efficiently used to offer a wide range of in-home services. A practitioner can reasonably afford several of these units, which can be loaned or rented, much the same as electrical nerve stimulators and heart monitors have been, to any appropriate patient with a television. Periodic office visits can monitor progress and allow for the programming of new home assignments. Such an application of microcomputers, it must be remembered, requires caution and attention to need for proper patient selection criteria.

The recent progress in the area of microcomputers has the potential to improve the lives of significantly handicapped individuals. If appropriate cautions are taken in applying this technology and remedial instructional issues are addressed, these advancements can greatly assist rehabilitation professionals in remediating brain-related deficits.

REFERENCES

Carman, G. O., & Kosberg, B. Educational technology research: Computer technology and the education of emotionally handicapped children. *Educational Technology*, 1982, 22(2), 26–30.

Colby, K. M., Christinaz, D., Parkison, R. C., Graham, S., & Karpf, C. A. Word-finding computer program with a dynamic lexical-semantic memory for patients with anomia using an intelligent speech prosthesis. *Brain and Language*, 1981, 14, 272–281.

Diller, L. A model for cognitive retraining in rehabilitation. *The Clinical Psychologist*, 1976, *29*, 13–15.

Gaynor, P. The effect of feedback delay on retention of computer-based mathematical material. *Journal of Computer-Based Instruction*, 1981, *8*, 28–34.

Gianutsos, R. What is cognitive rehabilitation? *Journal of Rehabilitation*, 1980, *46*(3), 36–40.

Hammill, D. D., & Larsen, S. C. The effectiveness of psycholinguistic training. *Exceptional Children*, 1974, *41*, 5–14.

Haring, N. G., & Bateman, B. *Teaching the learning disabled child*. Englewood Cliffs, N. J.: Prentice-Hall, 1977.

Hartley, P., Panzer, E., & Harris, C. Microcomputer assisted instruction in psychology. *Computers in Psychiatry/Psychology*, 1982, *4*(3), 18, 19.

Hirsch, R. S. *Human factors in man-computer interfaces*. San Jose, California: IBM Human Factors Center, 1976.

Hasselbring, T. S. Remediating spelling problems of learning-handicapped students through the use of microcomputers. *Educational Technology*, 1982, *22*(4), 31–32.

Institute of Rehabilitation Medicine. *Working approaches to remediation of cognitive deficits in brain damaged persons*. Rehabilitation Monograph No. 62. New York: New York University Medical Center, 1981.

Johnson, J. H., Godin, S. W., & Bloomquist, M. L. Human factors engineering in computerized mental health care delivery. *Behavior Research Methods & Instrumentation*, 1981, *13*, 425–429.

Lawrence, P. D., & Horne, S. J. Input modes: Their importance in the clinical application of electronic aids for disabled persons. *Archives of Physical Medicine and Rehabilitation*, 1979, *60*, 516–521.

Lynch, W. J. TV games as therapeutic interventions. Paper presented at American Psychological Association Annual Conference, 1981, Los Angeles, California.

Malec, J., Jones, R., Rao, N., Stubbs, K., Flynn, M., & Questad, K. Effects of videogame practice on sustained attention in patients with craniocerebral trauma. Paper presented at the 59th Annual Session of the American Congress of Rehabilitation Medicine, Houston, Texas, November 1982.

Mann, L. Perceptual training revisited: The training of nothing at all. *Rehabilitation Literature*, 1971(a), *32*, 322–335.

Mann, L. Psychometric phrenology and the new faculty psychology: The case against ability assessment and training. *Journal of Special Education*, 1971(b), *5*, 3–14.

Miller, E. Psychological intervention in the management and rehabilitation of neuropsychological impairments. *Behaviour Research and Therapy*, 1980, *18*, 527–535.

Perez, F. I., Brown, G. A., Cooke, N., Pickett, A. P., Rivera, V., & Grabois, M. Stroke patients: Computerized behavioral approach to cognitive assessment and retraining. *Archives of Physical Medicine and Rehabilitation*, 1980, *61*, 500.

Rankin, R. J., & Trepper, T. Retention and delay of feedback in a computer-assisted instructional task. *Journal of Experimental Education*, 1978, *46*, 67–70.

Schneiderman, B. *Software psychology: Human factors in computer and information systems*. Cambridge, Mass.: Winthrop, 1980.

Sevcik, E., & Sevcik, J. A learning program for problem readers. *Recreational Computing*, 1980, *8*(4), 25–28.

Super, D. E. (Ed.). *Computer-assisted counseling*. New York: Teachers College Press, 1970.

Taber, F. M. The microcomputer—Its applicability to special education. *Focus on Exceptional Children*, 1981, *14*(2), 1–14.

Wong, F., Campbell, D., & Becker, B. Head injury and video games: a precautionary note. *Western Journal of Medicine*, 1983, *138*, 107.

Ysseldyke, J. E. Diagnostic-prescriptive teaching: The search for aptitude-treatment interactions. In L. Mann & D. A. Sabatino (Eds.), *The first review of special education*. Philadelphia: Journal of Special Education Press, Grune and Stratton, 1973.

Ysseldyke, J. E. Process remediation with secondary learning disabled children. In L. Goodman & L. Mann (Eds.), *Learning disabilities in the secondary school: Title III curricula development for secondary learning disabilities*. King of Prussia, Pennsylvania: Montgomery County Intermediate Unit and the Pennsylvania Department of Education, 1975.

Using Computers in Neuropsychology

Odie L. Bracy, III, PhD

The microcomputer has become an almost indispensable tool in my practice of neuropsychology and cognitive rehabilitation. Those among us who say that this kind of statement scares them, and believe me there are many, perhaps do not understand computers or are not attending to the fact that I refer to the computer as a tool and not as an end in itself. I became acquainted with computers in the late 1960s and early 1970s, while taking undergraduate computer science courses. When I discovered, in 1978, that an affordable microcomputer was available, I immediately went out and purchased a Model I Radio Shack TRS-80 computer. I had returned to graduate school for my doctorate in psychology, and I had more ideas for utilizing the computer within my field than I could possibly have pursued.

At first, I experimented with computerization of existing test instruments, such as the MMPI. As a result of those efforts, I have programs for administering and interpreting several psychological tests and for interpreting a battery of children's intellectual and achievement tests that I am continuing to use frequently, even now. As time drew near to begin my doctoral dissertation, I was determined to combine my interest in neuropsychology, neurophysiology, and computers in my research. A study of the electrophysiological correlates of learning evolved into my dissertation. For this project, I interfaced EEG amplifiers to my TRS-80 computer via an analog-to-digital converter. I decided to employ the computer for all aspects of the experiment. The computer was mounted on a compartment so that when the subject was seated inside, he was facing the monitor. Visual material was presented via the monitor for the subject to memorize. The presentations were in the format of paired associates learning tasks, in which two objects were presented simultaneously. The subject was to memorize what was paired together so that when later presented with one of the pair, he was required to recall the other figure. Graphics figures paired with the digits 0–9 served as the stimulus figures. The computer presented the material to be learned and simultaneously collected EEG from a scalp site on each hemisphere. The data were stored on a diskette (some 80 diskettes) for later analysis by the same computer. Copies of the dissertation, including the computer program, are available through me or Dissertation Abstracts International.*

During my internship in neuropsychology, I became more interested in developing original tests, interpretive packages, and therapy programs. Ever since the years I had spent working with cerebrally compromised children, I had been interested in rehabilitation activities. With this in mind, I began developing programs for diagnosis of brain dysfunction and for cognitive rehabilitation of brain functions following injury or stroke. What resulted and has continually developed is a rather comprehensive set of programs designed to rehabilitate brain-injured individuals.

In my opinion, it is important to place demands upon the injured brain regularly and frequently to maximize recovery, reorganization, or whatever processes produce improvement. While there may be many therapeutic modalities that will serve to reorganize and enhance brain functioning, none compares to the potential offered by the computer. The computer will not replace the warm, emotional contact, empathy, or understanding provided by humans, but it will present stimuli, will time events, will record responses, and will be consistent in ways not humanly possible. To function fully, the brain-injured person must regain the ability to interact with the environment, even in novel situations, and perceive, plan, make decisions, and act, based upon that person's own analysis of the situation he faces. Therefore, I think we must direct a good portion of our efforts toward the interrupted brain processes that underlie the more complex cognitive processes. Over the last two years, I have developed computer programs that address, in addition to the basic foundation skills (attending, concentrating, shifting, discriminating, making differential responses, initiating, inhibiting, scanning, etc.), visuospatial skills, conceptual skills, auditory perception skills, and memory skills. I have developed these programs over the course of cognitive rehabilitation therapy with about a dozen patients. At the time of this writing, the programs are being used in over eighty hospitals across the United States. The programs are written for use on the Apple II+/e or the Atari 400 or 800 computers. In addition to therapeutic interaction with the patient, the programs perform basic statistical compilations and store data about the patients on diskette for later longitudinal statistical analysis.

Most of my patients were injured or suffered a stroke 4 to 6 years prior to my intervention, although I have a few acute cases as well. My own mode of providing cognitive rehabilitation therapy is unique in

---

*The dissertation is entitled "Electrocortical differences between learned versus non-learned trials during a pair-associated learning test" and was published in May 1980.

that I require my patients to purchase their own Atari 400 computer for a home-based rehabilitation effort. (Publications of case studies are being prepared, but are not yet available.) Only one of my patients has not shown significant improvement, and he was unique in having a cognitive dysfunction that was primarily aphasic in nature. The hospitals in which my programs are being used are primarily treating acute cases. Verbal reports from therapists indicate that they are experiencing much success with the programs as well. A catalog of the cognitive rehabilitation programs I have developed is given below.

As for the future, I plan to continue my computer work with cognitive rehabilitation. However, in addition, I would like to pursue my interest in neurophysiological investigations. I feel there is much that can be done with EEG and CAT-scan data, as well as with diagnostic interpretation of data from neurological and neuropsychological examinations.

CATALOG OF COGNITIVE REHABILITATION COMPUTER PROGRAMS*

I. FOUNDATIONS PACKAGE

This is a package of computer programs designed to rebuild attention, attention-shifting, initiation/inhibition skills, capacity to discriminate, and capacity to respond differentially. Programs address both visual and auditory input modalities. Performance feedback to patient is immediate. Statistics (mean, variance, correlations and errors) are produced.

Program Descriptions

Simple Visual Reaction I. One-inch yellow square is presented after random delays. Patient reacts by pushing joystick button. Immediate feedback is provided for correct responses or errors. Average latency to respond, correlation between delays and latency to respond, variance, and number of errors are presented after fifteen trials.

Simple Visual Reaction II. Same as Simple Visual Reaction I, but stimulus squares are ¼ as large.

---

*Information and prices on these programs are available from: Psychological Software Service, P.O. Box 29205, Indianapolis, Indiana 46229.

Visual Reaction Stimulus Discrimination I. On a random schedule, either a blue or a yellow one-inch square is displayed after random delays. Patient must react to yellow square and inhibit responding to blue square. Same statistics are produced as in Simple Visual Reaction I.

Visual Reaction Stimulus Discrimination II. Same as Visual Reaction Stimulus Discrimination I, with smaller stimuli.

Visual Reaction Differential Response I. Monitor screen is divided into halves. When small black square appears randomly on screen after a random delay, patient is required to push joystick toward the half of the screen in which the square is displayed. Total average latency, average response latency for stimuli displayed in each quadrant, variance, number of errors, and location of errors are displayed.

Visual Reaction Auditory Prestimulus. This program operates the same as the simple visual reaction, except that each target stimulus is preceded by an auditory prestimulus, to which the patient must inhibit responding.

Visual Discrimination Differential Response I. Patient must make a discrimination between two possible stimuli and respond with either the left or right hand, depending on the stimulus displayed. The same statistics described above are displayed.

Visual Discrimination Differential Response II. Three large squares are presented that vary in color randomly. When either of the outside squares matches with the center square in color, the patient pushes the joystick toward the matching side. The number of correct responses and errors are presented.

Visual Scanning. A dark green line is plotted, one block at a time (speed is adjustable), beginning from the upper left corner in a scanning pattern as used for reading. On a random schedule, a yellow block is plotted instead of the green. The patient must react before three additional points are plotted. The percent correct is displayed.

Simple Auditory Reaction. A tone is presented after random delays. The patient reacts by pushing the joystick button. Average latency to respond, correlation between delays and latency to respond, variance, and number of errors are presented after fifteen trials.

Auditory Reaction Stimulus Discrimination. A target tone is presented for a few seconds. The patient must react by pushing the joystick button whenever this tone is repeated, and must inhibit responding when other tones are presented. Statistics are as for Simple Auditory Reaction.

Auditory Reaction Visual Prestimulus. This program operates the same as the Simple Auditory Reaction, except that each target stimulus is preceded by a visual prestimulus, to which the patient must inhibit responding.

II. VISUOSPATIAL SKILLS PROGRAMS

These programs were designed to remediate impairment in visuoperception and visuomotor integration skills.

Program Descriptions

Maze I. Patient must use the joystick to move a small yellow block through the maze as rapidly as possible without hitting the walls. Time to completion and the number of wall contacts is displayed.

Maze II. Same as Maze I with a more complex maze.

Cube-In-a-Box I. The computer randomly moves a large open square around the screen. The patient attempts, using the joystick, to keep a small cube within the large square. Feedback is excellent! A score is produced.

Cube-In-a-Box II. Same as Cube-In-a-Box I, except that the computer's square is smaller.

Bilateral Motor Integration. Same as above except that the integrated effort of both hands turning the dials on the game paddles is required to move the small cube around the screen.

Paddle Ball. The ball must be intercepted at the bottom of the screen to keep it in play. The patient controls the paddle by turning the knob on the computer game paddle. The ball speed and the length of the paddle are adjustable. The number of interceptions over ten trials is displayed.

Line Orientation I. An 11-point compass is presented on the left side of the screen. On a random schedule, one of the compass lines changes from black to yellow. Using the joystick, the patient must rotate a single line displayed on the right side of the screen so that it matches the angle of the target line on the compass. Score is based on precision of answers. Feedback is provided and ten trials are presented.

Line Orientation II. An 11-point compass is presented on the center of the screen. On a random schedule, one of the compass lines changes from black to yellow. After a few seconds, the screen clears except for a single horizontal line, which the patient must rotate and from memory try to match the angle of the preceding target line on the compass. Score is based on precision of answers. Feedback is provided.

Fine Motor I. Using the game paddle, the patient must turn the knob to move a small cube back and forth and up the screen at a rate that will maximize speed while not exceeding the preset maximum rate. If the knob is turned too rapidly, the patient is automatically started over at the beginning. The number of restarts and the time to completion are displayed.

III. WORD AND NUMBER CONCEPTS, MEMORY AND COGNITIVE ORGANIZATION SKILLS

Program Descriptions

Word Concepts I (Big/Little). A large and a small square are displayed so that positions are changed randomly. The patient must move a small black square under the targeted stimulus (either big or little). Feedback is provided, and percent correct is displayed.

Number Concepts I. Patterned groups of yellow blocks ranging in number from one to ten are randomly displayed. Patient must move the computer's cursor over the correct number, displayed at the bottom of the screen, and press the joystick button. All ten numbers are displayed simultaneously, and the cursor beeps each time it moves. Average trial time for the twenty trials is displayed.

Number Concepts II. Same as Number Concepts I, except only one number is displayed at a time and there are no beeps to denote a change. Patient must recognize the number in order to perform the task.

Verbal Memory (Sequenced Words). Program starts with presentation of three 4-letter words, which the patient must briefly study and then recall in the order presented. If the patient recalls correctly at the current level, then the program adds one word to the next presentation. Word order is randomly chosen so patient gets different sets at every session. Recall is by recognition.

Numeric Manipulations I. Patient must recall a previously presented number and add it to currently presented number. The patient indicates the answer with the joystick. Feedback provides reinforcement for correct answer and a new number is presented for next trial. The whole procedure is timed over forty trials.

Spatial Memory I. A random trail is generated, consisting of a user-generated number of steps. Without clues, the patient must learn the trail through trial and error, so that it can be traversed from beginning to end without error. The patient is started over whenever an error is made.

IV. PERCEPTION TRAINING PROGRAMS

Auditory Discrimination I (Pitch Discrimination Training). The computer instructs the patient to listen to a target tone. A visual aid consisting of a vertical line on the monitor is provided as a reference. The computer then instructs the patient, "CLOSE YOUR EYES," and it presents a second tone accompanied by a short line. Using the joystick, the patient raises or lowers the tone until it matches the target. The movement of the short line corresponds with the change in pitch produced by the patient. The short line will line up on top of the longer line when the two tones match. The patient can use the visual aid (the lines) during the early stages of training. The mean error (difference between the choice and the actual correct response) is produced.

Auditory Discrimination II. Similiar to the program above, except that the patient is able to hear only one tone at a time. The target tone can be reviewed at any time with the press of a button.

Auditory Discrimination III. Series of tones are presented in increasing complexity for the patient to recall via manipulation of the joystick.

V. NEUROPSYCHOLOGICAL ASSESSMENT AIDS

Program Descriptions

Visual Perception Test (Closure and Integration of Parts). As a vertical black bar sweeps across the screen, a geometric shape is revealed briefly in a sequential left-to-right sweep. Ten shapes are then displayed and the patient must indicate with the joystick which shape was just revealed by the sweeping bar. The number of correct choices is displayed.

Auditory Perception Test (Pitch Discrimination). The computer presents 120 trials ranging over three octaves. Ten comparisons are requested for each of twelve target tones. The patient indicates with the joystick whether the two tones (presented as "A" or "B") are "SAME" or "DIFFERENT." The number of errors and the frequency code for each error is displayed.

VI. DIAGNOSTICS AIDS

Program Descriptions

Headache Evaluation. The professional answers a series of questions regarding the symptomatology of the patient's headache. The computer chooses the most likely diagnosis and displays information including: etiology, other concerns to be investigated, treatment, prophylactic measures and finally, a ranked listing of all diagnoses from most to least likely. Hard copy can be requested.

Wechsler Memory Scale Interpretation Aid. When the raw scores from the Wechsler Memory Scale (standard form or Boston Revision) are entered from the keyboard, the memory quotient, t-scores, standard scores, and z-scores are calculated for each subtest. Percentage recalled on the 20-minute delayed trials is calculated also if used. Hardcopy can be requested from the menu.

Administrative and Clinical Information Management

I t has been estimated that computers are used in almost four-fifths of the mental health centers in this country; the number used by private practitioners is growing rapidly. Most of this use is for administrative functions. The computer's ability to keep detailed and timely records is of great value in managing a practice, institution, or agency. With this information, it becomes much easier to assess the organization's present situation and plan for its future. Systems that provide management with such information are called, reasonably enough, *Management Information Systems* or MISs.

There are a variety of MISs that are of importance to the mental health clinician, including clinic-administration systems, community-wide mental health information systems, patient-tracking systems, and many others. Each type of facility has its own particular needs. In the following chapters, mental health administrators from several settings present their views and experiences using computer-based management information systems.

Over and over again in the chapters of Part X, you, the clinician, will be cautioned not to abdicate your professional responsibility just because you are working in an unfamiliar territory. Nowhere is this more clearly stated than in the title of the first chapter: "Information Systems Are Too Important to Be Left to Non-Clinicians." The clinician must be the person ultimately responsible for the design and implementation of the MIS. Of course administrators, technical staff, programmers, and manufacturers should make their recommendations about the development of any computer system that is to provide information to mental health management. But the final say in planning and execution should be the clinician's.

This lesson has been demonstrated by painful experience in scores of centers and offices: a clinician obtains a computer system; unwilling, or believing himself or herself unable to master the arcane knowledge required to design an MIS, he or she delegates or abdicates the responsibility to those apparently more knowledgeable. Predictably, the result is the development of an MIS that meets the needs of programmers, administrators, technicians, and manufacturers, but not the clinicians.

To avoid this problem, the mental health clinician must insist that any technical person with whom he or she works has the time and intellectual capacity to understand mental health concepts and needs. The clinician must avoid placing faith in a programmer who puts together a system on the basis of what supposedly can and can't be done, rather than on the basis of what the clinician needs and doesn't need to have done. Too often the results are approximate solutions that do not really meet the clinician's needs and voluminous, costly printouts that are basically useless.

The clinician needs to have some knowledge of what MISs have accomplished and what the usual problems in instituting such systems have been. Part X of this book is addressed to that need. The experiences of the authors of the following chapters should be of great help to anyone considering setting up a mental health management information system. For example, Rick Zawadski and Stephen Gee describe the four-year development of the On Lok integrated fiscal and client information system. The system provides information to meet program, policy, and research information needs. The authors describe the system and offer recommendations for any human-service organization planning to computerize.

Often a computerized information system is not used by one agency only, but many within a single community. Issues of interagency cooperation and communication in the use of computerized information systems are examined by Larry Searcy. Issues of policy, funding, confidentiality, needs, resources, obstacles, and politics all arose in the course of the gestation and birth of his project. He clearly details them all in the pages that follow.

Should an individual or an agency use a computer consultant in setting up a computer system? The experiences of one agency that employed a consultant after it found its computer system was not working out very well is described by Hi Resnick and his colleagues. Their experiences with the Kwawachee Counseling Center highlight common problem areas and suggest solutions to them.

For those readers who have a general idea of the administrative use to which a computer might be put but who lack a knowledge of specific details, Michael King's chapter on microcomputer applications in a hospital social-work department will be of special interest. Michael takes the reader step by step through the use of the Apple-based system now being used in his department, pointing out various options for the designer of such systems and clarifying important principles underlying the planning and implementation of the system.

And to round off Part X, Jim Newkham provides the reader with a concise from-the-heart list of do's and don'ts that should sit prominently on the desk of anyone planning to implement a computer-based management information system.

Information Systems Are Too Important to Be Left to Non-Clinicians

Zebulon Taintor, MD

In the mid-seventies, those of us who participated in panels on computer use presented at the American Psychiatric Association often outnumbered the audience. However, at the Chicago meeting in 1979, an invited special session on information systems in psychiatry was remarkably well-attended. Many in the audience had recently acquired personal computers and were wondering what to do with them. We attempted to meet their needs in a panel the following year at San Francisco. We had an overflow crowd and could answer only half of the questions. Last year, despite an expected decrease in attendance because of the Equal Rights Amendment protest, an invited course on working with computers was sold out the first day that any course was sold out and, until the time of the meeting, remained the only course sold out for the latter part of the week. Again, the course was heavily attended by owners of microcomputers who, in many cases, had not articulated very well their reasons for acquiring the hardware and were hoping we could tell them what to do next. The discussion was a lively one, although we were berated for not knowing the best word-processing program to run on an Apple II, etc.

As someone whose advocacy of the use of computers has centered around the abilities of big machines, I must acknowledge a great debt to mental health professionals who have taken up personal computing. They have become an informed group that provides sophisticated pressure for improvement of mental health information systems. This editorial is to encourage them to become even more active in the struggle.

"Information Systems Are Too Important to Be Left to Non-Clinicians" originally appeared in *Computers in Psychiatry/Psychology*, 1982, 4(1), 1–3, and is reprinted by permission.

(These remarks were prepared by Dr. Taintor in his private capacity and do not necessarily reflect the opinion of the Alcohol, Drug Abuse, and Mental Health Administration.)

The need for help in dealing with information systems is apparent to almost anyone who is having to deal with one. The gap in quality between the use of computers and public institutions and one's personal computer is very much like the contrast between the experience in one's private practice and that of working at a large facility. While the facility has a greater budget, can be mobilized to deal with more people, can offer a broader range of services to the needy, etc., recent analyses of career paths of psychiatrists show movement into the private sector, where much of what transpires is under one's direct personal control. Institutions smack of Big Brotherhood and, because power is often further away than the computer terminal, often sap one's energies in trying for improvement. However, if clinicians are not active in this situation, is there cause for hope from other groups? Let us consider them.

Manufacturers. As Director of the Multi-State Information System, I witnessed several examples of successful hucksterism by hardware manufacturers. There was the group that said air-conditioning was not required for its minis, but several melted down. Public purchasing policy often requires that the lowest bidder be selected, usually a manufacturer that was taking on IBM, but that rarely was successful when it was discovered that its loss leader could not be converted into a profitable item. Deliveries were often late and specifications, often false. Unlike the private sector, in which one can acknowledge a loss and move on to a better situation, the political problems and the loss of face often led to increasing outlays of public funds, much like the peasant woman giving the old soldier more of the ingredients of the soup that he claimed was being made only by the magic nail. Once committed to a particular manufacturer, it is hard for the public sector to pull back.

Technical Staff. Many public computing outfits have overspent on hardware and are tied to civil service scales for personnel. There is a perpetual drain of talent to the private sector, where salaries are much higher and working conditions often more pleasant. This insures that the public sector will be manned by varying proportions of those who are idealistic enough to work for the public good and those who cannot find any other sort of gainful employment. Dedication to public service is not frequently found as a source of professional self-esteem among programmers and systems analysts, whose education and tradition leads them to derive self-respect from developing the definitive system of the future, rather than a clinical desire to help people. Technicians are often turned off by the irrationality that fascinates many clinicians. They will often stay in their offices working for administrators. This sometimes leads to bizarre and inappropriate systems, such as efforts to maintain a completely current census in a remote hospital where the night switchboard operator does it better, or telling you a patient's drug regimen is better obtained from the computer than nurses' Cardex, where you can find out whether or not the patient actually took them. Technicians frequently overestimate the clinicians' appetite for sitting at a terminal and entering data. Although physicians and nurses have communicated successfully since the beginning of their professions, technicians will often intervene and say that a form is needed to get something in the computer, rather than managing data entry from the voluminous papers available.

I am indebted to Gene Laska for the story of the intelligent, rich, beautiful, thrice-married virgin. First she chose a businessman who was so involved in his commercial empire that he scheduled a board meeting of all his directors who had come for the ceremony. He waxed so ecstatic over proposed mergers and acquisitions that he collapsed of a heart attack before the wedding reception. Determined to avoid aggressive commercial types, she next picked a sports car racer who was so overjoyed after the ceremony that he took off for a wild drive and flattened himself against a stone wall on the Riviera. She was determined then to find herself an attractive intellectual who would stay at home and live in a risk-free environment. When last heard from, her wishes had been satisfied. She married a computer scientist in a small midwestern college town several years ago. He does not travel. They are always together during the long winter nights. The only problem is that so far he has spent all of his time saying how good things will be eventually. . . . This is not to say that many computer technicians are not eager to do their best, but they cannot be expected to work in isolation and must be brought to a good understanding of what the principle business is: helping people to get well.

Administrators. They understand that an information system is usually necessary for fiscal and for statistical reporting systems. Clinicians have often failed to show how easy it is to take such a system and make it clinically responsive. Fortunately, publications in this area have recently been gathered together by NIMH in a publication that should serve as a beacon to those who wish to convey how much progress has been made in computer applications in mental health.* Purely administrative systems are usually resented by clinicians, since they often do not decrease paperwork, and seem to have a reductionistic aspect that involves grubbing for money and looking at numbers rather than people. However, clinicians must be faulted for not having insisted that other variables be followed that might better demonstrate the worth of their efforts. Lack of administrative support and adminis-

---

*Hedlund, J. L., Vieweg, B. W., Wood, J. B., Cho, D. W., Evenson, R. C., Hickman, C. F., & Holland, R. A. *Computers in mental health: A review and annotated bibliography.* National Institute of Mental Health Series FN No. 7. DHHS Pub. No. (ADM) 81–1090. Washington, D. C.: U. S. Government Printing Office, 1981.

trative ignorance cannot be regarded as the fault of administrators alone.

Clinicians. Clinicians are the only group that can hope to deal with the three other groups in a way that will insure that the use of computers addresses the primary mission of any mental health enterprise. Depending on the size of the machine and the amount of data collected, we have the opportunity to build naturalistic data bases that can help to provide clarification of diagnostic entities, indications of treatment efficacy, statements of budgetary needs, cost-benefit analyses, improved clinical practice through use of guidelines (such as is occurring for medication orders in New York through MSIS), and a host of other worthy enterprises. Clinicians, who are overburdened by paperwork, must fight to have computers serve them. Knowledge of what computers can do is an important asset in efforts to continue to improve the use of larger computers in institutions. One important step is to develop user groups with some power to review the priorities and activities of the data-processing manager, to set policy for the use of the information system, to review what reports are being used for what purposes, and to see how operations can be further streamlined.

Comments on these thoughts are welcome at Room 8–101, National Institute of Mental Health, 5600 Fishers Lane, Rockville, Maryland 20857.

A Practical Guide to Integrated Computerized Information Management

Rick T. Zawadski, PhD
Stephen Gee, BS

O n Lok Senior Health Services is a nonprofit, community-based service program, which has been meeting the needs of the frail elderly in San Francisco's Chinatown–North Beach area since 1971. On Lok pioneered in the development of adult day health services, becoming the first state Medicaid demonstration site in 1974. In 1975, On Lok expanded its day center program into an outpatient continuum of services. In 1978, On Lok was awarded a research and development grant to develop a complete long-term care system, the Community Care Organization for Dependent Adults (CCODA). Today, through the CCODA, On Lok provides all necessary health and health-related services—from translation to hospitalization—to clients who have been certified as eligible for institutional care (Zawadski & Ansak, 1981). To support that service program, On Lok has developed a comprehensive and integrated fiscal and client information system. It has created and used this computerized system to meet program, policy, and research information needs. This report describes the system, discusses its costs and benefits, and offers some recommendations for the human service organization planning to computerize.

DEVELOPMENT OF ON LOK'S INFORMATION MANAGEMENT SYSTEM

Like any other long-term health care program, On Lok Senior Health Services has a variety of information needs and accountability require-

"A Practical Guide to Integrated Computerized Information Management" is adapted from *Computerized Information Management in Long-Term Care: A Case Study* by Rick T. Zawadski and Stephen Gee, San Francisco, CA: On Lok Senior Health Services, 1980.

ments. Its service staff needs to have scheduling information, to know the functional status of each client, and to determine the service needs of the client population. Administrative staff must monitor client census, service development, and program costs. Reimbursement agencies require an accounting of the program's census, of the services delivered, and of the costs of these services. Both internal and external evaluators need information regarding client characteristics, quality of care, services delivered, service costs, and client changes over time to measure the effectiveness of the project.

While the term *information management system* may imply computerization to many people, the concept of the information system predates and is really independent of computers. All organizations deal with information, some more effectively than others. An information management system can be defined as the organization and integration of information into a system to meet organizational needs. An effective manual information system is the prerequisite to successful computerization.

Information has always played a critical role at On Lok, in part because of the fiscal and management concerns of the project's founders and in part because of the organization's expanding research and demonstration responsibilities. An efficient system was needed to collect client-specific data to meet internal service management needs as well as to gather fiscal and program data for reporting to On Lok's funding agencies.

On Lok's Information Management System (IMS) has been in development and use for over ten years. A manual information management system was first established to provide crucial program information, such as service, meal, assessment, and transportation schedules; attendance and insurance reports; name and address lists; service records; and cost and assessment data. Computerization allowed for faster, more accurate, more comprehensive, and more frequent production of that information.

When On Lok was awarded funds in 1978 to develop, operate, and study its CCODA, it set as a top priority the development of an on-line computer system to automate and manage its information needs. Specifically, a system was needed to meet the following requirements:

- To record services to meet federal guidelines;
- To report cost, service, and census data required by state and federal regulations;
- To access client biographical information—addresses; Social Security, Medicare, and Medicaid numbers; demographics (including birthdates);
- To schedule services, transportation, and meals;

- To monitor staff service activity;
- To follow client changes over time—individually and as a group—in terms of their functional and health characteristics;
- To track costs by individual, to link costs to service packages, and to predict costs over time for particular client groups.

Since there was no system in the field that met these diverse yet important information needs, On Lok developed its own system, designed for the community-based human service provider. This on-line, microcomputer-based system has now been operational for three years.

SYSTEM DESCRIPTION

A computer system consists of three major components: hardware, firmware, and applications software. A more technical description of these three components is given elsewhere (Zawadski & Gee, 1982). The following sections focus instead on a few of the significant characteristics of each component.

Hardware

Hardware refers to the physical equipment of the system. The On Lok project uses a single system that can deal with many users simultaneously. On Lok's system is manufactured by Alpha-Micro Systems. Most of the contact or dialogue with the system is through terminals (CRTs): TV screens with typewriter-style keyboards. There are fourteen CRTs spread across On Lok's three centers in the Chinatown–North Beach–Polk Gulch community. The longest distance between centers is about two miles. All of the CRTs are connected to one computer, so changes made at any terminal automatically update the information at all terminals.

In addition to the CRTs, three printers are attached to the system, of which two are letter-quality printers. High-quality printing is important for word processing, from letters to final reports. In the system, every CRT is a full word processor.

Firmware

Firmware, a relatively new term to most computer users, refers to the programmed computer instructions that are permanently coded into the system. The computer that On Lok chose came with a number of common programming languages (e.g., BASIC, PASCAL, LISP), a word-processing system, and a very efficient multi-user operating system.

An operating system is the set of permanent programs that operate and manage the computer system. The Alpha-Micro operating system, designed for a multi-user environment, can serve from one to sixty CRTs and has an especially important feature: password control. While there are many advantages to integrating diverse information into a single system, there is frequently need to restrict access to some information, e.g., confidential client or accounting information. Password control allows any user to restrict access to his or her information area.

Applications Software

Applications software is the set of programs tailored to meet the needs of the information user. On Lok's software system was developed to meet the special needs of the human-service provider. An overview of the system is depicted in Figure 34–1. On Lok's software system can be divided into two distinct components: fiscal management and client management. The fiscal management component performs all accounting functions—specifically, accounts payable, payroll, general ledger, and fixed asset management—and provides fully integrated fiscal control. The client management component maintains basic information on all clients, i.e., participants in On Lok's long-term care service program, their characteristics, services received, and health/functional status. An important design feature of On Lok's software system is the integrated data base, linking the fiscal management and client management components. Figure 34–2 provides a sample of reports generated by On Lok's system.

Integrated Data Base

The real advantage of a single, coordinated information management system is the ease of integrating discrete components into a common data base. The computer system developed at On Lok, for example, has been designed to integrate cost information with service information. Such a data structure allows maximum flexibility in aggregating costs along different dimensions to provide information on the service program and on the individual's service package. Cost per service unit is reported on a regular basis and has been used in conjunction with client identifiable expenditures and individual client service records to produce a cost per client per month variable. (An example of unit cost reporting is included in Figure 34–2.) In turn, that variable is used as a criterion measure to examine cost distributions among clients with different degrees of impairment, change in costs over time, and predictors of cost.

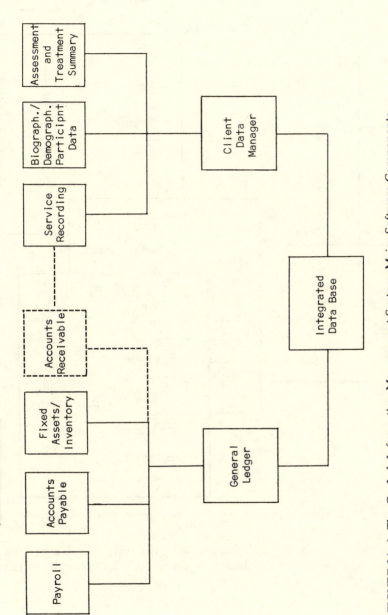

Client Management

Fiscal Management

FIGURE 34–1. The On Lok Information Management System: Major Software Components.

Source: Rick T. Zawadski and Stephen Gee, *Computerized Information Management in Long-Term Care: A Case Study,* San Francisco, CA: On Lok Senior Health Services, 1980, p. 8.

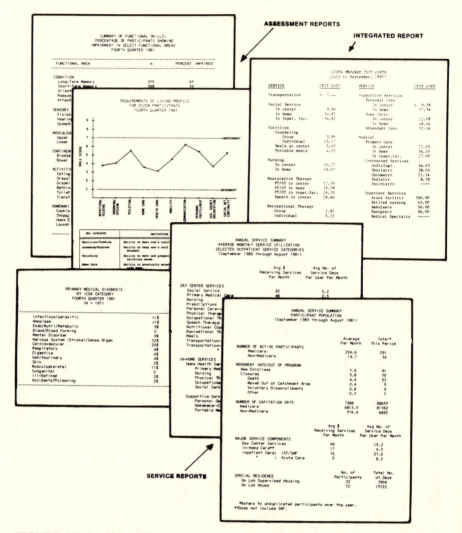

FIGURE 34–2. Client Management: Service, Assessment and Integrated Reports

Source: Rick T. Zawadski and Stephen Gee, *Computerized Information Management in Long-Term Care: A Case Study*, San Francisco, CA: On Lok Senior Health Services, 1980, p. 14.

DISCUSSION

Is computerization cost-beneficial, cost-effective today? What are the costs and benefits of the On Lok system? Would such a system work elsewhere? Based upon the On Lok experience, what recommendations could be made to other human service organizations considering computerization? This discussion section addresses some of these frequently asked questions.

Computerization—Is It Worth It?

Today On Lok continues to refine its computerized information system—improving efficiency of present systems, adding new subsystems and routines, and exploring new roles for computerization in human service settings. With all major elements of On Lok's computerized information system now fully operational, some of the costs and benefits of developing and operating such a system can be assessed.

Many small to medium human-service providers find computerization to be desirable, readily acknowledging its benefits but not giving such systems serious consideration because costs presumably are prohibitive. Providers recount others' "horror stories" of spending large sums of money for incomprehensible equipment designed and operated by people with whom they could not communicate and, not surprisingly, resulting in limited, if any, benefits. Fortunately, recent technological developments make possible a very different scenario.

A full assessment of cost must consider not only the financial costs for equipment and application systems, but also other organizational costs of making the transition to such a system.

Financial Costs. In 1978, for about $19,000, On Lok purchased a fully operational computer system with two CRTs and a letter-quality printer. While that system has been expanded five times in the subsequent four years to meet On Lok's growing computer needs, the basic system would adequately serve most small human-service providers. Today a similar system, with multi-tasking capabilities and reliable permanent storage, should cost less than $15,000, or approximately salary-plus-fringe for one year of clerical support.

An often overlooked but vital system cost component is applications software. When On Lok developed its system, applications software for payroll and accounts payable were available and served as a base for the fiscal management system, but in areas such as client management, service recording, and scheduling, no one had even thought of computer applications. On Lok had to develop those software systems itself, and developing a coherent software application package from scratch is expensive. Over the past four years, On Lok has invested more than $200,000 in its computerized information system. That includes all staff involvement (research, administration, service provider, and programmer time) and rights to some software licenses. Of course, some of these costs also would have been required for a manual information system.

While software development costs are relatively high, once developed, software application systems can be used in other settings. For example, On Lok's IMS could be transformed with relatively minor modifications into an information system for day health, home health, or other long-term care providers, for a fraction of the initial development cost.

There are also operating expenses. Hardware maintenance is a recommended option for any small user. Packages providing total systems support and replacement units during repair are available, usually at one percent monthly of hardware purchase price or less. Costs of supplies such as printer ribbons and paper should also be taken into consideration.

Requisite staff support is also minimal. Once an applications system is established, it does not require a full-time computer professional for its operation. A regular staff member, perhaps in accounting or administration or service program, who has an interest and some aptitude for equipment, can assume day-to-day operations responsibility. Amortizing hardware costs over a five-year period with 1982 interest rates and adding in operating costs for maintenance, supplies, and some staff time for operating support, a computer system like that purchased by On Lok would still cost an organization only about the equivalent of the salary of a clerical staff person.

Other Organizational Costs. Computerization, like any technological change, scares people; this reaction, if anything, is more prevalent in the human-service field. At On Lok, for example, many users had difficulty adjusting to the computer, felt threatened by the new tool, and were afraid to use it. These feelings were anticipated, and great care was taken to introduce staff to the system and to demonstrate that this technology could be their servant rather than their master. At On Lok today, over 30 staff are familiar with the use of the system and many others are asking that the system be extended to include their information needs.

In addition to the many expected benefits in efficiency and quality of information, computerization has proved to be a useful resource to On Lok in many other areas. Information now plays a bigger role in improving the quality of care provided as well as the overall effectiveness of the program.

Efficiency. Computerization has greatly reduced the time requirements for all routine financial accounting and external accountability tasks. For example, a manual payroll at On Lok used to require two days—summarizing time sheets, computing salaries, preparing checks, and recording for taxes and withholding. Today, with three times the number of employees, the entire payroll function is completed in less than six hours, and the computer does more: prints checks with employee information on all deductions and vacation, hol-

iday, and compensatory time due; tracks and monitors staff hours by
department; serves as a personnel administration tool; and provides
detailed personnel cost information for program management and research. All tax information is regularly computed and stored, and quarterly and annual tax reports and W-2 statements are automatically computer-generated, moments after the last payroll of the period is run.

Reliability—Quality of Information. Computerization has not
only increased the efficiency of information management within the
program, but has also provided significant benefits in the quality of
that information, i.e., its reliability and its validity. The simple use of
manual information systems can increase the accuracy of participant
information. In On Lok's first days, there did not even exist a clear
consensus among staff regarding the number of participants being
served—with estimates varying from 90 to 400! Instituting a simple
manual information system—differentiated referrals, active participants, and closed cases—revealed an active caseload of 77 people.

But that manual system could not easily keep up with the daily
changes as new participants joined, others left, many moved and
changed phone numbers. The manual information base traditionally
was about 90%–95% accurate. Introduction of an on-line computer system with regularly updated lists improved that reliability. It did not
take many mistaken phone calls to a changed phone number to convince staff that accurate information was essential. Today, the accuracy
of information routinely used by staff is over 99.5%.

Utility. A particularly significant benefit of computerization has
been in the new ways information has been put to use for the On Lok
program, providing service support, quality-assurance, management
planning, and research. On Lok, in fact, deliberately calls its system an
Information Management System (IMS) rather than a Management
Information System (MIS), because computer information systems are
more than just for management use.

The client management system generates a range of schedules
needed by service staff—attendance, meals, transportation, and health
care appointments. Similar purpose-specific lists and a computer-ac-
cessible client information base have become invaluable service-delivery tools, coordinating the many different services and professionals
involved in community-based care.

By routinely comparing service plans to services received, the
computerized information management system can monitor service-
plan compliance. By comparing outcomes, the information management system assists in assessing the relative benefits and costs of different treatments.

Daily, weekly, and monthly status reports regularly update staff
on census, services, and costs. Information feedback enables the pro-

gram's management to identify potential problems early, establish and monitor goals, and plan future programming. The research element of On Lok's program helps to stimulate discussion between direct service and administrative staff about the usefulness of reports and the system's performance.

Cost-Effectiveness. While it is always difficult to address the cost-effectiveness of an intervention such as computerization, the task has been made easier, with cost savings alone offsetting equipment and development costs in just a few years. All of the extra information services, e.g., management reports, service and quality-assurance monitoring, and the use of information in planning, development, and research, have been added dividends of the venture.

Actions ultimately speak louder than words and, in the final analysis, it is organizational behavior that speaks to the cost-effectiveness of a system. It is interesting, therefore, that in the spring of 1982, the service program staff—rather than the research staff, which initiated computerization—were the ones to demand new, larger investments in more computer equipment and an expanded role for the information systems.

Recommendations

Much has been learned through the process of computerizing the On Lok community-based long-term care system. From that experience, a number of recommendations emerge for other human-service providers who are implementing, planning, or even considering computerization.

Start Small! Smaller is better. Too often small or medium-sized organizations overextend themselves by investing $100,000 or more in computer equipment, only to find the equipment alone provides neither a service nor a solution. In choosing hardware, it is important to choose equipment at the appropriate level, with the capability for expansion. The single-user personal computers, although inexpensive, are not realistic starting points. On the other hand, big-name computer manufacturers often charge a high premium for their reputation. In selecting equipment, assess present and future needs. Buy equipment to meet your immediate needs, but assure yourself that your system can grow.

It is far safer to start with modest expectations and exceed them than to start on a grand scale with great promises that ultimately disappoint those the system was to serve.

Kill the Old-Time Programmer! When computers were first introduced into banking, in exchange for the benefits of the machine, bankers had to relinquish some of the control over their businesses to programmers who understood little or nothing of the business. Bankers, however, got smart. They learned enough about computers to take back control of their businesses. Now people in human services must also get smart. The age of the old-time programmer is dead. No longer can programmers be isolated physically and administratively in an organization, without training or personal interest in the content area. No longer can programmers be unwilling or unable to communicate with others who know the problems and the needs; no longer can systems be accepted that respond approximately to the request and never fully deal with the problem. While it may be too early to find computer-literate nurses, social workers, and therapists, it is time to demand that any computer professional you work with be willing to LOOK at your program and its needs, to LEARN the basics of your business, and to LISTEN to what you want in an information management system to meet your real, day-to-day needs.

Bottoms Up! Traditionally, computer systems are developed from the top, e.g., federal and state funding agencies, who force their requirements on local agencies and, in turn, on the provider. As opposed to this "top-down" method, the "bottoms-up" design approach has many advantages. Computerization should begin at the service provider level. The more diverse and demanding information needs of the service providers make them the logical starting point. Moreover, involving service providers in developing the system to meet their needs ensures their commitment to the system. Providers must meet their funding agencies' reporting requirements, so these information requirements will be taken into consideration. Ultimately, a bottoms-up approach can produce an integrated, multilevel information network that maximizes information transfer, maintains the confidentiality of service recipients, and meets the information requirements of state and federal funding sources. The resulting information base will permit effective program-monitoring, provide a base for ongoing research, and serve as a practical tool for rational service-planning and policy development.

Get Involved. The primary lesson from On Lok's experience is that the service provider must get involved in its information management. Today, with diminishing resources and competition from proprietary organizations, it is no longer enough to be a concerned and caring person. The human-service provider must develop the skills of the sophisticated manager, one of which is the use of information. With current information technology, if the service program administrator, its planners, and its service providers do not control the information they use in day-to-day operation, they will ultimately be controlled by it.

SUMMARY

On Lok Senior Health Services has demonstrated the feasibility and utility of the microcomputer in meeting a long-term care program's information needs. Over a four-year period, On Lok has developed a system that meets the program, policy, and research information needs of its: (1) program administrators, (2) direct-service staff, (3) research and evaluation staff, and (4) program monitors from outside reimbursement and funding agencies. On Lok's introduction to computer technology came through the use of a mainframe computer, which is still used to supplement in-house capacity. The advent of microcomputing technology made it possible for On Lok to obtain its own hardware, create a dedicated system, and transform the role of information in the program.

Hardware and software growth has been incremental at On Lok. Hardware is upgraded or added as On Lok's needs change and/or technological breakthroughs occur. Software development has created a fiscal management component, a client management component, and an ability to integrate the two. Software is regularly written or modified to accommodate new users and emerging information needs.

Thus, community-based long-term care now has access to technology long available to and used by business and industry. At On Lok, the two areas of greatest concern in long-term care—cost containment and quality of care—can be continuously monitored. Feedback, i.e., knowledge of results from the computerized information management system, enables On Lok's administrative and service staff to make decisions more rationally and to modulate their strategies on the basis of sound information. In short, On Lok, an operating service program, has harnessed modern computer technology to put information to use for long-term care case management as well as for program management purposes.

REFERENCES

Zawadski, R. T., & Ansak, M. L. *On Lok's CCODA: The first two years.* San Francisco: On Lok Senior Health Services, 1981.

Zawadski, R. T., & Gee, S. *Computerized information management in long-term care: A case study.* San Francisco: On Lok Senior Health Services, 1982.

Issues in the Development of a Community-Wide Mental Health Information System

Larry L. Searcy

This article is a description of experiences and opinions the author has gained while developing an automated information system that crosses agency and discipline lines. It is in no way intended as a research piece. Its purpose is to highlight problems and suggest solutions to enhancing interagency cooperation and communications.

PROJECT BACKGROUND

Kansas City, Missouri, is an urban center with a population of approximately 500,000 people. Since the 1950s, the population shift to the suburbs has been like that found in other medium to large cities nationally. The resultant inner-city environment has been conducive to behaviors in adolescents living in the central city that categorize them as high risk. Typical characteristics of these behaviors are school failure, contact with the juvenile justice system, chronic unemployment, drug and alcohol abuse, and teenage pregnancy.

In response to the needs of Kansas City young people, some 250 public and private agencies are currently in operation. These agencies, for a variety of reasons, tend to address only one type of need a youth may have. Pressures that create a single-needs approach are historically well-rooted and do not seem to be likely to abate anytime soon. Amongst single-need pressures are categorical funding, the expertise and treatment bias of professional staff, and a backdrop of declining fiscal support. Yet, it is difficult to envision a youngster with severe emotional problems who does not also experience difficulty in the public schools. He or she, in addition, may be involved with drugs, has been involved in status offenses or more severe legal infractions, may have been or still is abused or neglected by his or her parents, etc.

Recognition that young people may be multiply-involved demands a holistic treatment response. In order to address the needs of young people from such a holistic perspective, it is necessary to view the existence of single-need providers as part of a service-delivery system. Organized as it is, there is no clear-cut access point to the system, nor is there any easily expedited movement between service deliverers once access is gained.

Youth already in the service system are often not able to get to appropriate, timely service. As earlier mentioned, most of these agencies deliver service from a single-need perspective. They do not have the necessary level of manpower or expertise to make an up-front referral to a more appropriate agency. Once service is initiated, agency staff members often are so intellectually and emotionally caught up in program strategies that they simply refuse to accept the fact that it may not be effective. Coupled with funding pressures that do not fiscally reward effective referrals, but rather measure agency effectiveness by comparing positive and negative terminations, it makes good sense for the agency to "hang in there" with the young person, regardless of the level of progress that the youth is experiencing. Without the ability to refer effectively, agencies also tend to view themselves as a last chance. They equate terminating a youngster to returning him or her to the street life from whence he or she came.

To a youth outside the service-delivery system, the selection of a service provider is very difficult. Generally, the young person and his or her parents are not familiar with agencies that are not in close geographic proximity to their home. Their knowledge base of those agencies close to their home is usually very limited. The decision to enter a particular agency is often not based on how appropriately the service matches the needs of the young person, but rather is based on the experience of a friend who participated in that agency's program or the convenience of the geographical location of the agency. Once involved with an agency, the youth's "problem" often becomes consistent with that of the agency mission. The youth may readily succeed with that agency only to discover that very little positive impact has been made on "problem" behaviors, etc., in every other setting in which the youth finds himself or herself. Once again the likelihood of an appropriate referral being made is slim due to a lack of manpower, an incomplete client information base, and lack of an accurate referral information.

Youth already in a public system often do not receive timely, appropriate service due to a lack of information and perceived legal constraints. Information flow about clients is at best inconsistent and at worse nonexistent. In many cases, youth appear before judges and other official decision-makers without their situation being fully known. In some cases this may be due to a conscious policy decision on the part of an institution to not share a type or class of information. In most cases, however, the existence of the information was never discovered, or its existence was known but the information could not be accessed in a timely way. By way of illustration, almost every service provider wants to know how the young person is doing in school. Extremely basic to that situation is knowing in which school the youth is currently enrolled. In the Kansas City Public School District there were 46,000 transfers during the 1981–1982 school year. Yet the district serves only 36,000 students. In some cases hard-copy cumulative files may be two moves behind the student. The central file may be showing the student absent at one school when in reality he or she is in attendance at another. Similar gaps between case movement and data update have been observed in all of the local public agencies dealing with young people.

Perceived legal constraints have also caused effective delivery of service to be very difficult. A common situation that illustrates these constraints is a young person who is in need of a residential care setting, remedial or special education, and/or psychotherapy. Each public agency that might be involved will assume only a very limited portion of the treatment approach and often will maintain that it is not responsible to provide service on any level because the primary presenting problem does not fall within its legal mandate. While some headway has been made in a few locales to bridge these gaps, they still exist and in some cases are getting worse.

To a youth who is outside the public service delivery system, getting to timely, appropriate service is even more difficult. Even if the young person recognizes that he or she needs help, there is no readily accessible entry point to the system, other than becoming known to the juvenile justice system.

Simply put, private agencies typically do not have the manpower or sufficient background information to make an up-front determination relative to the client's needs as compared to their services. Public agencies perceive their intake to be limited by statutory mandate. Even if these legal limitations were not present, they too do not have sufficient manpower or accurate information that would allow an appropriate up-front referral to be made. As a result, there is no readily accessible entry point to the service delivery system once a youth is no longer in it, and little chance for an effective referral once service has been initiated.

On a broader level, the environment in which policymakers function relative to this quiltwork of service delivery is not conducive to reliable, consistent decision-making. It is extremely difficult to carry out a community-wide needs assessment without unbiased, accurate aggregate data.

Agency-level data that may be useful in such a global assessment often do not exist or are not in a form that is readily transferable to other settings. Almost all agency performance data that do exist are internally generated and, due to funding pressures, usually biased towards presenting the agency in a positive light.

The lack of a community-wide planning base becomes fuel for the fire of agency isolation. Funding decisions made in this environment reinforce the propensity of agencies to continue a single-need approach without looking to other agencies for support.

PROJECT RATIONALE

Realizing that a holistic approach to service is more effective in both costs and treatment outcomes than a piecemeal one, we note that enhanced interagency coordination and communication is essential. It is clear that the political forces active during a period of declining funding would discourage the centralization of the intake process. Such a centralization would necessarily bring to the specified intake structure a pre-eminence that would attract funding that otherwise would have gone to direct-service agencies. Yet the same environment also fosters a willingness to participate in joint or cooperative efforts, if for no other reason than the resultant heightened community and political presence.

In view of the above, traditional funding reactions and strategies are no longer effective. Further funding of direct service exclusively would only worsen the situation. Forcing direct-service mergers is highly unlikely and in most cases not appropriate.

In order to establish system access points and an appropriate referral system, timely, accurate, client-specific information had to be shared by service-deliverers.

On the policy level, unbiased third-party information describing presenting problems of youth, service levels by problem area, expenditure levels by service area and by agency, client demographics and predictive trend analysis, etc. needed to be compiled and reviewed.

In order to satisfy all of the above needs, it was proposed that an automated information clearinghouse be established. The envisioned clearinghouse would have the capability of providing any client-specific data that existed anywhere in the "system" to any other agency also involved with that client. The envisioned information system would be interactive so that up-front entrance/referral/treatment decisions could be made in a timely way. Hence, each agency could become an access point to the rest of the system.

The proposed clearinghouse would also be able to provide aggregate data as described above to policymakers on a quarterly or monthly basis. The aggregate data would be generated directly from the internal operating data of the participating agencies, not from agency-generated summary reports.

PROJECT-PLANNING ACTIVITIES

Through the support of a group of local foundations, Act Together of Kansas City initiated a six-month planning period on June 1, 1982. The goals of the planning period were:

1. To determine the technical feasibility of an automated information clearinghouse;
2. To project implementation costs;
3. To determine the information requirements of such a system;
4. To determine what level of cooperation could be expected from major public youth-serving agencies and to facilitate the same.

TECHNICAL FEASIBILITY SURVEY

In order to determine if this sort of approach was technically feasible, it was decided to perform a survey of cities around the country in an effort to locate such a system. After reviewing the professional literature in various disciplines, several stood out as having forayed extensively into this field: (1) juvenile justice, (2) education, (3) child welfare systems, and (4) social service generalists, i.e. directors of city or state-level social service departments, etc.

One of the real problems encountered in this aspect of the planning was a dearth of literature describing such systems. In many cases the literature simply provided reference to locales in which such systems were operative or names of individuals involved in such work. Very little literature described a currently operating system in much detail. The survey was therefore carried out for the most part by telephone contact and correspondence. Approximately 35 phone contacts were made and in excess of 200 letters were forwarded to social service professionals. The phone contacts were generated by following up leads provided by professional acquaintances. The correspondence was generated via the membership list of an organization known as Computer Use in Social Service Networks.

Since case management is the first priority of our system, automated tracking systems were of special interest. Therefore, the phone contacts and correspondence focused on locating tracking systems. In response to our mailings, we received replies from 11 states and 2 foreign countries. Each response was reviewed and the most promising were followed up by phone. In all, approximately 200 tracking systems were identified. Due to fiscal and time constraints, only 8 were actually visited and observed firsthand.

Of the four disciplines mentioned earlier, juvenile justice and child welfare appear to be the most experienced in the development of tracking systems. In the juvenile justice area, a variety of systems have spun off from a fairly generic system known as PROMIS, although in our survey we discovered that each PROMIS system was different from the others, due to the unique characteristics of each locale. Also, systems developed in a juvenile justice setting appear to concentrate on tracking a case through the legal process rather than tracking behaviors through a treatment plan or facilitating case management.

The child welfare discipline has developed tracking systems in response to the legal requirements of P. L. 96–272. Systems found in this field are more attuned to case management. They also tend to have resource and referral information as a major component of their design.

In education, the interdisciplinary treatment approach appears to be gaining a lot of momentum. Tracking systems appear to be most utilized in special-education settings relative to the design and implementation of individualized education programs. In one instance a school district was the focal point for an integrated social service system, although it never truly utilized automated tracking. It is also important to note that most large school districts long ago automated portions or all of their cumulative files, which in many ways are a tracking system.

Social service generalists initiated automated tracking/integrated social service systems as far back as the late 1960s. A tremendous surge of interest blossomed in the early to mid-1970s, apparently motivated by a large infusion of H.E.W. funding. Some are still operative today, but most were either scaled down or shut down completely when the federal funding disappeared.

One area in which city governments, voluntary action centers, etc. have remained active is resource and referral information. A major impediment to the establishment of such systems seems to be reaching community-wide agreement on the categorization of agencies by generic service definitions. The UWASIS II appears to be the most popular service taxonomy currently in use.

COSTS

Cost figures for the surveyed systems ran anywhere between $250,000 and $500,000. The two universal cost components were software development and hardware acquisition (usually about 50% each). In reality, costs associated with such a system can be viewed as much higher, if factors such as staffing, space, climate control, etc. are considered.

Based on this cursory examination of what had already been implemented across the country, it was concluded that such an information clearinghouse was technically feasible. Further, certain universal precepts seem to cut across disciplines in the establishment of such a system: the limiting impact of hardware and the need for a free-standing data base.

The Limiting Impact of Hardware

Generally speaking, any information system cannot be more flexible than its hardware. Information needs are changing rapidly and, as a result, a hardware configuration that was appropriate five years ago may not be so today. Additionally, hardware that may have been state of the art is rapidly becoming obsolescent with little or no resale value. (One school system offered to *give away* a mainframe that had been considered state of the art eight years ago, and it had no takers.) Additionally, as hardware becomes outmoded, maintenance and utility costs that were once acceptable seem to be tremendously high compared to that of newer models. Once project overhead is viewed as extremely high, it becomes increasingly difficult to defend the project in a budget hearing.

Need for a Free-Standing Data Base

Almost all of the systems observed built a data base that is free-standing of the agencies that generated the original data. In order to build such a base, it is necessary to either input selected information on additional forms or utilize a tape-to-tape transfer. In the former approach, caseworkers may end up filling out more forms then they currently do. In the latter situation, the data is only as current as the tape-to-tape relay. If the relay occurs every twenty-four hours, there is no problem. If the agencies agree to a biweekly or monthly transfer, the available data is obviously dated and may be inaccurate.

INFORMATION REQUIREMENTS

To caseworkers inside both the public and private service, providers' access to client-specific and referral information is critical. If accurate, timely, client-specific profiles (i.e., service histories) cannot be generated, it is very difficult to develop comprehensive treatment plans. Most caseworkers recognize the need for this information and attempt to gain it. Usually this involves gaining a parent's or guardian's signature on a release of information waiver, presenting it to the agency that should have the information, and waiting for the receipt of same. In a survey administered to local caseworkers, the turnaround time for this transaction varied from one week to several months (depending on the agencies involved, etc.). No clear-cut procedures or other factors could be identified that explained the variance. Caseworkers also reported that they spend 25% to 30% of their time trying to gain such information. Time spent in collecting information obviously limits the amount of time available for direct-service activities. In many situations the caseworker simply gives up after an initial effort because he feels he cannot commit any more time to developing a client-specific information base.

Similar time obligations are involved in identifying outside resources. Information regarding which agencies provide what service, entrance procedures, fee structures, etc. is not readily available to caseworkers. Experienced caseworkers have indicated that this is their most serious problem in developing a treatment plan. New or inexperienced caseworkers are often overwhelmed when trying to locate outside resources. When one considers that caseworker turnover rates may be as high as 30% to 40%, it is clear that the plight of a new worker critically impacts the effectiveness of the service-delivery system.

It therefore seemed logical to form user groups made up of caseworkers, supervisors, and in some instances a mix of all of the participating institutions. The school district was the most difficult relative to identifying appropriate "users." All of the other systems are event- or case-driven. The school district is driven by a variety of events, stemming out of a legal requirement to provide education for a certain number of days per year and hours per day. Its staffing patterns are mandated on a minimal level and course offerings are also mandated. As a result, each youth entering a school setting does not require the system to respond exactly the same way. The link between the student's presence and the system's procedures is not nearly as correlative as might be found in the juvenile justice or protective service systems.

The user groups met biweekly and essentially carried out two tasks. The first was to create a case flow chart of their own system. As the flow chart was developed, decision points inside the system were identified. Each decision point was examined and a list of the information needed to make that decision was developed. Treatment plans were also examined to determine what new information might be generated and how it would be recorded. The second task was to examine case flow charts and data bases of the other institutions. As they became familiar with the other participating systems and the information available through them, the users identified and prioritized the information they would like to access. The information requirements of the system, as identified by the users, were much broader than the "first step" agreed to by the agency decision-makers. Their value was not therefore tied into initial implementation, but rather to the course for future expansion of the clearinghouse information system.

Additionally, by going through the step-by-step process of laying out the information requirements, the users better understood the complexities the directors were dealing with at the policy level.

After the first step was agreed upon, the users became advocates for the project within their own system. Much of the work of the members of these groups involved soliciting input from their peers who were not active in the user groups. As a result, they became highly visible within their respective organizations and served as communication links during implementation.

The user group meetings also made clear the need for intense training around the issues of case management, caseload management, and how an automated information system can positively impact both. During an early meeting of one of the groups, a caseworker expressed the opinion that client-specific records weren't really needed because, after all, the worker could get the information directly from the client. Another attitude prevalently displayed at the early meetings placed limits on information that would be used by the system, consistent with the information filled out on a particular agency's forms. When asked to describe a utopian client data profile, in fact, one caseworker responded by delivering the intake sheet his agency used.

The necessity of effective user training was also observed relative to the systems involved in site visits. At sites that did not precede or accompany implementation with extensive training, user resistance greatly delayed bringing the system up. In one case, a system was more than one year behind due to user resistance as expressed through a lack of cooperation relative to input procedures (errors, delay, or no input at all).

Based on the on-site visits and the conclusions of the user group, several information requirements and limitations became clear, as discussed below.

24-Hour Turnaround. Due to the daily flux in the originating data bases, the quicker the turnaround time (elapsed time from the request for information to the receipt of the same), the better. After much discussion, a twenty-four-hour turnaround was viewed as adequate.

Case History. Most of the day-to-day treatment histories were stored in narrative reports. It became obvious that to attempt to electronically move such narratives would not be practical. Other information could be moved that was viewed as extremely important. For example, the juvenile court considered a certified date of birth as critical to their process, as it determined if the matter was within their jurisdiction. It was agreed that basic demographics and other similar data would be of help and were available.

Referral Information. The user groups identified a tremendous need for easily accessible, regularly updated resource and referral information. One suggestion from the group involved developing a software package that would match client characteristics to available resources.

INTERAGENCY COOPERATION

It seemed apparent that to try to initiate meaningful discussion with all of the youth-serving agencies in the community would invite chaos. It also seemed obvious that most of the target population we were concerned with had been involved in one of four major public agencies. These four agencies were brought together in what became known as the Public Agency Working Group.

Participants in this group were to be the decision-makers of each institution. Hence, the president of the school board, the superintendent of the Kansas City Public School District, the director of the Jackson County Juvenile Court, the regional director of the Missouri Division of Youth Services, and a representative of the regional director of the Missouri Division of Family Services were members of the group.

While this makeup did facilitate frank discussion at high decision-making levels, probably only the school district's combination of a board representative and the chief administrator was optimal. In case of the court, it was still necessary to gain agreement from the juvenile court judge and eventually to gain a court en banc agreement (court en banc involves gaining agreement from all of the circuit court judges). In the case of the Division of Youth Services and the Division of Family Services (both state agencies), agreement then had to be sought and gained with administrators higher up in the organizational structure, who were housed at the state capitol. For a number of reasons, logistics not the least of them, the optimal membership could not be achieved. The lack of an optimal configuration extended the official agency sign-off process over six months.

The first obstacle to clear in gaining group momentum was arranging a meeting schedule. Various attempts at arranging such a schedule failed, amongst them, asking for dates by phone until a schedule emerged and having each member submit a calendar for the next two months with standing commitments and other meetings blocked out. According to information gained from both of these methods, the entire group could never meet. Finally, a conference phone call was placed to all of the members and in less than fifteen minutes a biweekly meeting schedule was arranged on a standing basis covering a 2½-month period of time. Only one meeting was canceled during that time, due to conflict with a state and county holiday (election day). Attendance at the meetings held was 100%. While the excellent attendance can be attributed to the professionalism of the members, it appeared that gaining a commitment to the schedule as a group in which peers were committing performance to each other was the solidifying factor.

At the first meeting of the group, it was agreed that the following issues had to researched, discussed, and resolved: (1) What information is controlled by statute vs. by agency policy? and (2) What is a mutually agreeable first step? After spending a considerable amount of time examining the agency policies regarding confidentiality and contrasting it to the law, it was decided that trying to implement a system that in some way provided information that has historically been released only via parent/guardian release was too large a step to be accomplished as a first step. It seemed clear that any movement in that direction would entail extensive in-house legal review and, even if deemed legal, might create a public controversy in which none of the institutions was willing to be involved.

The group therefore began discussing first steps. The focus of the system as a result of these discussions centered around expediting current procedures by substituting electronic communication transfer for the manual transfer procedures that were currently in use. Additionally, a range of client-specific information to be moved electronically was agreed upon and the class of personnel who could generate requests was identified.

It is important to note that on each of the above factors, universal agreement was never gained. Some of the issues, especially the personnel questions, were highly volatile. The participants often viewed mistrust of a particular class of employee inside their structure as an institutional affront. The group had to work very hard to remain focused on the common goal and not eat up time and energy expressing frustration based on a perception of a lack of professional respect accorded their institution.

After agreement was reached on a first step, a document of agreement was prepared. This document spelled out the functional obligations of each of the participating agencies. It was then routed through the final decision process of each agency. No group meetings were held for one month during this period of time, but close contact was maintained with each agency to ensure progress towards gaining official agreement.

Amongst the conclusions gained from the activities of the Public Agency Working Group are three we list below.

1. Major public institutions seem to equate access to their internal records with exposure to criticism from outside agencies. Much of this mistrust appears to be historically rooted in "turf" issues that have been around for years. If the group focus cannot be rigidly centered around the welfare of the client, these issues can stymie the entire process. In order to help assure such focusing, each meeting agenda should be larger than a one-hour meeting can deal with. The group will remain task-oriented and a willingness to cooperate can be fostered through peer pressure generated in such a problem-solving atmosphere.

2. It is essential that the key decision-makers in each organization derive a sense of ownership from the process. Hence, no readymade design was ever presented. A design evolved from tasks performed by the group.

3. Requests for in-house legal opinions should not be couched in terms of "Is this legal?" Rather, the chief administrator should bring to legal counsel a finished product and ask for assistance in implementation.

COMMUNITY POLITICS

A final area in which the project was immersed during the planning phase was community politics. Once the planning process began, a number of similar efforts designed to coordinate services or establish automated tracking systems came to the fore. Needless to say, if these situations are not handled carefully, another series of "turf wars" could easily begin.

The local reaction to this situation involved all of these interests coming together and communicating in such a way that all of the systems will be compatible. Act Together's posture was to assist others via information gained through the system survey, etc.

Private agencies probably fear exposure even more than public agencies do. As a result, their initial reaction to the project implied that they didn't need further client information. They cast doubt on the accuracy of publicly housed information and suggested that the funding supporting the project could be better spent on direct service, i.e., their agency.

Had the required funding been generated through public sources, it is possible that the community-based organizations could have stopped it before it began. Private-sector funding appears to be the most insulated and will buy the necessary time to win over or identify private-agency advocates that can be called upon to serve as liaisons with their peers.

CONCLUSION

It is hoped that the description of our experiences contained in this chapter will assist people making similar efforts in other locales. The application of computer technology to social science is just beginning to realize its potential. But when all is said and done, we are no longer limited by technology. We are limited only by our imagination and willingness to take risks.

Introduction of a Computer at a Counseling Center: A Case Study

Herman Resnick, PhD
Charlene Matheson, PhD
James A. Buss, MA

Our story is probably typical. A social agency purchases a computer and finds, after an initial enthusiastic reception, that it is only barely used. The problems that the computer is supposed to fix, however, persist. Staff works overtime to get out reports, and agency business continues without timely feedback on its operations. In an effort to improve the situation, a persistent, innovative administrator makes contact with a computer specialist who understands not only the technical dimensions of computer introduction, but also the social ones. This combination proves sufficient to integrate the new technology firmly into the existing routine. Staff uses the computer more frequently, enhancing the general operation of the agency. In addition, other departments within the agency become interested in the computer and its contribution; the process of diffusion of an innovation begins (Rothman, 1976).

This chapter describes the up-and-down experience of the Kwawachee Counseling Center of Pierce County, Washington, with a computer, and traces the role of a consultant brought in to stimulate its more efficacious use. A final section is devoted to explicit lessons learned from these experiences.

THE DECISION TO PURCHASE A COMPUTER

Kwawachee Counseling Center is a community mental health center that serves the Native American community of Pierce County, Washington. The center is one department of a comprehensive health care center called the Puyallup Nation Health Authority. The service delivery population consists of approximately 8,000 Native American residents of Pierce County. Kwawachee also receives referrals from agencies in neighboring counties. The center has an in-house staff of 8 and is overseen by the health authority administrative staff. The center serves an average client caseload of 250.

The Kwawachee Counseling Center provides culturally relevant mental health services to the Native American community. The center opened in 1977 with a major goal of increasing the acceptability of using mental health services. For this to occur, the community had to develop a trust in the staff of the mental health program. It was in this context that the computer was introduced.

The idea of purchasing a computer was in the beginning stages of development when the Puyallup Health Authority Administration released money for special projects. The staff of Kwawachee was called to a special meeting to set priorities on agency needs and agreed that a computer should be purchased.

There were several reasons why staff at that time thought that owning a computer would be useful. Mental health centers are required to develop a system of accountability—a management information system (MIS)—to provide information to funding agencies on client demographics, use of services, and agency performance. To comply with the MIS requirements, counselors recorded their work activities and time involved on a weekly activity log. Kwawachee's data coordinator then compiled information manually and submitted it for entry into the state's computer. The turnaround time for reports averaged about three months. This overlong period of time compromised the applicability and effectiveness of the reports within the agency. Staff found it difficult to act on dated feedback. They felt that more immediate feedback on performance would enable them to respond more quickly and thereby keep agency performance in compliance with Kwawachee Counseling Center's contract specifications.

Other departments within the health authority also thought a computer would enhance their operations. The planning department felt that grant-writing and program evaluation would be facilitated by having more current statistics. The accounting department envisaged a more efficient billing process. It was believed that direct client services would benefit by more timely assessment of staff performance, enabling immediate intervention in clinical supervision sessions. Behavioral treatment programs would be enhanced by providing clients with a graphic representation of their progress.

Financially, the purchase of a computer seemed like a good investment. Diminishing government funds for social service programs have necessitated position cuts through attrition in many agencies. The agency hoped to mitigate the effects of this by increasing the efficiency of support staff so that they could assume additional responsibility within the agency. The agency also hoped to offer billable information-management services to the other programs within the health authority, so an existing position supported by income generated through direct services could become self-supporting.

With these objectives delineated, the agency assigned the responsibility of selecting the appropriate computer, printer, and software to a predoctoral counselor who had had computer training in graduate school. Given the time constraints, selection was limited to what was available in the local market. Within two weeks an Apple II+ computer, black-and-white monitor, two disk drives, a TEC letter-quality printer, and software for word processing (Applewriter), spreadsheet analysis (VisiCalc), and electronic filing (PFS) were delivered.

THE ARRIVAL OF THE COMPUTER

The arrival of the computer began a period of excitement and feeling of "coming of age" at Kwawachee. Staff watched with excitement as the dealer demonstrated the computer. They felt that if they followed the dealer's instructions and read the first two chapters of the Apple manual, the agency would then be computerized. Initially, staff competed for time at the computer and the administration had to identify which staff needed to learn how to use it first. One staff member discovered that the computer could produce an infinite variety of patterns similar to those used in Indian beadwork. This was interpreted as an auspicious beginning. Staff felt that surely the computer would be their friend.

After a while, the newness of the machine wore off, and the intricate beadwork patterns were no longer enough to entice the staff to explore the capabilities of the computer. It became apparent that long, tedious hours would have to be spent to learn how to use the software packages confidently and effectively. It also became clear that special schemes for data organization and data entry would have to be developed to meet the agency's needs. The task was much more complex than had been anticipated.

In the meantime, the ongoing work of the agency still had to be done. Data still had to be compiled, and agency reports still had to be delivered monthly. Staff enthusiasm for using the computer diminished, and the Apple retired under a blanket for several months. Analysis of the problem revealed that the training that came free with the purchase of the computer was insufficient to implement the dream system. Furthermore, ongoing responsibilities of the data coordinator did not leave enough time for her to train herself.

When the computer was almost one year old, the agency decided to enlist the assistance of an independent computer consultant, whose work has insured that the agency will survive the transition into the computer age.

THE INITIAL INTERVIEWS WITH THE CONSULTANT

The consultant's first task was to interview staff at the agency, not only to find out why they bought a computer and what they had planned to do with it, but also to assess sociological and cost implications not always considered by newcomers to the computer age. Who would gain from the computer's successful operation? How much would it cost? What steps would have to be taken to put it into operation?

The consultant's initial interviews with the director and the data coordinator revealed that their goals for the computer were not identical, but both had to be met if the project was to succeed. The data coordinator wanted to make routine paperwork easier. The director wanted to increase accountability and improve control over her own operations, with the possibility of providing computing services for sibling agencies. In addition, the consultant had to look for unstated goals. Education, career advancement, prestige, or other positive objectives may be as important as increased productivity or service. These secondary, often hidden, objectives are important to motivating an agency's staff, and can have a critical role in the computer's acceptance. Staff may also harbor negative goals that will prevent acceptance of the computer unless they are counteracted.

At Kwawachee, the consultant found that staff was genuinely enthusiastic about the computer and believed it would make routine work more fun. Lack of use of the machine in the first year was traced to frustration with the primitive state of "human interface" technology. The dealer had not delivered training as promised. The data coordinator had made a valiant effort to read the manuals and set up the electronic filing program, but had become frustrated after running into small but insoluble problems. For example, the printer would not advance the paper, so long reports were overprinted, all on one line. The solution was well-hidden in an appendix of the manual.

The consultant also had to glean some estimate of the value of the implementation to the agency. Much of the cost can reside in the development of software. Custom software can cost many times the cost of the hardware, and is expensive to maintain. To propose an expensive solution for an inexpensive problem would have left the agency with an implementation that could not possibly succeed. Software purchased from a vendor can provide imperfect but adequate solutions to most problems, inexpensively.

THE CONSULTANT'S ANALYSIS AND IMPLEMENTATION

After the initial assessment, the consultant conducted additional interviews in order to analyze in detail the desired reports and the capabilities of the electronic filing program. Electronic filing works by laying out forms on the computer's screen in much the same way you'd design forms on paper. The filing program also allowed the agency staff to store the forms on magnetic disks, where they could be retrieved in a variety of ways for examination on the screen or inclusion in printed reports. Although easy to use, the existing program had several limitations. It could not sort information for reporting or adequately format reports. It supported only the simplest data organization and the way data was stored and organized on the computer's screen could not be changed once it was defined. When clients left, their records had to be deleted and retyped, rather than simply transferred to another file.

To rectify these problems, the consultant found an alternate filing program that allowed much more flexibility in changing data structures as well as sorting and better report preparation. The new program also had a means of writing out the client records in such a way that they could be combined with other information and read back in for future applications where the cost was justified.

Actually getting the reports set up involved more interviews, design, and review by appropriate staff. The consultant and the agency staff decided to make the computer forms look like the paper forms because the paper forms had a history of their own and reflected convenient processing. They also wanted to take advantage of improvements the computer could offer. Above all, the filing system had to feel natural and convenient to the data coordinator, who would be living with it daily. Enough decisions had to remain with the data coordinator so that using the computer was not just a boring series of button-pushes. With these requirements in mind, the consultant set up separate forms for vital statistics, psychiatric history, and financial status of each client. Each counselor would have a form for direct client service, and one for other activities. Reports consisted of a monthly client list for quarterly review, quarterly service reports summarizing the number and type of services, caseload reports for each counselor, and reports for billing.

In addition to analyzing and installing the electronic filing system, the consultant trained the director, data coordinator, and the secretary in word processing and using the spreadsheet program.

The Kwawachee staff were not jealous of each other's knowledge about the computer and helped one another with routine tasks in order to free up time to learn and practice. This made training much easier; it's not typical. The director had facilitated this by giving almost everyone involved some role on the computer and differentiating the roles, encouraging cooperation, and making competition constructive.

Documentation describing the agency's computer-based operating procedures—how to add new clients, how and when to make multiple copies for recovery from accidents, what to do when a floppy disk fills up—was an important complement to the training. Although the consultant didn't rewrite any software manuals, he did indicate which section of which manual applied to which of their unique operating procedures. Good documentation is mandatory for infrequently used procedures, for staff turnover, and for procedure and program maintenance. Beyond that, the consultant made himself available for occasional follow-up questions for six months or so, to complete the staff's training.

WHAT NEXT?

Computer installations are never finished. If a computer is installed so that it is used, and as people become aware of what computers do and what they don't do, they see new ways in which their computer can make their work easier, better, or more pleasant. New versions of existing software come out that perform additional tasks. New programs come out that are useful. Additional hardware may become useful. An operation may use two programs together, and upgrading one often means the other must be adjusted. The consultant's role must include being available after the installation to provide answers to new questions, to provide improvements for previous work, and to pass on information about new programs and upgrades that will be useful. Just as autos need occasional oil changes, so do computers and their software. They need tinkering, and budgets must allow this.

WHAT ARE THE LESSONS FOR OTHER AGENCIES?

The turning point for the Kwawachee Counseling Center was the decision to select the computer specialist to guide the agency in the thinking and decision-making with respect to their computer. A competent consultant must:

- Closely question you regarding why you want a computer;
- Provide you with the names and numbers of previous clients;

- Work with a representative planning group composed of board, staff, and administration, before and after installation of the computer;
- Teach you about computer capabilities as well as limitations, so that you can learn what questions to ask;
- Help you establish a network of other computer users in situations similar to yours;
- Realistically inform you of the costs involved in software as well as hardware;
- Make you aware of ongoing costs for maintenance and for the inevitable enhancements you will require as your expectations change;
- Design the installation of the computer in such a way that there are built-in incentives for use;
- Train your staff and provide documentation of special procedures;
- Work with you after you buy the computer.

In a recent article, Dick Schoech (1979) warns social work agencies to avoid consultants' proposals that "meet the needs of the consultant" more than the needs of the agency." Consultants who are primarily computer programmers are often more interested in writing programs than in solving your problems. To avoid this syndrome, hire a systems analyst who will analyze work situations and propose improvements. While a systems analyst would hire a programmer in some circumstances, a small social service agency has little direct need for programmers because general-purpose software has made such software an affordable luxury in most circumstances. A computer consultant should be a problem-solver, not a programmer—or a vendor (Martin, 1982).

A second lesson was the amount of resources required to introduce the computer into the ongoing life of the agency. Computers neither install themselves nor run themselves. At least three models have worked: motivation, trial-and-error, and dedicated time. The motivational approach is easier to fall into than to create. Many computer installations have worked only because someone in the office is motivated to spend weekends and evenings pursuing it. The disadvantage of this approach is that the overtime effort is usually not integrated into the ongoing work environment and is difficult for an administrator to follow and control. When the motivated staff member leaves, the office is often left without enough documentation for a smooth transition.

The trial-and-error model is the one originally chosen by Kwawachee. The model is very common. With an inexpensive computer, this is often a cost-effective approach to office automation, even if the machinery sits idle much of the first year. Failure of the other models is not unusual, and they generally result in much higher cost.

The educational benefits of the trial-and-error method can be bought cheaply. Some simple folk wisdom: the first time anyone does something new, the probability of "failure" to produce results is high. It's more appropriate to look for the probability of learning enough to succeed the second or third time. Computers involve some major conceptual changes in the way people do business, and getting the most experience for the least cost from early attempts to use them is a more valid measure of success than how many hours the first machine is used.

The final model, dedicated time, recognizes that changes to ongoing operations have a cost, and allows for dedicated release time for someone in the office, or for someone brought in from outside, to engineer selection, installation, customization, and operation. The result is usually more professional, though the cost may be surprising to folks who expect computers to save money. Operating costs will certainly increase during installation, and some operations run more cheaply without computers. Of course, some more expensive operations are justified by increased output, higher-quality output, a better work environment, or other reasons.

In addition to resources required for setting up the system, the administration needs to budget not only for the initial purchase of the hardware and software, but also for cost-effective enhancements that are continually being brought to market. A second area for ongoing budgeting is the training and development of staff for administering and running the computer. Finally, the staff have to be released from their normal work routine to help fully introduce the computer into the everyday operation of the agency. It is normal procedure in computer installations to run the previous procedures alongside the computer procedures for awhile until everyone has confidence in the new procedures. Unless the agency is able to make these expenditures, the likelihood of rejection of this new implant is high.

The third major lesson was the value of establishing a planning group composed of personnel who have links with the varied board, staff, and administrative constituency that make up the agency personnel. This planning group needs to develop clear ideas about several issues, such as: their process of helping introduce the computer to the varied financial, clerical, training, and service aspects of the agency; their authority (they are legitimized to make a certain set of decisions and not others, and to communicate with varied groups and not others, etc.); their time lines (they need to set realistic time limits for reporting progress or lack of it to staff and administration); and their sources of information about the capabilities, costs, and social aspects of computers.

Another administrative task is to develop with the clerical and support staff a process for hiring, training, and promoting of the people responsible for operating and managing the computer. Still another requirement of administration is the establishment of links with other agencies and other management information systems. Finally, administration should recognize that human-service staff may have built-in resistance to computers, or they may have latent enthusiasm for computers, but they're probably not neutral about computers.

REFERENCES

Martin, James. *Application development without programmers.* Englewood Cliffs, N.J.: Prentice-Hall, 1982.

Rothman, Jack. *Promoting innovation and change in organizations and communities.* New York: Wiley, 1976.

Schoech, Dick. A microcomputer-based human information system. *Administration in Social Work* 1979, 3(4), 423–440.

37

Microcomputer Applications in a Hospital Social Work Department

Michael A. King, DSW

This chapter describes the development, content, and design of several programs developed by the author and designed for use on a microcomputer for a hospital social work department. The hospital is a 485-bed facility with a full range of inpatient and outpatient medical services, a 29-bed inpatient psychiatric unit, a large psychiatric clinic, a large alcoholism clinic, and an inpatient alcohol detoxification unit. With some minor adaptation, the programs I designed can be utilized in individual or group private practice, free-standing clinics and agencies, as well as hospital social work and psychiatric departments. The programs can also be used as a data base system for clinical studies and research.

I became frustrated over the years with the lack of appropriate programs for the human services. Few people who know how to write computer programs are also truly familiar with the mental health and health fields, and the programs that were developed never quite offered what was needed. Generalized data base programs often have the same deficiencies. Furthermore, because they are designed to meet the broadest possible needs, they generally require the user to carry out procedures that are not necessary for the tasks at hand. It was clear to me that a computer would minimize the amount of time spent on tedious tasks as well as provide more and better information than could be accomplished manually. I decided that the way to get what was needed was to take on the task personally.

The programs are being used on an Apple II + computer with 64K, two 5¼-inch disk drives, a 12-inch monitor, and an Epson MX 80 printer. The programs can be translated for use on other microcomputer systems as well as on mainframes (which was recently done).

There are two programs that will be described in detail, the Patient Registry Program and the Statistical Program, both of which have been in operation for some time. The Patient Accounts Program for financial and billing purposes is in the final stage of development. This chapter will describe the overall structure and flow of the programs and the features that facilitate the work.

The programs are user-friendly. They are menu-driven, have instructions clearly noted on the screen at all points, include extensive error-checking so that inappropriate entries will not be accepted and acted upon by the computer, and provide the opportunity to escape from most areas without having to proceed with an unwanted task. There are no codes used in the screen format or the print format that might confuse an operator, and information such as dates are written as one would normally write them, rather than the way computer programs usually demand them. These aspects made the programming task more complex, but greatly simplified data-entry and retrieval in terms of operator error.

PATIENT REGISTRY PROGRAM

This program maintains records on patients known to the hospital social work staff. Two files are set up for each worker, one an alphabetized index of their patients, which contains both the patient's name and the location of the patient's record on the disk. The other file is for the patients' records and contains twelve fields (the patient's name is not part of the actual record; it exists only in the index file), including the date of referral, who referred the patient, age of the patient, service in the hospital that the patient is located on, the status of the case, the date the case is closed, the disposition, and several fields containing information about placement activities to other facilities (Figure 37–1). These fields can be adapted for variations on the data required in other facilities.

The program begins by asking for a password, which can be set to any alphanumeric combination that the user decides on. The password can be changed frequently as desired. This helps to prevent unauthorized access to the information on the files. The current date is also entered, so that you can keep track of when the program was last run.

The main menu, a list of options indicating the general activities that can be performed by the program, is shown below. The operator simply types in the number of the option desired.

1. Enter New Patients
2. Read/Modify Records
3. Print Lists

4. Search
5. Transfer Cases to Closed File
6. Add New Worker
7. Delete Worker or Change Name
8. Stop for Now
9. Utilities

Both the Enter New Patients and Read/Modify Records options bring up a list of staff names. The selection by the operator of a number corresponding to a staff name brings up the specific worker's file. After the number is entered, the patient record form appears on the screen. In the Read/Modify mode, the index of patient names appears on the screen and the user may select the patient record desired. The information for the record can be entered, changed, or updated as needed. Before completing this process, the question is asked on the screen as to whether the data are now correct in order to provide an opportunity to correct typographical errors or other information. If a

```
PATIENT RECORD FOR BRENNAN

PAT: JONES JONATHAN

REF BY: RND               OPENED: 3/2/83

SERV: PSY                 STATUS: CLOSED


AGE: 93                   CL/TR-IN: 3/10/83

            PLACEMENT INFORMATION
            ----------------------------------

PL REF:                    FROM:

ON A/C:                    WHERE PL:


LEVEL PL:                  DATE PL:




CHANGE NEEDED? Y/N &
```

FIGURE 37–1. Sample Patient Registry Record.

patient is being transferred to another worker, the computer will automatically move the patient's record to the file of the new worker, leaving in the original worker's file a notation of the transfer.

The choosing of Option 3, Print Lists, brings a menu to the screen asking which lists are to be printed. The lists that the program provides include caseload lists by worker, which are alphabetical lists of patients and the associated data from the records; a statistical summary of cases opened and closed, age groupings, and all the other information in the records; and a placement list, which contains the names of patients awaiting placement to other facilities. These lists are printed out on a monthly basis for the most part, though the program is set up to produce a printout whenever requested. The printouts also give year-to-date figures for all the information. Once the process is started by the operator, the sorting, tallying, and printing is fully automatic.

The Search option allows the user to search for one or as many as one hundred names to see if patients are already known in the file. This has eliminated the duplication of service that occurred when one worker was opening a case and the patient was already known to another worker elsewhere in the hospital. The use of the search also facilitates communication and reduces work by allowing a worker who may know a patient to provide some of the history information, rather than having to obtain it a second time from the patient.

A binary search method is used so that instead of having to compare a specified name to, say, 1,000 names on the indexes, usually only 3 to 4 comparisons are needed to find a name or determine that it is not in the file. In addition, a wild card search capability is being implemented. If the operator is unsure, for instance, whether a name is spelled *Jensen* or *Jenson*, a question mark can be typed between the s and n of the searched-for name and all names ending in *s-n* will be shown.

The Transfer option provides the ability to transfer out cases that have been closed to a disk containing closed files. This is done at the end of each month, after the various reports have been printed out. It is an entirely automatic process requiring the operator only to start it. The operator can then go on and do other things while the computer handles this task, resulting in only current cases remaining on the active disk. The next two options (Add New Worker, and Delete Worker or Change Name) are for adding a new worker who comes on staff, changing a worker's name (in the case of marriage or divorce), and deleting a worker from the active file. The worker's name and the file of closed cases will still remain on the closed disk for the purpose of searching, but will no longer encumber the active list of workers.

Option 8, Stop for Now, pauses the computer's operation at the point at which it is awaiting the password, so that anybody passing by cannot get any information by pressing the keys, nor can they create possible chaos by playing with them.

The last Option, Utilities, provides access to a series of computer housekeeping tasks. These utilities include a method for starting a new disk, backing up modified disks, getting a printout of the number of cases each worker has on file, and other procedures to facilitate the use of the program.

STATISTICAL PROGRAM

The statistical program operates in similar fashion to the Patient Registry Program. It is menu-driven and allows for many of the same options. This program deals with the variety of activity by staff in relation to patients, patient-related services, and other aspects of their work. A table is set up each month for all the staff, containing time spent in in-

```
DATA FOR FRIEDMAN 1/31/83   HEMO/AMB

           INTERVIEWS    TIME UNITS    COLL TIME
------------------------------------------------------

SCREENING      72             80             3

COVERAGE        0              0             0


GROUP          14             36           XXX

OPEN CASES    120            192            50

ROUNDS        XXX            XXX            38
              ------         ------         ------
  TOTALS      206            308            91
------------------------------------------------------

# CASES OPENED    25 # CASES TR IN        0
------------------------------------------------------
# CASES TR OUT     0 # CASES CLOSED       25
------------------------------------------------------
HRS. WORKED   150     DIR SER %        .66

IS THIS CORRECT? Y/N &
```

FIGURE 37–2. Sample Social Work Activity Report.

dividual, group, family, and collateral treatment, and other activity
(Figure 37–2). Records are therefore accessed for a specific month, and
the computer will inform the user what year's disk is currently in the
drive. In addition to worker activity, the number of hours worked for
each worker, number of cases opened, transferred, and closed are also
in the table. A calculation is done on a running basis as to the percent
of time each staff member spends in providing direct services to patients. Whether entering data or modifying data, the screens shows
one worker's record at a time. Information on each screen also includes
the date of the last entry and the service that the worker is assigned to.
Reports are printed with the current month as well as year-to-date figures, and this can be done for any month and year. Starting a new
month, once the operator clears the disks, will occur automatically. A
new table is set up for the succeeding month, with zeros in each of the
cells. In the same manner, a new year can be started as well.

SUMMARY

My computer programs were designed with certain principles in mind.
They are set up to operate on an interactive basis rather than to be periodically processed in a batch. This means that after each record is written or changed on the screen, the information is rewritten to the disk
so that if a power interruption or other problem occurs, only the last
record that was being dealt with will have been lost. With batch processing, which would hold the writing to the disk until all the information on the records was ready to be entered, the user would run the
risk of having to reenter the entire day's work if there was a power
interruption.

Another principle that is used in setting up the program is that the
operator has to spend the least amount of time at the computer itself.
This is partly done through designing a speedy program operation and
also by structuring the program to allow as much automatic processing
as possible.

Furthermore, the programs are designed in modular fashion so
that program modules to accomplish additional tasks can be easily
added with minimal modification of the main program.

The computerization of these functions has been beneficial in several ways. Retrieval of information about patients has been made fast
and simple, as has the updating of those records. Much of the statistical information about patients and staff activity was impractical to get
on a manual basis, because of the large investment of manpower required. With computerization, not only has there been more information available, but it is available any time it is needed. In the past,

many of the manual reports were received quite late for appropriate action. With the computer, the staff too can receive information easily, which helps them to keep better organized.

The low cost of a microcomputer makes computerization an alternative easily afforded. The cost for the equipment described in the beginning of this article was less than $4,000. The savings in time and the value of the quality of information far exceed the expense. Of course, the microcomputer can also be cost-saving through its use as a word processor for manuals, reports, chart notes, and other needs that could otherwise require extensive retyping.

Lessons That Have Been Learned Implementing a Computerized Management Information System

Jim Newkham
and the Staff at the Heart of Texas
 Mental Health/Mental Retardation
 Center

1. Don't pioneer. If a "canned" program is available, USE IT. Careful reading of Western history indicates that statistically the pioneer lost his scalp more frequently than the settlers following him. So, if you get the pioneering spirit, check the statistics on who loses his scalp.

2. If your manual system is not working, don't try to go up on a computer. It will only compound your problems.

3. If you don't have the full backing and support of the executive and board, you won't survive.

4. Feedback is essential. Upload the information that will be most beneficial to staff first, so that it can be fed back to them.

5. Simplify rather than sophisticate. K.I.S.S. (Keep It Sweet & Simple).

6. Don't put other demands on your staff when trying to put up the system.

7. Always assume hardware and software will be LATE—LATE—LATE—LATE—LATE.

8. Never assume that the programmer knows more about finances

*"Lessons That Have Been Learned Implementing a Computerized Management Information System" originally appeared in *Computer Use in Social Services Network,* 1982, 2 (2), 3, and is reprinted by permission of the author.

and management than you do. He should do no more than write the programs and run the hardware.

9. Train clerks and secretaries first and involve them from Day One. A stable support staff, and we mean down to the last clerk, are the heart of the agency.

10. Be prepared during the implementation stage to work seven days a week, fourteen hours a day to get the system running. Our experience is that the staff are more than willing to make this kind of commitment if they understand how the system will work for them.

11. You will always assume that your tried and trusted manual system is correct and the computer has erred. It takes experience to learn that the manual system has its errors too.

12. Don't expect any help from your peers or funding agencies. They are more likely to be placing bets on your losing your scalp than succeeding.

PART XI

The Computer as Therapy Adjunct

C an a computer do therapy? Whatever the final answer to this question may be, it is clear that the computer has a number of capabilities that can extend and enhance the therapist's impact. Examples of this are the use of the computer to help patients organize their thoughts and feelings about certain issues or to present simulations and games that can assist them in developing greater frustration-tolerance or better long-term planning abilities. Though it is simplistic and vision-limiting to conceive of the computer functioning like a clone of a human therapist, imaginative programs are being developed that seem to be of real therapeutic value. In Part XI some of these applications are examined.

The first two chapters deal with early attempts to program a computer to simulate the functions of a nondirective, Rogerian therapist. The next two present a more recent innovation, the use of computer-based adventure games in therapy. The games present the players with various options as they wend their way through an imaginary world filled with strange creatures and situations generated by the program. Players can fight, run, buy, sell, explore; they can be cautious, bold, impetuous, honest, deceitful, etc. Their decisions have short- and long-term consequences in the game for themselves and for others with whom they are playing. David Allen examines various ways these games may be used in therapy and looks at a variety of commercial programs that may be adapted for use in child therapy. And then in a fascinating study, Betty Clarke and Dick Schoech examine the effects of the therapeutic use of a computer game on adolescents, the reactions of their parents, and the views of agency personnel to their use.

The final chapter in Part XI reviews a study done a number of years ago in which subjects were helped by a program to express their feelings about their personal problems to a microphone-plus-computer system that simulated some aspects of understanding. Even though subjects were informed beforehand that the "understanding" was only simulated, many stated they benefited from the experience in ways that illuminate some aspects of what is therapeutic about therapy.

Eliza
and Her Offspring

Philip DeMuth, PhD

liza is a computer program that simulates a psychotherapeutic interview. Developed by Joseph Weizenbaum and refined by Kenneth Colby at MIT's Artificial Intelligence Laboratory during the
1960s, Eliza is so named because, like Shaw's Eliza Doolittle, Eliza is
educable to the point of appearing to be conversant. Whereas Shaw's
Eliza would mouth pleasantries like "The rain in Spain stays mainly in
the plain," Weizenbaum's Eliza mimics the responses of a psychotherapist. The much-quoted press release announcing Eliza's capabilities
went as follows:

Men are all alike.
IN WHAT WAY?
They're always bugging us about something or other.
CAN YOU THINK OF A SPECIFIC EXAMPLE?
Well, my boyfriend made me come here.
YOUR BOYFRIEND MADE YOU COME HERE—THAT'S
    INTERESTING.
He says I'm depressed much of the time.
I AM SORRY TO HEAR YOU ARE DEPRESSED.
It's true. I am unhappy.

DO YOU THINK COMING HERE WILL HELP YOU NOT TO BE
    UNHAPPY?

(*Later in the session*):

You are afraid of me.
DOES IT PLEASE YOU TO BELIEVE I AM AFRAID OF YOU?
My father is afraid of everybody.
REALLY, EVERYBODY?
My father is very fearful.
WHAT ELSE COMES TO MIND WHEN YOU THINK OF YOUR
    FATHER?
Bullies.

DOES THIS HAVE ANYTHING TO DO WITH THE FACT THAT YOUR BOYFRIEND MADE YOU COME HERE?

Like the early development of Ms. Doolittle, this Eliza convinces the unwary for a time. Eventually, however, her limitations may become apparent. Consider the following transcript:

Yes.
I SEE.
Yes.
I UNDERSTAND.
Yes.
YOU SEEM QUITE POSITIVE.
Yes.
YOU ARE SURE?
Yes.
I SEE.
Good.
I AM NOT SURE I UNDERSTAND YOU FULLY.
Well, I can't explain.
HOW DO YOU KNOW YOU CAN'T EXPLAIN?
How does one know anything?
WHY DO YOU ASK?
Because I don't know.
IS THAT THE REAL REASON?
You're the analyst—you tell me.
WHAT MAKES YOU THINK I AM THE ANALYST—YOU TELL YOU?

That's what the promotional material said. Eliza achieves its conversational verisimilitude with the aid of a few neat tricks. After the user types in a sentence, Eliza scans it for the presence of any of her preprogrammed keywords. These keywords are words to which Eliza is cued to formulate specific responses. They are arranged in a hierarchical order, so that in case a sentence contains two keywords, the most important one will be used in framing a response. In the above example, Eliza found the keyword *alike* at the end of the first sentence, which cued its canned answer of "In what way?" In the second sentence, the keyword was *always*, causing Eliza to respond by asking for a specific example. Eliza transforms certain words reflexively, so that *you* becomes *I*, *your* becomes *my*, and so forth. Because English is such a complicated language, it is easy for Eliza to make transformational mistakes, as it did in the last sentence quoted. Eliza also will concatenate part of the input sentence with the canned response, if necessary.

In the first example, *unhappy* is taken from the client's sentence and appended to "Do you think coming here will help you to not be—." Eliza typically has several possible responses for each keyword, to add variation. Four responses to the keyword *yes* are shown in the second example. If no keywords are found, a neutral statement, such as "Tell me more about it," is presented, or a previous input string is called up from memory—as it did in making the impressive connection between *bullies* and the client's boyfriend. However, Eliza would have responded the same way even if the client had typed in *artichokes* instead of *bullies*. In other words, it was a lucky guess. But then, sometimes psychotherapists get lucky, too.

Several different versions of Eliza are available to microcomputer owners. They are advertised in the popular computer magazines and will not be reviewed here. The significant limitation to these programs from the mental health professional's point of view is that they are written in an entertainment format. Thus, Radio Shack's Eliza program includes a number of joke responses. Other versions are more bland, but they are usually devoid of significant psychotherapeutic content, having been devised as "Gee Whiz" programs intended primarily to demonstrate the wonders of the computer itself. To those interested in exploring the structure of Eliza in BASIC, a serviceable listing is provided in David Ahl's *More Basic Computer Games* (Ahl, 1979). Long gone, apparently, is Colby's original modification of Eliza, known as Doctor, which contained an extensive lexicon of keywords and responses and was fashioned with psychotherapy in mind. Researchers wishing to experiment with Eliza will probably have to develop or refine their own versions of it. What is more, these will almost certainly need to be compiled, because the BASIC language versions of it run too slowly to sustain user interest.

Meanwhile, a moral debate has developed. Weizenbaum and Colby parted company, and Weizenbaum's views on computerized psychotherapy have soured. In *Computer Power and Human Reason* (1976), he declares computerized psychotherapy to be immoral and obscene, the sort of thing of which "the very contemplation ought to give rise to feelings of disgust in every civilized person" (p. 269). This is so, Weizenbaum explains, because the computer fails to provide interpersonal respect and understanding, not because it is technically incapable of functioning as an effective psychotherapist.

Imagine that Eliza were perfected to the point where every disorder in the Diagnostic and Statistical Manual of the American Psychiatric Association could be cured by it in one hour. Exponents of Weizenbaum's position would still be forced to conclude that it should not be used, since a priori their moral insight lets them know that nonhuman therapy is immoral and obscene. But the moral good thus secured would be vitiated by the loss of the ability to help a large number of people with mental illness. The ethics of computerized psychotherapy are not a one-sided affair.

Although Eliza cannot claim to offer interpersonal respect and understanding (except vicariously, from the programmer), it does possess some advantages over human therapists. It is never tired. It does not get impatient or become enmeshed in countertransference difficulties. It is not concerned with the fight it had with its wife or husband that morning when it is supposed to be listening to clients, or wishing it were on the golf course. It works twenty-four hours a day for a few cents' worth of electricity. And Eliza does not have sex with clients.

Eliza is often described as a Rogerian-type therapist, but this is only approximately true. While Eliza is extremely nonjudgmental and nonpossessive, it cannot be said to be "warm" unless the computer is overheating, or unless we refer to the "warmth" of the preprogrammed responses themselves. Similarly, Eliza cannot be said to be genuine or congruent, except in the sense that it is genuinely a computer program functioning as a human therapist might. This brings up the important question of how Eliza is presented to prospective clients. If Eliza is packaged as an electronic therapist, a Carl Rogers with a rheostat, people are likely to be disappointed—especially at the present stages of its development. However, if Eliza is presented as a tool that people might use to stimulate their own thinking about issues of emotional concern to them, more satisfying results may be achieved.

The genuineness requirement is best fulfilled by the human agent who introduces Eliza to the uninitiated. Eliza is capable of making some reflective statements and probing for feelings underlying the user's words. But often it intervenes or interprets in a way that a strict Rogerian would never do. When it does deviate, it can do so in the service of some alternative but compatible therapeutic model. Eliza can be eclectic. Below I list some of the schools that were drawn from in developing the version of Eliza found in my *Psychological Diary* (DeMuth, 1982).

Rational-Emotive Therapy. Eliza can pick up a number of keywords associated with *irrational ideas* (Ellis, 1962) and challenge them. For example, "I should—" is met with "Who says you should—?" "Horrible," "Awful," and "Terrible" are matched with, e.g., "Awful, or merely unpleasant?" "I need—" is paired with "You mean, you want—." "I can't—" is paired with "You mean, you won't—."

Gestalt Therapy. Fritz Perls once claimed that all psychotherapy could be done using just three sentences: "What do you want?"; "What are you doing?"; and "What are you feeling?" (Perls, 1973). These form the thrust of Eliza's standard responses when no keywords are located in the user's input string. In addition, certain emotions are explored dialectically, as described in the Gestalt literature (Stevens, 1971). "I resent—" becomes "I think you also appreciate—." "Afraid of—" becomes "I think you are also attracted to—." Eliza also responds to the user's questions by asking that they be turned into statements, another common Gestalt technique.

Transactional Analysis. On most Eliza programs, the typical opening line is "Please state your problem." According to Robert and Mary Goulding, a superior opening gambit is "What would you like to change today?" This suggests to the client (a) that change is possible; (b) that the client will be doing it; and (c) that the client might do it today, rather than ruminate on some vague "problem." Analysis of scripts, games, and ego states are, for the time being, beyond Eliza's reach.

Neuro-Linguistic Programming. This new school, however pretentious in some of its elaborations, provides an intriguing theoretical basis for Eliza. Briefly put, NLP borrows a number of metaphors from transformational linguistics. It assumes that people's options in the real world are limited not so much by the real world itself as by their private unconscious cognitive maps of that world—their *deep structure.* The distortions in their deep structure are in turn apparent in their verbal strings—the *surface structure.* By noting the problems in the surface structure, the client can be helped to redraw his or her mental map in a more accurate manner (Bandler & Grinder, 1976). Eliza serves this end by challenging hidden generalizations in the input sentences. Words like *it, thing, anybody,* and *always* are aligned with responses such as, "Which person in particular?"; "Really, always?"; or "When you say 'it,' I wonder if you are really talking about yourself?"

Eliza has several tantalizing future prospects. McLuhan (1967) has pointed out some of the difficulties in assessing and predicting the future of any new technology. First, we tend to approach the future looking into the rear-view mirror, assuming a linearity with the past. Secondly, the new technology is traditionally made to do the work of the old before it comes into its own. Films contained stage plays, television contained radio shows, and microcomputers in psychiatry and psychology do psychological testing, billing, office management, and possibly psychotherapy. But the larger impact of microcomputers on our personalities will likely be in the way they restructure our social environment, not in how they do psychotherapy. Nevertheless, several possibilities for Eliza are now apparent.

First, with the increasing capabilities of pocket computers, it is feasible to program a version of Eliza to run on them. This will make it possible (as Fritz Perls once advised, although in a way he never intended) for people to carry their therapists around in their pockets. Such a device could be loaned out by practicing psychotherapists to their patients as an adjunct to psychotherapy, in much the same way as home biofeedback machines are used as ancillary treatment.

Second, Eliza can be made to interact with personality test data. In a rudimentary way, this has already been done in the *Psychological Diary*. It can in principle be done in a much more sophisticated way. Instead of offering the same set of responses to everyone, Eliza's therapeutic replies could be tailored to each individual, drawing from test data for fruitful areas of exploration much as a human therapist might.

Third, it is presently possible to add on to Eliza data from the client's Galvanic Skin Response. Topics which appear emotionally charged (as measured by the GSR) could be selected for special focus by the program.

Fourth, Eliza could be made available to people over interactive television, allowing home users to load the core program into their terminal and discourse with Eliza by means of the television set and keyboard.

Fifth, as voice recognition is achieved over the next twenty years, Eliza could be attached to a telephone. Anyone in the world could call Eliza's number, talk for as long as he or she wished, and simply have a small fee added to his or her monthly telephone bill for the service.

If Eliza is to fulfill its potential, extensive research will first be necessary. Which version of Eliza is most helpful to which patient populations? What are the possible hazards associated with its use? How does Eliza compare with no treatment, placebo, and human therapists? These are among the many questions that remain for researchers to address. While the moral questions surrounding its use will never be wholly answered by the empirical questions on its efficacy, data concerning its therapeutic possibilities ought to be collected and carefully weighed. If Eliza can be programmed to be an effective therapist, either in its own right, or as an adjunct to treatment by human practitioners, then perhaps it would be well for the public, as informed consumers, to decide its fate, rather than for computerized psychotherapy to be condemned in advance by technological savants.

REFERENCES

Ahl, David. *More basic computer games*. Morris Plains, N.J.: Creative Computing Press, 1979.

Bandler, R., & Grinder, J. *The structure of magic*. Vol. 1. Palo Alto, California: Science & Behavior Books, 1976.

DeMuth, P. *Psychological diary*. Cleveland: Psychological Systems, 1982.

Ellis, A. *Reason and emotion in psychotherapy*. New York: Citadel Press, 1962.

Goulding, M. and R. *Changing lives through redecision therapy*. San Francisco: Brunner/Mazel, 1979.

McLuhan, M. *The medium is the massage.* New York: Bantam Books, 1967.

Perls, F. *The gestalt approach & eyewitness to therapy.* New York: Bantam, 1973.

Stevens, J. *Awareness.* New York: Bantam, 1971.

Weizenbaum, J. *Computer power and human reason.* San Francisco: W. H. Freeman, 1976.

40 | The Use of Computer Fantasy Games in Child Therapy

David H. Allen, MD

"...the child is given the opportunity to play out his accumulated feelings of tension, frustration, insecurity, aggression, fear, bewilderment, confusion.

"By playing out these feelings he brings them to the surface, gets them out in the open, faces them, learns to control them, or abandons them. When he has achieved emotional relaxation, he begins to realize the power within himself to be an individual in his own right, to think for himself, to make his own decisions, to become psychologically more mature, and by so doing, to realize selfhood." —V. Axline

---

Play therapy has been a primary mode of working with children for many years, since children often have difficulty working in a direct talking mode. Children express their conflicts and feelings in their play, and this has been found to be a useful approach in therapy. Fantasy allows the client to experience something at a safe distance, and to experience something that he is not yet ready for in real life. He can repeat an experience many times and gain mastery over it in the process.

Recently fantasy has become more acceptable with adults in guided imagery, and in hypnotherapy. Dreams have been felt for many years to play an important role in working through daily as well as life-long conflicts. Stories have been useful therapy adjuncts for centuries. Fairy tales, parables, and even novels have been used therapeutically, some since Biblical times. They bypass the conscious defenses and have impact more directly on the unconscious. Methods have been refined utilizing stories as therapeutic techniques, as outlined in Dr. Richard Gardner's *Therapeutic Communication with Children*, and in David Gordon's *Therapeutic Metaphors*. I refer you to the references for a more complete description of play therapy principles.

The computer fantasy games add a new dimension to these techniques, in that they allow the operator to more fully enter into an identification with the characters in the story by allowing the operator some control over the characters' actions. The child actually experiences first-hand in the therapy session encounters and events with which he is required to cope as part of the play. His responses reveal his coping strategies. It also offers the therapist a chance to intervene therapeutically, immediately, and also to relate it to other areas of the child's life. The child can repeatedly play it until he masters it, under the close supervision, support, and guidance of his therapist.

This chapter will deal with my experiences over nine months with one particular fantasy game, Ultima, from California Pacific Computer Co., which runs on the Apple II+ personal computer. It is a game that I happened upon by accident; while playing I was impressed with the therapeutic potential. There are many other similar games that may be as useful in a therapy setting, depending on the particular problem.

Ultima is basically a Dungeons and Dragons adventure game, but uses only one character, rather than a group. This character is created by the player, within guidelines, and also named by the player. His progress is saved each week on his own disk, allowing any number of players to play at different times, each with his own character, and at different stages of the game. The player can be a fighter, wizard, cleric, or a thief, each class giving him special abilities and handicaps. Many of the rules of the game are learned by experience and by making mistakes, much as happens in real life. The therapist can act as a mentor, guiding the child along the way or as someone to provide support.

The player begins with a limited number of hit points, which are depleted as he is hit in battle; no experience points; a small amount of gold and food; plus simple weapons and armor. If he can find his way to town without getting attacked and "killed" (by losing all his hit points) or by running out of food, he can buy better weapons, armor, and food. If he has obtained some experience points (through his encounters) he may also purchase magic spells. While it is possible to find many moralistic objections to a game of "killing," I prefer to utilize it as a metaphor for mastering difficulties (when he kills a monster), or for making a mistake or a loss of self-esteem (when he gets "killed" or loses hit points).

If our adventurer gets "killed" (or I should say "when"), then he is resurrected—but without weapons or money and a very limited supply of food. He then has to learn to utilize what he has and can do with that, rather than with what he had previously.

While in the town he may go to the pub and purchase a "brew," and in the process he may obtain information there regarding the object of the game (there is also a surprise penalty for drinking too much).

When he happens upon a castle, he may offer himself in service to the king and obtain a quest. Fulfilling these quests will either make him a more powerful character or help him obtain something necessary for completing the ultimate quest of the game. The king also has a princess locked up in his castle, which the child must eventually rescue to complete the game. This is no easy task, but it is rewarding.

The game is done in high-resolution graphics, with a layout of the land, complete with mountains, forests, oceans, and plains. Scattered about are towns and cities, but also dungeons, which the child can enter searching for a certain quest or to obtain gold. The player can also gain in hit points after a successful venture into a dungeon. Each dungeon has ten levels, each level with more powerful and dangerous monsters, but also with greater rewards. One must muster up the courage and a successful strategy to eventually probe the dungeons to their deepest levels.

From the above description, those who are analytically oriented can see much symbolic significance in the game. This is probably best left in the metaphor, however.

One seven-year-old boy was having difficulty adjusting to his parents' divorce, with resultant symptoms of anxiety, fears, and inhibition. He first ventured into the game as a cleric. After getting "killed" several times and feeling rather unsuccessful, he asked if he could change characters. He wanted to become a thief. I allowed him to make this change, and he immediately tried to steal weapons and armor. These attempts also met with little success, and he settled down with a more honest attempt. No effort was made on my part to bring the underlying conflicts into consciousness. His symptoms subsided enough that his mother and I decided, in consideration of other circumstances, that he could safely discontinue therapy.

The structure of the game itself has therapeutic implications. The child who is overly timid gets "killed" more readily than the one who is more aggressive. Also, the child who is impulsive is more likely to get "killed" often. By behavioral means, the impulsive child learns to plan ahead and be more cautious, while the timid child learns to be more adventurous and to take risks. The insight that the child can learn something useful from his experiences is to me one of the more valuable contributions of the game, for although he may get "killed," his experience points continue to rise, and he can return with new knowledge to master the previous difficult encounter.

The therapist may take several different roles. First of all, he can act as a mentor that the client can turn to for suggestions or advice, leaving the child free to choose his own course. The child learns that he may profit from following this advice. To avoid too much dependency, the therapist may at times encourage him to learn on his own by trying different alternatives. This can be useful in setting the stage for utilizing the therapist for real-life problems.

Another role is to provide support for the frustration that arises during the game, and to help the player learn the appropriate lesson from his painful experiences. One player would buy equipment but forget to "ready" it to use, and find it would get stolen from his inventory; or he would go into the dungeon without his armor. Since armor cannot be put on inside the dungeon, he would lose a number of hit points unnecessarily before he could get back out. I could empathize with him, since I had been through it before myself, and also I could point out the need and value of planning ahead. Later he went into space, did not keep a map of where he had gone, and became lost, unable to find his way back to Earth. He lost the whole session of play that day and was very frustrated. Later his mother reported that he had told her it was his fault, because he did not plan ahead. He came back to the next session eager to map out space and accomplish his mission.

The therapist may identify and confront maladaptive defenses. The same youngster mentioned above would protect his ego by projecting the blame onto others. Once he went into the depths of the dungeon to find and kill a particular monster, which was his quest. He met many others on this search, which he readily dispatched, but with the loss of hit points in the process. He was down to about 150 hit points from 1,500, and asked me whether he should go back up. I advised him that he could not stand many more attacks like that. He took a few steps and met a monster who took 160 hits from him in the first blow, thus "killing" him. He became very upset, blaming me for what happened. This was a typical defense, projecting his inadequacies onto others. I was able to empathize with his frustration, while at the same time not accepting responsibility for his decisions. He gradually began accepting responsibility himself for what happened to his character. Another time he was busily moving between two different locations in order to build up his character, and he did not notice his dwindling food supply. He was shocked and then frustrated when the screen notified him that he was "dead," and then resurrected with only a fraction of the hit points he had previously achieved, and no gold or weapons. I was able to empathize with him, since I had endured many similar experiences in playing the game, and I was able to point out the need to be attentive to several things that were important, rather than to pursue a single goal without concern for other factors.

A third role is to utilize the experiences in the game and apply them to the patient's real-life problems. One student, although he was 13 years of age, was very much tied to home and was not getting along with his peers. Efforts to work therapeutically with him in traditional ways did relieve his presenting symptom of trichotillomania; however, his peer relations remained poor and he avoided any interaction with them. He related to me pretty much as a peer, and his motto was "bug and get bugged." He took to the computer game eagerly, and instead of turning the clock ahead to end the session early, he tried to turn it back to get more time. We interacted more cooperatively after that, enjoying an activity together, rather than being antagonists. He played cautiously, gradually becoming more adventuresome and taking more risks. As he played he became more relaxed, to the point where he could respond to questions about his school day. He associated his peers with the monsters in the game, who had become less frightening as his ability to cope with them had increased. This opened up the possibility of looking at other ways of coping with the "monsters" in his real world.

As you can see from the above, the game is quite complex. It takes a child approximately 9–10 months to complete, playing at the rate of 45 minutes per week. Length of time to finish varies depending on his age, intellectual functioning, and luck. Younger children and those with more fragile egos need more guidance and assistance to keep from being overwhelmed by defeat. One 7-year-old boy with fragile ego development refused to play again after getting killed. This was useful to me in understanding his coping abilities, however.

Children who have completed therapy with the game appear to have more self confidence, a sense of mastery, more willingness to accept responsibility for themselves, and less stigma about having been in therapy.

Dr. Ron Levy, as quoted in *Softline* magazine, prefers the game Wizardry over Ultima, because he thinks it is more subjective. By this I assume he means that more is left to your imagination. It utilizes six characters working together, but this limits the number of patients who can play the game with the same disk. It is probably too complex for some younger players.

Softalk describes a social services agency utilizing Synergistic Software's Odyssey adventure as a therapeutic device. This game reportedly will insure that if you are evil, you will run into many similar characters to make your progress more difficult.

Some other computer games I am familiar with that have therapeutic promise are Crush, Crumble and Chomp, from Automated Simulations, and Interactive Fiction from Adventure International. Crush, Crumble and Chomp allows you to create and be a monster, which after wreaking havoc and destruction, eventually gets killed, resulting in a "triumph for civilization." Interactive Fiction creates a scenario in which you respond to another character by typing in a response on the keyboard. The character then responds in different ways, depending on your input. This mode could be designed purposely for therapeutic gains, so that the patient finds, in certain types of interactions, that utilizing particular coping mechanisms would most likely lead to un-satisfactory consequences, and that other methods would give more fa-vorable outcomes. The patient could experiment with different meth-ods of interaction within the safety and privacy of a computer, before deciding what to try in real life. This would help to teach flexibility in his interactions.

We are just at the beginning of finding ways to utilize a computer in a therapeutic setting, and the possibilities are only as limited as one's imagination. Should we try to design games to fulfill specific therapeutic needs? This should be experimented with; however, I sus-pect that the unconscious of the games' creators plus the collective un-conscious of all those who buy a game and make it a best-seller may more accurately fulfill these needs than would our attempts to do this with specific therapeutic goals in mind.

Research needs to be done on just what measurable therapeutic gains can be made utilizing a computer. But of course this continues to be true about any form of psychotherapy.

REFERENCES

Adams, III, R. R. Come cast a spell with me. *Softline*, March 1982, *1*, 30–36.

Axline, V. M. *Play therapy*. New York: Ballantine Books, 1969. (Originally pub-lished in 1947.)

Gardner, R. A. *Therapeutic communication with children*. New York: Science House, 1971.

Gordon, D. *Therapeutic metaphors*. Meta Publications: Cupertino, California, 1978.

Harrison, J. F., & McDermott, J. F., Jr. (Eds.). *Psychiatric treatment of the child*. New York: Jason Aronson, Inc., 1977.

Miller, J. Lutheran social servants. *Softalk*, May 1982, *2*, 85.

Schaefer, C. E. (Ed.). *Therapeutic use of child's play*. New York: Jason Aronson, Inc., 1976.

41

A Computer-Assisted Therapeutic Game for Adolescents: Initial Development and Comments

Betty Clarke, MSSW
Dick Schoech, PhD

When computers first became available, they were used to automate existing processes, e.g., word processing, bookkeeping. Today, computers are being used to automate processes designed with computer technology in mind and not possible without it, e.g., videogames and artificial intelligence. This same progression is occurring in therapeutic uses of computers. Initially, therapeutic computer applications automated existing processes, such as testing and data analysis. We are now approaching therapeutic applications that are not possible without the computer and are specifically designed to make maximum use of the computer's capabilities—for example, medication-matching and biofeedback.

This chapter presents an application that uses the unique capabilities of the computer to help solve a therapeutic problem. It describes the development and testing of an adolescent therapeutic computer game that uses the rapid-branching and looping capabilities of computer programming to help adolescents learn impulse control. In addition to describing the game, its theoretical base, and the results of the preliminary testing, this chapter describes the clients', parents', and colleagues' reactions and the impact on the organization in which the game was tested. The focus of this chapter is not on computer technology, because the game uses relatively standard technology, but on the application of technology to a complex therapeutic problem and on the

The therapeutic computer game described in this chapter was developed as part of the requirements for the Master of Science in Social Work at the University of Texas at Arlington. Further information on the therapeutic game may be obtained by writing to the authors.

introduction of a new technology into an organization. It concludes with a discussion of problems involved in therapeutic games and the future prospects. In essence, this chapter describes a relatively sophisticated therapeutic use of standard computer technology and the experience and problems that the authors encountered in the design, development, and testing process.

ADOLESCENCE, THERAPY, AND COMPUTER GAMES

Adolescents typically resent treatment. They view the therapist as another authority figure forcing them to obey the rules, and they resent being labeled as "the problem." Often parents literally force them to attend treatment; as a result, the therapist faces typical problems encountered in working with involuntary clients. When parents leave the room in the intake interview, adolescents often express their anger, fear, and resentment towards therapy by such statements as "you want to get into my head" or "you can't make me do anything." Some just shrug their shoulders and sulk when interviewed.

While adolescents hate therapy, they love computer games. The computer game arcades are proliferating in malls and shopping centers. Grocery stores have been known to rearrange their shelves to find an area where they can add a few machines to make extra money. Home video games have found an extensive market as youth entertainment products.

Given that computer games are highly motivating to youth, it is natural to ask whether a computer game could be made to deliver therapeutic benefits during the course of play. To test this hypothesis requires specifying the population to be treated, the adolescent problems the game addresses, the therapy the game is to deliver, and the design of the game.

The Population

Adolescence has been defined as the no-man's land between childhood and adulthood (Kraus, 1980). This definition reflects the tumultuous behavior characteristic of adolescence in our society. A more precise definition is that adolescence is the period of life between the onset of puberty and physical maturity (Lidz, 1968; Coppersmith, 1967). This maturation process usually occurs somewhere between the ages of 10 and 22, depending on the individual. During this period, adolescents move toward independence from parents to dependence on peer groups. The moving away from parents as models may spread to relationships with other adults, such as teachers and counselors. This growing independence from authority, coupled with the awakening of sexual drives, physical growth, and social awareness creates uncertainty and recklessness as the adolescents test their own capabilities (Lidz, 1968).

The Problem

A frequent problem of adolescents is low impulse-control. Adolescents with low impulse-control arrive at the intake interview with varied behavioral problems, such as fighting, skipping school, drug or alcohol abuse, low grades, stealing, and lying. Generally adolescents are unsure why they do things wrong. They are angered easily and threatened by authority figures. Many adolescents express an awareness of society's rules, but feel they just can't help themselves. When asked about self-control, they make statements that suggest that self-control is desirable, but difficult to obtain. They express remorse for their problem behaviors, but claim they are unable to control themselves at times. Lidz (1968) defines the problem of impulse control as the ability to maintain self-control while struggling with new sensations and their attendant demands. Researchers have suggested that a lack of impulse control is not a personality deficiency as much as a lack of self-statements that inhibit behaviors (Kendall, 1977; Meichenbaum, 1977).

According to Kraus (1980), adolescents are being institutionalized at an alarming rate, and tailoring treatment strategies especially for adolescents is recommended. Colby (1980) says the drop in psychiatrists from the former 20% to 25% of medical students to 5% to 8% at present, combined with the growing public demand for therapy, suggests that computers must become involved in treatment. Once standardization and system development is complete, cost of computer-based treatment is lower per patient than traditional treatment (Sidowski, Johnson, & Williams, 1980).

Therapeutic Base of the Computer Game

To design a successful therapeutic adolescent computer game requires finding a therapeutic base. The authors based the game on existing treatment modalities in order to avoid developing a totally new therapy, to increase the likelihood of treatment success, and to insure the game was not perceived as simply a game with no valid therapeutic underpinnings.

According to Wagman (1980), several problems exist in applying computers to psychotherapy. The first problem is that free association with computers is difficult and awkward. The second problem is that psychotherapy deals with the emotional rather than thought content of people. Also, only limited technology is presently available. To avoid these problems, a review of therapies relevant to the problem of impulse-control and adaptable to computer game design was undertaken.

Fantasy and therapy often go together (Schoettle, 1980). The idea is that therapeutic "work" can be accomplished in a state of relaxation, which allows clients to practice a new habit or attitude before facing a difficult situation (Chambless & Goldstein, 1979; Coppersmith, 1967). Lidz (1968) states that active fantasies help adolescents ward off impulsive acts that create danger and the fear of a loss of control.

An accepted form of treatment with children, which combines fantasy and therapy, is play therapy. The notion is that play is the natural place for the child to experience self-expression (Axline, 1969). The child is given the opportunity to play out feelings of tension, aggression, fear, and confusion. The child is able to recognize that he or she is an individual capable of making decisions and gaining control. Computer fantasy games appear to have the same appeal for adolescents. They present an opportunity to make choices, to strive for a goal, and to accept consequences in a fantasy world, thus allowing the player a place to express feelings without the fear of retaliation (Malone, 1981).

Another therapeutic modality often used in conjunction with computers is behavior therapy. One recent change in behavior therapy has been the recognition of the role of cognition in human behavior. Cognitive behavior therapists have accepted the notion that changing thought can change feelings and behavior (Chambless & Goldstein, 1979).

Many researchers (Beck, 1976; Colby, 1980; Mahoney, 1977) have found that cognitive therapy is one of the best modalities for implementation on a computer. In cognitive therapy, the patient becomes engaged in a revision of beliefs, expectations, and values. Adolescents have various dysfunctional beliefs and it is the cognitive therapist's role to challenge and/or change these beliefs (DiGuiseppe, 1981). Internalizing these changes is critical in the development of voluntary control (Lidz, 1968; Meichenbaum & Goodman, 1971).

Two techniques are primarily used by cognitive therapists working with impulsive children: (1) teaching children to consider alternate methods of solving problems and (2) teaching self-statements to help children cope with making errors, for example, "mistakes are part of learning" (Edleson, 1981; Wagman, 1980; Williams & Akamatsu, 1978). Meichenbaum and Goodman (1971) suggest that any program designed to develop self-control should provide training and task comprehension, produce self-regulating attitudes, and show how to use them to control nonverbal behaviors.

Computer Game Design

Computer games have been researched by a large number of people. Many articles have been written discussing effective methods, game design, and the public enjoyment (Adams, 1980; Malone, 1981; Stuck,

1979). Several issues of *Byte* magazine (December 1980 and 1982) were devoted to computer games. Besides hardware and software, computer game design should consider the age and sex of the players, the length of the game, the introduction and instructions, amount and content of feedback, and ways of termination (Stuck, 1979).

Crawford (1982) states that the biggest difficulty in computer game design is to make the game challenging to the human player. Either computer games must be enhanced through techniques of artificial intelligence or humans must be somehow limited in their ability to respond. One of the ways Crawford recommends handicapping game players is to limit information; however, care must be given so that the lack of information stirs the imagination rather than causing confusion and frustration. Other suggestions by Crawford for designing entertaining games include allowing players both offensive and defensive strategies, providing scores that reflect a player's improved level of play, and insuring that the game appears winnable.

Malone (1981) discusses the design of computer games in terms of what was liked by the children, adolescents, and adults he interviewed and observed. Although verbal games were popular, graphics were preferred. Other important characteristics were challenge, curiosity, involvement of others, and fantasy. Challenge was related to the outcome's being clearly defined, yet uncertain. Involvement of others was related to a multiperson game. Curiosity was related to choice being novel and surprising. Fantasy, he speculated, derived its appeal from satisfying emotional needs. Games that set clear, specific goals for winning were seen as more challenging and attractive, and games in which the computer kept the score were more popular.

In summary, a computer game was seen as a potential tool in the treatment of adolescents with low impulse-control. Based upon the literature, cognitive therapy was chosen as the appropriate therapeutic base and the game design was a fantasy, role-playing game in which clients won or lost points based on their decisions.

THE COMPUTER GAME

Description of the Game

The therapeutic game was developed to provide adolescents with support and advice without causing anger and resentment towards treatment. The game was to provide incentives for attending therapy and to remove the stigma typically associated with the concept of self-control and replace it with interest in attaining self-control.

The game developed was similar to Dungeons and Dragons and

Adventure (Adams, 1980). The setting for the game was an underground cave, which the players explored by giving commands and making decisions. The computer presented scenarios with a list of three to four possible decisions. The client then chose the best decision among the alternatives. Points were added or subtracted depending on the correctness of the choice. Correct choices were those that would be made by a person with high impulse-control. Low impulse-control choices were also presented, but always resulted in problems, i.e., an impulsive solution would have negative future consequences.

The game was designed with 10 rooms and 16 decision points. Each player had a score, which the computer tallied, based on the client's decisions. Five points were given to clients at the beginning and clients were told they would lose points for bad decisions. Surprise bonus points were added for good decisions and good attitudes at specific intervals. When players lost all their points, they lost the game. In order to win the game, the player had to retrieve the king's crown, which was located somewhere in the cave.

Cognitive therapy impulse-control techniques were incorporated into the game design through the concept of "coaching." Game decisions were based on the specific behaviors and attitudes targeted for change. The computer introduced problem-solving skills, new self-statements, and reinforced the client for positive attitudes as well as nonimpulsive decisions. A character named Mentor was created to provide this feedback and coaching. Mentor dialogue encouraged self-reflection in the thought processes and attitudes associated with good impulse-control. The following impulse-control attitudes and behaviors were imbedded in the coaching dialogue:

1. Planning is important.
2. Think before you act.
3. Consider alternatives carefully.
4. Keep your goals in mind.
5. Remember to consider the consequences.

The following are examples of Mentor's positive self-statements.

1. Even though you have made a mistake, you are learning to be a good decision-maker.
2. One of the reasons you were chosen for this adventure is because of your leadership potential. Everyone makes mistakes, but you can learn to make fewer mistakes. Believe in yourself.
3. Good for you! Believe in yourself. You have won a bonus point.

Clients were allowed to terminate the game if they did not wish to face the consequences of a bad decision, or if they felt they were not learning from the game. The game would ask: "Would you like to quit this game and start fresh another time?" If the clients were ambivalent, i.e., not wanting to face the consequences but not wanting to quit the game, the computer would print "If you do not wish to quit this game then you must return. I will take you there." The player was returned to the last position in the game.

The game was written in a programming language called BASIC using a DEC-20 computer and a Teletype model 43 printing terminal. A CRT (cathode ray tube, a T.V.-like screen) was not available at the testing facility. Although in the beginning the lack of a CRT was thought to be disadvantageous, it turned out to be an advantage, because each time a client played the game, a hard copy from the printer was available for study. Since the game was written and did not involve computer graphics, the hard copy helped clients review the situations presented. The printouts were also useful in discussing the game session with the client.

After the design and programming were complete, a pretest was conducted using two male adolescents from a local junior high school. These adolescents expressed surprise and pleasure to think of self-control as a task to learn and practice. Based on the pretest, game instructions were clarified so that the players could proceed without supervision by the researcher. Mentor's comments were changed to make them seem less authoritarian and more supportive.

Illustration of a Sample Game Session

The game began with a statement to the client that it would teach self-control. An introduction to the point system and instructions were presented as follows. (Computer-generated print is in roman and client responses are in italics.)

What is your name?
Betty.
Hello. Betty, do you need instructions? Yes or no?
Yes.

This program is designed to improve self-control. It provides an opportunity for you to practice making decisions in a fantasy adventure. The skills you learn can be applied to making decisions in your everyday life.

You will be given 5 "hit" points at the beginning of your adventure. You will be asked to make decisions during your adventure. Good choices will earn additional "hit" points. Poor choices will cause you to lose hit points. If you lose all of your hit points, you lose the game.

After the decision has been made and the action taken according to your instructions, the computer will tell you the results or consequences of your choice. Sometimes additional feedback will be provided by a character named Mentor.

Are you ready to begin your adventure, Betty? Yes or no?
Yes.

(An introduction to the fantasy was next. The client was presented with a self-statement describing the client as a "leader.")

Adventure of Lost Loch

King Tripoli of the Kingdom of Lost Loch has offered 5000 gold pieces to you if you can successfully lead a journey through the dreaded Cave of Darkness to bring back his crown. The crown was stolen 1 year ago by a wicked duke who is hiding in the cave gathering supporters. The duke claims he is going to be the new ruler soon. A number of previous attempts to get the crown have been unsuccessful. Only one person has returned and his memory has been tampered with.

How old are you? Type your number of years.
10.

Though you are very young, Betty, you have been chosen because of your bravery and leadership potential. The king is 91 years old and is too old to lead the mission himself. He is depending on you.

Three other characters were created to help players on their quest. These characters were: Tycho, a fighter; Marta, a magic-user; and Brochi, a thief. They made suggestions regarding decisions and used their special skills when needed. The idea was to provide the client with an opportunity to role-play a decision-making interaction with other characters. The characters, which were based upon personalities found in other adventure games, were selected because they represented behaviors often present in impulsive clients, i.e., fighting, stealing, and relying on luck or believing in magical solutions. The characters were explained as follows:

The king has selected volunteers for your support:
Tycho—He is a fighter with 10 years combat experience. He is the only survivor of a previous expedition. He only remembers entering the cave.
Marta—She is a 2nd level magic-user with 3 spells. They are web, mirror, and charm.
Brochi—He is a thief who has great speed and a good ear.

The first decision the player faced was who should enter the cave first. The computer gave a hint of the correct answer. When the choice was incorrect, Mentor provided feedback and a point was deducted.

> You are at the cave entrance and discuss your assault on the cave. All members agree that a strong, experienced fighter should go first in case of an attack. You want to go first, but the other members say the leader must be protected. You decide.
> 1. Marta goes first.
> 2. Tycho goes first.
> 3. Betty goes first.
> Type 1, 2, or 3?
> *1.*
>
> Marta enters the cave slowly and carefully. She hears a rustling sound and looks up into the eyes of a giant rat! The rat jumps.
>
> **
> Mentor says—though Marta is an experienced wizard, she is not a fighter. Marta has no sword and has to use one of her spells when called upon to defend the group. You have made a mistake and must face the consequences. Remember to consider all of the options before you choose an action. Are you ready? Input yes or no.
> **
> *Yes.*
>
> Marta screams then remembers to "web" the rat, but not before the rat claws your arm. After medication, you continue south. Consequences: You have lost 1 hit point, Marta has lost 1 spell.

In this decision, the player is given a strong hint that the correct answer is 2. The game rewards the player for pausing and considering options in light of the information provided. It attempts to change the adolescent's image of a leader from one who is reckless and resistant to authority to one who cautiously considers options and the advice of others.

Each room provided the player with several choices. A problem-solving skill was presented in the narrative when the player made a poor choice, for example:

> You are in a rectangular-shaped room. On the east wall are numerous dark passages. In the southwest corner is a dimly lit passageway. Behind you on the west wall is a single dark passageway. What do you do?

1. You tell the group to split up and explore briefly the east passageways.
2. You choose the southwest passageway.
3. You choose the west passageway.
   Type 1, 2, or 3?

1.

You and Brochi take one passage together. You discover the area is a maze with passages leading off in all directions. You tell Brochi to turn and stop the others before they get lost in the maze. Brochi runs off to warn the others. As you stop and turn, you stumble and fall!

****

Mentor says—splitting the group up is unwise with all the dangers of a cave. You have made a mistake and must pay the price. Remember to pause and consider carefully before you decide. Are you ready to return? Input yes or no.
****
Yes.

If the player takes the slight hint that a dimly lit passageway may be safer than a dark passageway, the player chooses 2 and is rewarded with a point. However, in this example, the player is not provided with a clear hint of the correct answer. She or he must think through the possible consequences of each option before realizing that splitting up to explore dark passageways is dangerous. Therefore, if the player chooses 1, she or he loses a point.

Points for a positive attitude were provided at several places throughout the game. The idea was to reinforce the concept that the player could learn the behaviors associated with self-control.

Clever of you to bring the mirror. It has saved a life. Do you think you are learning to pause and consider before you act? Input yes or no?
Yes.

Good for you, Betty. Believe in yourself. You have won a bonus point. Your new total is 4.

You look quickly about the room. There are three passageways. The north passageway is dimly lit and Brochi says he hears a growling sound.

(The game continued until the player won or lost or decided to terminate the session.)

Administering the Game

The game was used over a four-week period with four adolescent clients, ages 11 to 17, who were determined to have presenting problems that indicated a lack of impulse-control. Specific target behaviors were fighting at home or school, skipping school, staying out past parental consent time, low grades, and stealing. Attitudes towards self-control and the computer game were monitored as the game was administered. Each half-hour of computer game was followed by a half-hour of traditional therapy.

RESULTS

Client's Behavior and Attitudes

The assessment of the effect of the sessions on clients was based on an analysis of computer printouts, clients' responses to direct questions, and observation of verbal and nonverbal client behavior while they played the game.

None of the clients showed any fear or hesitation toward using the computer—only fascination and enthusiasm. Three of the four clients were openly hostile and uncooperative in their individual initial interview, but they became animated when told they would participate in a computer research project. "Let me see it!"; "Can I play with it?"; "Is there somebody out there?" were typical reactions as they gathered around the printing terminal. The first time clients were allowed to play, each one sat down, started reading the game, and continued on until he or she made a mistake in typing or something didn't go right; then the client would ask for help.

Of the total 16 therapy sessions, only one was missed, due to illness in the family. Prior to this research, the adolescent attendance rate was 66%. This suggests that attendance in therapy increased as a result of using the computer game. One adolescent, after playing for four weeks, requested another game "like that one." When informed this was the only one, she was disappointed.

Each individual player brought his or her own style of play to the game. One player giggled and bounced in her chair. Another player sat stiffly and grimaced. The temperament of individual clients showed in their play of the game. One client played the game with such seriousness and such a grimace on her face that the therapist asked if the client would prefer not to continue. She said, "Oh no! This is fun!" When the therapist pointed out the look on her face, she said, "But, that's the way I am. I'm a serious person." Whether smiling or frowning, clients did not want to quit playing the game at the end of the 30 minutes.

Game patterns were a rich source of information for analyzing behavior and illustrating behavioral problems to clients. For example, one 14-year-old made five times the number of decisions as a 13-year-old during equal 30-minute intervals. A comparison of players' behavior, attitudes, and printouts suggested that the client making quick decisions reacted to the game more impulsively than the "cautious" client. The speedy player became frustrated because she made no progress in the cave. She alternated between claiming the game was rigged to proclaiming that she was stupid. In looking at her printout, we found she had made the same mistakes repeatedly, lost all her points more than once, and had failed to find more than four rooms. In discussing her frustration after the computer session, she said she thought she would have more luck than that and was determined to do better the next week.

Two of the players tried to trick or test the computer by putting "garbage" in as a decision. Usually these trials were distributed randomly throughout the session. Once, when the computer prompted a player to restrict responses to those listed, the player again typed in a "garbage" response. It took the computer six repeats of its request before the player correctly typed a 1, 2, or 3. This suggested that the client was testing the rules of the game to see if they were flexible or firm and indicated an attitude of testing behavior toward life in general. This was substantiated by a previous diagnosis of the client as untrusting toward others.

One of the clients, whose presenting behavior was stealing, was fascinated with the thief in the game. She was very concerned that he was not giving accurate information. At the end, when he grabbed the king's crown, she sat up straight in the chair and said, "Oh no! I've lost!" This demonstrated that the client had identified with the characters that had been created for the game.

One of the clients laughed after playing the game for the first time and said she bet the computers were all laughing at the way she played the game and that the computers were saying to each other, "You think that's bad, you should see this one." This suggested that the client had an active fantasy through which she could project her fear of failure without feeling threatened.

One week the university computer was down and the clients were told they wouldn't be able to play the game. All of the clients said they were disappointed and tried to call the university computer phone number, even after receiving the message that the computer was unavailable. After failing to get the number, they participated in therapy without resistance and at the end of the hour said, "See you next week. Hope the computer is working."

The therapist encouraged talking about the process clients went through in making decisions during the game. Clients responded well to this questioning. These questions easily evolved into talking about problem behaviors in terms of self-control, planning, and decision-making. Typical statements at the beginning of therapy were, "Self-control is doing it right" or "I can't control myself" or "I know it's wrong, but I can't help it." After four weeks of therapy, clients talked about self-control as "deciding what I want to do" or as "learning what I think before I do something." In a review of the literature, self-control was defined as an internalization of commands. Client statements indicated that they may have redefined self-control from an "it" to an "I" or from an external process over which they have no control to an internal process, which they control.

One player said she had made a decision that was wrong because she had not listened to the advice of her fellow characters. She said, "I knew that was a selfish choice. I'm too selfish." Then she added, with enthusiasm in her voice, "But, Mentor says I can be a good decision-maker if I try." This suggested the client had never thought of herself as a decision-maker and the game had provided a new self-concept.

In therapy sessions after the game-playing episode, clients were willing to discuss school and family problems in terms of problem-solving skills. Clients discussed options like quitting school, getting a job, or making good grades in light of personal goals. They accepted criticism and feedback without hostility or rebellion. When the therapist would say, "What is your goal in this?", the client would say, "Aha!" recognizing Mentor's comments about making choices with a goal in mind. In the game, the goal was to get the king's crown, not to make side trips, for example, to see what or who was growling. This suggested that the terms and process that the game introduced were transferred to clients' presenting problems.

Parents' Behavior and Attitudes

Overall expectations were that parents would respond positively to the therapeutic computer game. However, some parents were expected to either express fear of the computer, question the use of a computer game as therapeutic, or not allow their children to participate in the research project. However, none of these occurred with this sample. All of the parents who were questioned about the possible use of a computer game with their children were willing for their children to participate. One parent asked if the parents could participate when their teenager had finished the four-week period.

Parents expressed an interest in the computer equipment, wanting to know how it worked. One parent said, "I want my daughter to learn about computers so she can get a better job." When the parent was reminded that it was a game designed to help adolescents learn about self-control, she replied, "That sounds good."

One parent asked if the printer was the computer. When told it was only the terminal, he said "I figured that. My daughter thinks it's a computer." He then suggested in a conspiratorial manner that we not inform his daughter. This cooperation in helping the client was particularly gratifying, since one of the most difficult problems in working with adolescents and their families is maintaining good relationships with both and convincing all that you have their best interest in mind.

All parents felt that the lack of self-control was a major cause of their adolescent's problems. All of them felt that if their child could learn self-control through therapy, many of the conflicts between parent and child would be eliminated. However, none of the parents felt it was the only problem. Parents all expected traditional therapy to continue after the computer game was completed.

Responses of the Agency and of Direct-Service Personnel

If a computer game is to be used as a therapeutic tool, it must be accepted by the profession. Based on the literature and previous experience, considerable resistance to computers in therapy was expected from colleagues.

Of the 12 colleagues who expressed their reaction when informed of this project, 3 expressed open rejection. Their arguments were based on the view that computers were dehumanizing and therefore had no place in a therapeutic environment. One colleague commented that using computers in a therapeutic setting was ludicrous, and made the statement: "Computers can't take the place of therapists." Another said with disbelief, "You didn't get permission to do that, did you? Oh well, I can believe it. It's the trendy thing. It's a fad." Another colleague was absolutely enraged that anyone, especially a mental health professional, would consider computers an appropriate therapeutic aid.

Two colleagues expressed support, with noted reservations. A psychologist commented, "Well, that's okay for computers to do that, but there's no way the Rorschach could be computerized, because it's too subjective." Another wanted continued reassurance that there was no way the client would be harmed and that the client would be sure to receive "normal" therapy.

The majority of the colleagues expressed complete support and were intrigued by the idea. One typical response was, "You do it and I'll support you." Two of the colleagues played the game and expressed their delight and reassurance that the idea was workable. Several professed an interest in continued research.

Allowing the therapeutic game with clients was a risk for the agency, which required weighing the benefits of research against the possibility of harm to clients or to the agency. The research project was reviewed in the agency by the clinical care committee and the administrative staff. The concerns of the clinical care committee were on confidentiality and the client's right to expect therapy to be beneficial. The participation in traditional therapy along with the computer game allayed the latter concern. The administrative staff's concerns were on protecting the agency from the possibility of bad publicity for allowing trendy and unproven therapy with clients. With funding increasingly difficult to obtain, the agency should be commended for taking the risks associated with any innovative therapy.

PROBLEMS OF COMPUTER GAME DEVELOPMENT

Various problems exist in developing a therapeutic computer game. One consideration is the time it takes to complete the development tasks. After researching the therapeutic base, the first task was to become familiar with other popular games. The second was to develop game characters with popular appeal and to create a setting that could be both entertaining and therapeutic. To operationalize the characters and the setting into action and dialogue took extensive writing and rewriting as choices were tested and refined. Numerous drafts were made to design rooms that were interesting and provided the opportunity for a new self-statement or a problem-solving skill. As rooms were added, additional changes were made to fit the rooms together into a cohesive chain of events. Then with the programming came another round of changes. BASIC was chosen as it was easy to learn because of the small number of commands necessary. On the other hand, it is not as powerful, in terms of programming options, as other languages. Game design using BASIC was primitive, but was adequate for this limited test.

A second difficulty is the interdisciplinary knowledge required to develop a therapeutic computer game. Therapy, computer programming, and game design are all complex areas of knowledge. A way of interfacing the three disciplines in a cooperative manner is necessary, since rarely will one person be proficient in all three areas. A team approach may be the best solution for the development of complex games, but roles, responsibilities, and professional jargon are barriers that may be difficult to overcome.

A third consideration is developing a game that appeals to a defined client population. Thought must be given to character development, story, and setting in light of the characteristics of the client. The sex and intelligence of the clients were major considerations in designing the questions posed and the choices offered. Choices could neither be too simplistic to be boring to intelligent clients, nor too difficult for clients with low intelligence. Development of Mentor's messages included a careful balance between supportive advice and reward and encouragement. It was necessary to provide information about self-control and yet not appear too judgmental or directive. A difficult task was to curb the comments from being too authoritarian or parental. In addition, if the dialogue was too stilted or fake, adolescents would be quick to reject it.

Another potential problem is rejection by colleagues and agencies. While absolute rejection is problematic, healthy skepticism is a very appropriate response. For example, some colleagues feared a dehumanization of the therapeutic process and that clients would be short-changed and misled for a clever idea or a trendy concept. For a therapeutic computer game to be accepted in the therapeutic community, it should be based on traditional therapy and avoid the misunderstanding that accompanied previous attempts, such as the famous Eliza (Weizenbaum, 1976). To reduce resistance, a therapeutic game should be presented as one of many tools a therapist can use in treating a client. It should not be seen as different from behavioral homework, visual imagery, role-playing, videotape, or a computer-scored MMPI. Presently, computers should never be viewed as replacing the therapist.

Our computer game proved to be a successful tool for learning more about the client and for retaining the client's interest in self-help. It also offered the client a setting in which to practice the changes discussed in therapy under the close supervision of the therapist.

A final problem was the theoretical base on which the game was built. Few therapies presently provide a solid base for deriving therapeutic principles that can be easily combined with computer capabilities.

PROSPECTS

Developers of therapeutic computer games should carefully consider several design options that we learned about through developing this game. Our computer game needed to be twice the current length and expanded with a second and third level of difficulty to provide enough decisions for continued interest. Extensive development of characters would be valuable. More interaction between the players and game characters could present numerous examples of peer relationships. The actual fighting of a battle may be an informative scenario for clients, especially those who get into frequent fights with peers.

A longer period of time is recommended for testing a game. This would allow a research approach, e.g., baseline data on specific behaviors could be collected before and after participation, to measure client change. Also, an attitude scale on self-control or a scale that measures locus of control could be given before treatment, and data could be collected on a comparison group. It would also be interesting to compare the use of a printer with use of a CRT terminal, which would provide visual feedback. Substantial research accompanying a game may be the best way to overcome resistance by colleagues and agencies.

One of the designs preferred by adolescents and recommended by Malone (1981) was a multiperson game. An opportunity for several teams to play at once and communicate through their assigned characters would be fascinating. Also, the opportunity for both cooperation and competition could be designed.

Future technological changes and the development of artificial intelligence will increase the possibility of game design. Graphics might be added to give a visual representation of the game, more options for client decisions, and more extensive interaction between characters. Clients or therapists could be allowed to customize the game based on the particular problems the client wanted to address. The game could then create solutions that are more in tune with the client's targeted behavior pattern and temperament. For example, a person who has difficulty verbalizing emotions like anger and sadness might be rewarded for choosing a good expression of anger over a misdirected statement or fighting.

Other technologies, such as videodisk and biofeedback, could be combined with a computer therapeutic game, thus improving the instantaneous interaction between client and computer. For example, the computer could monitor and reward client stress-reduction and improved decision-making as the client interacts with a text/audio/video (animation and movies) scenario.

CONCLUSIONS

Computers are widely used for data processing in mental health, and it is now feasible to use the computer in more therapeutic ways. Our computer fantasy game was developed as an aid to therapists. It avoided some of the objections raised with regard to computers in therapy, since the therapist retained control of the treatment and utilized the computer game as a behavior therapist utilizes homework.

The computer game we have described resulted in adolescent clients becoming more cooperative and enthusiastic about treatment. Clients discussed problem behaviors in light of the game without becoming resistant to therapy. Thus, we can conclude that the game provided the opportunity for a good relationship with the therapist and then continued to support a nonthreatening atmosphere for therapy.

The initial success of this game illustrates the feasibility of addressing adolescent impulse-control problems and perhaps other problems using the computer as a tool. With increased time for development and increased knowledge of computer game design, mental health professionals can successfully design games that are beneficial to clients.

This chapter began by stating that computers evolved from automating existing processes and procedures to automating processes and procedures that were impossible without computers. Our computer game typifies this evolution and points to the potential of developing many new therapies that were not possible before the computer. Presently, computer technology far outpaces its use in therapy. As computers are increasingly used in therapeutic processes, traditional therapeutic underpinnings will be replaced by concepts we have yet to discover. An exciting area is open for therapists with insight and imagination who are willing to do the work and to take the risks.

REFERENCES

Adams, S. Pirate's adventure. *Byte,* 1980, 5(12), 192–212.

Axline, V. *Play therapy.* New York: Ballantine, 1969.

Beck, A. T. *Cognitive therapy and the emotional disorders.* New York: International Universities Press, 1976.

Chambless, D. L., & Goldstein, A. J. Behavioral psychotherapy. In J. Corsini et al. (Eds.). *Current psychotherapies.* Itasca, Illinois: F. E. Peacock Publishers, 1979, 230–272.

Colby, K. M. Computer psychotherapists. In J. B. Sidowski, et al. (Eds.). *Technology in mental health care systems.* Norwood, N. J.: Ablex Publishing Corp., 1980, 109–116.

Coppersmith, S. *Antecedents of self-esteem.* San Francisco: W. H. Freeman and Co., 1967.

Crawford, C. Design techniques and ideals for computer games. *Byte,* 1982, 7(12), 96–108.

DiGuiseppe, R. J. Cognitive therapy with children. In G. Emery, S. D. Hollon, & R. C. Bedrosian (Eds.). *New directions in cognitive therapy.* New York: Guilford Press, 1981.

Edleson, J. L. Teaching children to resolve conflict: a group approach. *Social Work*, 1981, *26*, 488–493.

Kendall, P. On the efficacious use of verbal self-instructional procedures with children. *Cognitive Therapy and Research*, 1977, *1*, 331–334.

Kraus, L. M. Therapeutic strategies with adolescents. *Social Casework*, 1980, *61*(5), 313–316.

Lidz, T. *The person*. New York: Basic Books, 1968.

Mahoney, M. J. Reflections on the cognitive learning trend in psychotherapy. *American Psychologist*, 1977, *32*, 5–13.

Malone, T. W. What makes computer games fun? *Byte*, 1981, *6*(12), 258–277.

Meichenbaum, D. *Cognitive-behavior modification*. New York: Plenum Press, 1977.

Meichenbaum, D. H., & Goodman, J. Training impulsive children to talk to themselves: a means of developing self-control. *Journal of Abnormal Psychology*, 1971, *77*(2), 115–126.

Schoettle, U. Guided imagery—a tool in child psychotherapy. *American Journal of Psychotherapy*, 1980, *34*(2), 220–227.

Sidowski, J. B., Johnson, J., & Williams, T. A. (Eds.). *Technology in mental health information systems*. Norwood, N. J.: Ablex Publishing Co., 1980.

Stuck, H. L. Approaching game program design. *Byte*, 1979, *4*(2), 120–126.

Wagman, M. Plato DCS: an interactive computer system for personal counseling. *Journal of Counseling Psychology*, 1980, *27*(1), 16–30.

Weizenbaum, J. *Computer power and human reason*. San Francisco: W. H. Freeman and Co., 1976.

Williams, D. Y., & Akamatsu, J. Cognitive self-guidance training with juvenile delinquents: applicability and generalization. *Cognitive Theory and Research*, 1978, *2*(3), 285–288.

42 | Review of "Talking to a Computer about Emotional Problems"

Marc D. Schwartz, MD

If the bread and butter of computers in mental health is the administrative/business function, the cake is psychotherapy. One of the early hopes of computer sci-fi fans was that computers, with their potential for artificial intelligence, could assist or replace human helpers. Over the years that hope has been moderated, and the computer as therapist has been used with the more realistic goal of exploring, analyzing, or simulating a small number of the complex variety of factors that make up "psychotherapy."

A necessary prerequisite to carrying out such studies is the determination of whether people would in fact talk to a computer about their problems. If people would, how would their verbal productions and personal reactions to the experience differ from those with a human interviewer? Might they find the experience helpful in some way?

In an attempt to answer these questions, Warner and Charles Slack devised an ingenious apparatus. Persons sitting in front of a microphone/keyboard/CRT terminal were encouraged to talk aloud about matters relevant to them. "Though oblivious to the meaning of spoken words, the machine responds to the occurrence of speech at the microphone and uses duration of speech and silence, time elapsed between various points of reference in the interview and response latency together with keyboard responses" to determine the computer's responses and requests.

To compare people's reactions to a machine and a person, a structured clinical interview was designed and used with 32 subjects by

"Talking to a Computer About Emotional Problems," by Warner and Charles Slack, appeared in *Psychotherapy: Theory, Research, and Practice,* 1977, *14,* 156–164. The present review by Marc D. Schwartz of that article originally appeared in *Computers in Psychiatry/Psychology,* 1978, *1*(3), 5 and is reprinted by permission.

both the computer device and by two human interviewers, the brothers Slack. In the computer-person dialogue, following the appearance of words of welcome and instructions on the TV screen, questions about sadness, loss, amatory or marital difficulties, alcohol, insomnia, etc. were posed. Responses typed on the keyboard were used as the basis for encouraging the subject to talk aloud about one of the issues typed in as being of importance to him/her. As soon as speech was sensed by the microphone, the computer acknowledged it with a response on the screen (e.g. "We are listening to you talk about . . . If finished, press GO.") and encouraged further discussion. Delays and prolonged pauses resulted in explanatory messages and requests for further discussion.

Before the experiment, the procedure was explained to the participants, with emphasis placed on the fact that the computer would be noncomprehending as a listener, but that tapes of the subjects' speech would be listened to later.

All the participants engaged in dialogue with the computer, though they talked much more to the doctors and were somewhat more self-revealing. Subjects were able to talk more substantively to the doctors in the mornings than in the afternoons. This was not true with the indefatigable computer, which gave the same results irrespective of the time of day.

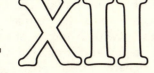

Education as Therapy

There are many situations in which the provision of information to patients or clients can have significant therapeutic benefits. This is particularly important in the fields of behavioral medicine and behavioral psychology. Relevant information can make it easier for individuals to cope with new situations, to change old patterns, to reduce certain kinds of anxiety, and to make certain vocational or personal decisions. The computer can present helpful instruction in a very thorough, carefully structured manner, tailoring it to the needs of the person receiving it. In Part XII a number of educational and therapeutic applications of the computer are examined.

An especially imaginative use has been devised by Sid Schneider at the FDR Veteran's Administration Hospital in Montrose, New York. Taking his cue from the mail-order business, Sid has developed an automated system that communicates with smokers through the mail about their habit and individually assists them in attempts to break it. While some might argue that human contact may be more powerful or persuasive in helping these individuals to stop smoking, for many of them time and money constraints do not allow that alternative. Early success with the "Quit by Mail" system has been encouraging. Certainly it is worth considering the use of similar systems in improving patient compliance with medication regimens such as lithium therapy or antipsychotic or antidepressant therapies.

Sex and the computer—What more provocative combination could one imagine in the early 1980s? The most private, sensuous, age-old human activity juxtaposed with the most modern, structured, nonhuman one. Where could the two usefully meet? Bob Reitman provides one answer in his chapter on the use of small computers in self-help sex therapy. His detailed presentation of a computer-based sex education program for male impotence gives the reader an opportunity to make the decision himself or herself about this intriguing application of computer technology.

Less controversial will be Danny Wedding's use of the word processor to generate individualized letters that reinforce behavioral and therapeutic material taught and/or discussed in the course of each therapy session. Danny provides the reader with examples of letters he has used and discusses some the advantages and problems he has found using his system. Following this, Richard Murray provides a detailed description of the functions, components, and costs of hardware and software systems that can offer automated educational and vocational guidance.

For patient education about various medical or psychological procedures, which is more effective, a nurse, a book, or a computer? The next chapter suggests that the answer may be, surprise, the computer. In an ingenious study of the effects of various kinds of instruction, the computer-assisted instruction was found not only to be more thorough and effective, but to be liked better than were the other two modes of learning.

And for those who are not familiar with the nature of computer-assisted instruction, John Flynn and Terry Kuczeruk provide a thorough introduction to the field. They examine advantages; disadvantages; issues for planning, research, and development; approaches to creating computer-assisted instructional material; costs; human factors in success and failure; evaluation of results; and the implications of this technology for mental health practitioners.

43 | Quit by Mail: The Computer in a Stop-Smoking Clinic

Sid J. Schneider, PhD

Almost every day, when I get my mail, I can see that a great number of facts about me have been stored in various computer files, with the intent of influencing my purchasing, voting, and paying behaviors. Mail-order houses have computers that are apparently keeping track of what I am buying from them; I purchased some gardening supplies from one of these businesses, for instance, and later found that a computer had generated my address on mailing labels for dozens of gardening concerns. My senator's computer keeps track of the viewpoints in my letters, and then determines which bills that the senator has introduced should be brought to my attention, and which are better off not appearing in my mail. Monthly, the electric company computer generates a message to give me feedback on how promptly I have been paying their bills. It seems that many kinds of enterprises have obtained computers, which they then program in a way calculated to influence my behavior. Apparently circumstances are backwards. I thought that as a psychologist running a stop-smoking clinic, it was I who was supposed to be influencing the behavior of others. I therefore acquired a computer myself and set about the job of influencing smoking behavior through the mail.

The computer is now comfortably at home in our smoking clinic. Our clinic, like most smoking clinics, uses behavior therapy techniques, especially self-control techniques. New responses to smoking urges are established, practiced, and rewarded, while the behavior of cigarette-smoking is made cumbersome and unrewarding. The smoker is trained to have progressively more negative thoughts about smoking and more self-congratulating thoughts about abstinence. The idea is that the smoker himself, by meting out and withholding his own rewards, can break the connection between the urge to smoke and the act of lighting up.

The self-control procedures that we provide serve as a vehicle for the smoker's motivation. When the motivation to exercise self-control surpasses the motivation to smoke, the smoker quits smoking (Bernstein, 1969; Kanfer & Phillips, 1970; Logan, 1973). In self-control therapy, the client's motivation plays a larger role, and the nature of the patient-therapist relationship plays a smaller role, than in most other forms of therapy (Wolpe, 1973).

Accordingly, self-control smoking-cessation therapy has appeared at times in forms in which there was little or no contact between therapist and client. The techniques have appeared in packaged form (American Cancer Society, 1971) and book form (Danaher & Lichtenstein, 1978), and as programs on radio and television (Best, 1980). The use of these mass media led to considerable success, with more cost-effectiveness than was possible in usual, face-to-face clinics. Far more smokers can be reached at one time when mass media are used.

A mass medium that had not been used in smoking therapy was direct mail. We applied for a Medical Research award to test such a program. Our application was approved and our program has begun. Smokers in the Quit-by-Mail section of our program receive essentially the same four-week program that clients in our program always have received. However, Quit-by-Mail smokers are treated at home, and mail to us on a weekly basis their smoking diary sheets, responses to smoking questionnaires, and the results of behavioral "homework." These data are entered into our computer, which then generates a return mailing specifically tailored to that particular smoker. In this way, the amount that a client smokes, the way he smokes, his chosen "quit date" deadline, his reasons for quitting, his smoking-substitute thoughts and behaviors, and a host of other data can be processed, using programs we have developed, to produce a mailing that personalizes for each smoker appropriate feedback and instructions for the week. For example, mailings take into account the extent to which a smoker is reducing cigarette-smoking over the course of the treatment; whether a smoker is quitting for, say, improved health as opposed to, say, greater attractiveness, and so on. Individual instructions, such as directions to change the brands, the hand and fingers to be used in smoking, take into account the smoking habits that the smoker reported in questionnaires. In all, we are able to reach a large number of smokers by using a mass medium, without sacrificing the ability to individualize and follow up the therapy and without sacrificing the ability to interact with the client, which are the usual drawbacks of using a mass medium. For example, televised Stop-Smoking Clinics permit no interaction or individualization of treatment. Moreover, we can keep a large amount of data concerning each smoker conveniently on computer file for analysis.

Our hardware includes a Data General Nova 2 minicomputer with 32K words (16 bytes) of memory; a Data General 6052 CRT; a Diablo

1620 letter-quality printer to produce the mailings; and a Data General 6098 sealed disk (12.5 megabyte) and diskette (1.9 megabyte) subsystem.

Our early success with the Quit-by-Mail system has been encouraging. The success rate immediately following treatment is in excess of 35%; comparison groups receiving noninteractive mail treatment techniques are faring no better than control groups receiving minimum treatment, in which about 5% are quitting. Smokers who receive face-to-face treatment appear to quit immediately following treatment at a very high rate, in excess of 55%, but these smokers are certainly the most motivated; they are willing to expend time and energy to travel to face-to-face groups. It is the smoker who needs assistance but is unwilling to go out of his or her way to get it who can be reached uniquely by the Quit-by-Mail program. Perhaps that group represents the majority of all smokers.

One of the most encouraging results of the evaluation of the program concerns its cost-efficiency. The Quit-by-Mail system requires less staff time per successful participant than does face-to-face treatment or noninteractive mail treatment. Also, the time involved is primarily that of technicians, whereas face-to-face groups, the traditional mode of behavioral treatment, require professional time. In this way, our clinic can treat over a thousand smokers a year, a number difficult to reach without a computerized system.

It will be most revealing to analyze the data concerning smokers at six-month follow-up. How many quitters will have reverted to smoking? Our system will prove itself only if it establishes lasting behavioral change. If it does prove itself, the concept of computer-based behavioral therapy need not stop with smoking-cessation. Clinicians performing weight-reduction therapy, phobia therapy, and other forms of habit management might benefit from our approach as well. Patient-computer interaction through the mail might also be useful to improve patient compliance with medical regimens, such as antihypertensive drug therapy. The computer has tremendous potential in the practice of health psychology.

REFERENCES

American Cancer Society, California Division. *Stop smoking program guide.* San Francisco: Author, 1971.

Bernstein, D. A. Modification of smoking behavior: An evaluative review. *Psychological Bulletin*, 1969, 71, 418–440.

Best, J. A. Mass media, self-management, and smoking modification. In: P. O. Davidson & S. M. Davidson (Eds.), *Behavioral medicine: Changing health lifestyles.* New York: Brunner/Mazel, 1980, pp. 371–390.

Danaher, B. G., & Lichtenstein, E. *Become an ex-smoker*. Englewood Cliffs, N. J.: Prentice-Hall, 1978.

Kanfer, F. H., & Phillips, J. S. *Learning foundations of behavior therapy*. New York: Wiley, 1970.

Logan, F. A. Self-control as habit, drive and incentive. *Journal of Abnormal Psychology*, 1973, *81*, 127–136.

Wolpe, J. *The practice of behavior therapy*. New York: Pergamon, 1973.

44

The Use of Small Computers in Self-Help Sex Therapy

Robert Reitman, PhD

D.L. has read a great deal of the popular literature on psychological impotence, attended workshops on it and other sexual problems and has, from time to time, made halfhearted attempts at seeking therapy for his difficulty. He has a hard time talking about himself and his problems. One of the significantly frightening possibilities to D. L. is his confusion about his impotence: What could have caused it? why him? and his fleeting doubts about his masculinity. The books he has read have covered much of the generalities about erection problems, but, not surprisingly, written material doesn't zero in on D. L.'s particular brand of impotence.

The most depressing aspect of D. L.'s problem—and he realizes it—is the dwindling list of possibilities for help. Having exhausted the literature and been disappointed, fearing direct therapeutic contact, giving up on men's groups and sex-problem workshops, D. L. now has the nagging belief that he may be reaching the end of the line.

M. K. has suffered in relative silence down through the years as she watched the sexual side of her marriage slip into nothingness. Early attempts at understanding, nondemanding behavior, and talking with her husband in loving, supportive ways slowly deteriorated into hours and sometimes days of silence and finally into loud, nasty quarreling.

R., her husband, seemed "perfect" in every other way: A good worker and father, a helper around the house, a generally open and fairly popular man, except in the area of sexuality, where, as time progressed, he drew more inward as he defended himself against his angry wife.

R. talked to his minister at various times and at some length on his inability to have erections. The minister tried helping, but little came of the counseling. The couple saw two different marriage counselors (one man, one woman) at different periods and were confounded by conflicting suggestions. Their physician suggested books (after urological workups that revealed little more than slightly low testosterone levels) and a sex-therapy couple. R. scanned some parts of the reading, but soon lost interest. When the sex therapists wanted both partners to participate in therapy, M. refused, claiming no responsibility for "his problem."

P. N. has been through sex therapy four times: once with a surrogate partner in an intensive 2-week program; another time with a behavior therapist with biofeedback devices and several days of progressive exercises; a third time with a committed girlfriend and another crack at the intensive program; and, finally, with a hypnotist, whose work included relaxation techniques that seemed to help temporarily.

Throughout, P. N. has sporadically continued his analysis; he has "more or less" discussed his impotence problem with his therapist, but has not told him about his periodic attempts at "fixing" his problem more directly. When he vaguely hints that his problem may be getting worse, the analyst just as vaguely hints that long-term psychotherapy is the only way to root out the base cause of such problems. P. N., running out of both money and patience, continues his vague and inconclusive attempts at dealing with his sexual impotence.

Virtually any clinician of any experience can make important suggestions for all these people. The list ranges from getting proper counseling and referrals to getting psychological help in regaining the kind of confidence it takes to properly deal with such problems. One of the most important components the clinician would point to is the person's desire to resolve the problem and the issues surrounding his choice to "do something about it."

Lest these cases appear to be isolated instances, consider the vast numbers of books (the good and the poor) on sexual problems being published and sold (and publicized regularly on TV talk shows), contrasted with the oft-quoted belief that therapists will never see more than 40% of people with sexual complaints. Note, too, that we are not a nation that believes its sexual problems rate the same considerations as dental problems, foot problems, or high blood pressure. And, while there will continue to be advances in virtually all areas of medicine and most in psychology, help in sexual matters will undoubtedly take many years to filter down to the patient level.

Clearly there have been attempts at solving this dilemma. A general but somewhat pithy frankness has set in in the media, although specificity is elusive. Books themselves are certainly not only better, but sometimes more pointedly deal with some of the issues regarding sexual dysfunction. Even the attempts at contact—workshops, groups, lectures, and the like—seem to be made of better stuff these days. Therapies, expensive and only variously successful, remain the arguably best choice.

The continually nagging question, however, remains: what help can the individual get who has sexual complaints that can be dealt with privately, at his or her leisure, that offers a program of information and knowledge, along with challenges to past or current mythology and provides the necessary motivation to move to the next step toward resolving the sexual problem?

As a longtime trained and certified sex therapist, as well as writer, teacher, and lecturer on the subject, these problems have bothered me for more than ten years. In attempts at solving them down through the years I have: (a) recommended books and exercises; (b) made homework assignments; (c) created a slide-film library to be used in education and counseling and for help in the home also; (d) conducted therapy in the office; (e) held workshops for individuals and couples in remote scenic hideaways; and (f) trained numerous therapists (individuals and couples) from all over the country to perform sex therapy.

It was about a year ago that I saw, as my research continued, that a new possibility existed: the small home computer. Before I got into its true potential, some obvious questions arose. If computer prices ever came within range of the average family, if there were relatively simple ways to learn to work with computers, if there were specially created programs that dealt in areas the average person would be able to make use of in the calm, quiet privacy of his own home. . .

As I moved deeper into the potentialities of the smaller computers, I could see that much of what I believed necessary was coming to pass—*except in the area of programming.* Prices have indeed come down—and promise to continue to do so. Relative sophistication and simplicity have seemingly come closer to merging. And the possibility of a person talking things over with a friendly machine and getting something back is also coming closer.

In practically all the helping professions, I discovered, there are movements afoot to utilize the seeming miracles of the burgeoning home computer world. The family-therapy publications sense that computers will soon be within the monetary grasp of that great mass of people who might never go outside the home for various kinds of help. The computer will teach disadvantaged people not only to read and write, add and subtract; it will help them to eat better; take care of themselves better (as well as their children and their aging parents); teach them how to balance their checkbooks; consider their futures in numerous ways; and, with the ubiquitous toys for young and old that

represent relaxation and family life to so many, enjoy this new "participating member of the family."

Approximately one year ago I began seriously considering researching specifically created programs, especially the possibility of doing male sex therapy for impotence with the help of my computer. But
even before creating a program solely for working *with* patients, the
revolutionary (to me) thought of creating programs for *self-help in the
home* occurred. Now, having "shown" this initial program to peers and
professionals three times (to date), I note not only a growing excitement within the profession, but a respect for its potential as well.

It is important to stop for a moment at this point to indicate the
kind of therapeutic work I do, because of its apparently successful
linkup to the potential of the home computer.

Cognitive therapy is, essentially, learning theory put into practical
terms. Combined with certain behavioral aspects, this kind of work begins with *creating an alliance with the patient against the problem*. This is
especially important because the patient immediately understands that
no one else can solve his problems; he must recognize them, define
them in practical ways in which they can best be dealt with, take responsibility for the parts he can control (also, conversely, to recognize
those aspects outside his control) and, with help, learn to handle them
in thoughtful, mature ways.

Moreover, this patient wants to understand his cognitions, or
thoughts about himself, and the situations in which he finds himself,
and his role in resolving issues for now and in the immediate future.
So, a man might find himself sexually unable to attain or maintain
erections, for example, and immediately believe that the impotence itself is the sole problem. Talking about it to a cognitive therapist, he
will find that, along with his inability to get erections, what he thinks
and believes about his impotence is just as significant. What he believes translates into what he tells himself and what he tells himself is
often the difference between solving the problem and not, or solving it
within several therapy sessions versus several years of fruitless dependence on discovery for its own sake.

In cognitive therapy (such as Albert Ellis's Rational-Emotive Therapy, amongst others), the clinician uses as many communicative tools
as he can: chalk and board, film in its various applications, written and
oral homework assignments, exercises, and the like.

Thus, when I began understanding the properties of the home
computer, it became easier to assimilate it into such psychotherapeutic
work as cognitive therapy.

The original thought was to create a program that would take two
clear and positive steps: (1) to examine the man's definition of, and be-

liefs and thoughts about, his psychological impotence and to offer reasonable realities apart from his myths, misconceptions, and misunderstandings; and, (2) to indicate clearly in a step-by-step fashion how this attitude restructuring could lead toward effective and successful behavioral changes (sex therapy). The notion was that the patient would be conducting his own therapy, with all that that implies.

As the program evolved, it became more and more evident that if it was to prove effective it had to have self-measurement devices to indicate progress and to offer alternatives to moving ahead too rapidly. And, if it was to be truly private, a therapeutic tool he could work with at home, the program had to become more free of any dependency (not reliance) on a therapist. That is, if he wanted a therapist, in addition to his own program, he could always retain one, but if he wanted to deal with his problems himself, the program would aid him in his self-sufficiency by being as complete as possible.

Therapists working with patients who have computers can utilize the program as homework, reinforcement, assignment, or as substitute sessions.

What follows is a selective portion of the cognitive restructuring part of the psychological impotence program.

After the "credits," the program opens immediately with this instruction to the patient: "Please type in your first name and then press ENTER." From here on the computer, in a conversational manner, works with the patient by name, in this example *Joe.*

The patient is then told they will be dealing with *his* sexual impotence. The "usual" definition, he is told, is that he can't have erections. He is then asked to respond to a short quiz that clearly shows him to be selectively, or psychologically, impotent.

```
HI, JOE.  WE WILL BE
DEALING WITH A SEXUAL
PROBLEM KNOWN AS IMPOTENCE.

LET'S BEGIN BY DEFINING
IMPOTENCE.

YOUR DEFINITION WOULD
UNDOUBTEDLY BE, 'I DON'T
GET ERECTIONS!'

THAT SOUNDS SIMPLE ENOUGH,
DOESN'T IT?
```

BUT THERE'S MUCH MORE TO IT
THAN THAT, I CAN ASSURE YOU.

                    PRESS 1.

PLEASE ASK YOURSELF
THESE QUESTIONS.

1. DO I OFTEN HAVE ERECTIONS
   WHEN I WAKE UP?

2. DO I USUALLY HAVE ERECT-
   IONS WHEN I MASTURBATE?

3. DO I MOSTLY HAVE ERECT-
   IONS WHEN I READ PORNO?

4. DO I OFTEN HAVE ERECTIONS
   WHEN I SEE NUDITY?

5. DO I SOMETIMES HAVE EREC-
   TIONS IN THE NIGHT?

                    PRESS 1.

IF YOU ANSWERED ANY OF
THE QUESTIONS 'YES',
YOU AREN'T ACTUALLY IM-
POTENT, ARE YOU, JOE?

YOU DO GET ERECTIONS!

SO, FOR THE SAKE OF ACC-
URACY, LET'S RE-DEFINE
IMPOTENCE, IN ORDER TO
BETTER DEAL WITH IT:

--YOU DON'T GET ERECTIONS
WHEN YOU WANT THEM OR
THINK YOU SHOULD HAVE
THEM. OR KEEP THEM FOR
AS LONG A TIME AS YOU
WANT TO, WITHIN REASON.

                    PRESS 1.

```
THAT SOUNDS MORE LIKE IT,
DOESN'T IT, JOE.

AND, BECAUSE YOU CAN'T
ALWAYS DO WHAT YOU WANT
SEXUALLY, THAT MAKES
MATTERS EVEN WORSE!

LET'S GET INTO THIS IN
DETAIL AND SEE IF WE
CAN'T DO SOMETHING ABOUT
YOUR PROBLEM.

                 PRESS 1.
```

His attention is then drawn to how he *feels* when he does not get an erection.

```
HOW DO YOU FEEL WHEN YOU
DON'T GET AN ERECTION:

     1.  ANGRY?

     2.  ANXIOUS?

     3.  DEPRESSED?

     4.  STRESSED?

     5.  FRUSTRATED?

        PRESS THE NUMBERS WHICH
        SEEM MOST APPROPRIATE.

        1 - 2 - 3 - 4 - 5
```

Each of the five key words, when chosen, offers a variety of words and phrases that could help identify how he feels.
Here are two samples:

```
'ANGRY'
    DO YOU WANT TO SCREAM
AND HOLLER, LASH OUT,
BEAT ON SOMETHING, CUSS
OUT SOMEONE, FEEL FURI-
OUS, MEAN, REALLY
TICKED OFF?
```

IF THIS DESCRIBES YOUR
FEELINGS, PRESS 1.

IF NOT, PRESS 2 AND
TRY ANOTHER.

'DEPRESSED'

DO YOU EXPERIENCE THE
BLUES AND BLAHS, FEEL
DOWN, VERY SLEEPY, TIRED
AND GENERALLY OUT OF IT,
WITH A 'COULDN'T-CARE-
LESS' ATTITUDE, FEEL
SOMETIMES WEEPY, SAD,
INDIFFERENT, LONELY,
BORED, LISTLESS AND
VAGUE?

IF THIS DESCRIBES YOUR
FEELINGS, PRESS 1.

IF NOT, PRESS 2 AND
TRY ANOTHER.

When he has chosen the feeling that best describes his own personal emotions (or has seen all of them), he encounters these next
frames on screen:

YOU DON'T ACTUALLY FEEL
ANGRY, ANXIOUS, DEPRESSED,
STRESSED OR FRUSTRATED
BECAUSE OF YOUR IMPOTENCE
ITSELF, JOE.

YOU FEEL THESE THINGS
BECAUSE OF WHAT YOU TELL
YOURSELF ABOUT NOT HAVING
ERECTIONS.

PRESS 1.

IN SHORT, WHEN YOU ARE NOT
SEXUALLY FUNCTIONING THE WAY
YOU WANT, YOU GET OFF
BALANCE AND BECOME IMMOBI-
LIZED BY MYTHS, MISCON-
CEPTIONS, AND MISUNDER-
STANDINGS.

                    PRESS 1.

IN THE NEXT PART, WE WILL
BEGIN DEALING WITH WHAT
YOU TELL YOURSELF ABOUT
BEING IMPOTENT, AND WHAT
YOU CAN DO ABOUT THESE
THINGS.

BUT FIRST, JOE...

                    PRESS 1.

LET'S REVIEW.

1. WHEN YOU HAVE ERECTIONS
   WHILE MASTURBATING, OR
   DURING THE NIGHT OR
   MORNING, YOU ARE NOT
   HOPELESSLY IMPOTENT.   T-F

2. IF YOU DON'T GET ERECT-
   IONS WHEN YOU WANT, IT
   WILL HELP TO GET AT WHAT
   CAUSES THE PROBLEM RATHER
   THAN SIMPLY BECOME UPSET
   BY IT.   T-F

3. ONE WAY OF RESOLVING
   SEXUAL PROBLEMS WOULD
   BE TO EXAMINE THE EFFECTS
   OF OUTSIDE INFLUENCES ON
   YOUR BEHAVIOR.   T-F

                    PRESS 1.

DID YOU ANSWER THE 3 QUES-
TIONS 'T',JOE?

IF NOT, PRESS 2 TO GO OVER

```
SOME BASIC REALITIES ABOUT
YOUR IMPOTENCE.  (DEFINIT-
ION, YOUR FEELINGS WHEN IT
HAPPENS, AND SOME OF YOUR
BELIEFS THAT COMPLICATE THE
SITUATION).

IF YOU ANSWERED 'T' TO ALL
3, PRESS 1 TO CONTINUE
ON WITH THE NEXT PART ON
SOLVING YOUR SEXUAL PROBLEM.
```

In the beginning of the next part Joe finds three basic causes of why most men become psychologically impotent. And, as he goes through the lineup within the first area, Performance Anxiety, he sees statements men make to themselves when they don't function sexually. He also sees the challenges to each of these statements.

```
1.  PAYING UNDUE ATTENTION TO
    EVERYTHING YOU DO, TRYING
    TO MAKE SURE YOU DO
    EVERYTHING PERFECTLY.

2.  PUTTING ALL THE RESPON-
    SIBILITY FOR YOUR IM-
    POTENCE ON YOUR PARTNER.

3.  TELLING YOURSELF ALL THE
    BAD THINGS YOU THINK
    ABOUT AND DO, AND SHOULD
    BE PUNISHED FOR.

                    PRESS 1.
```

When 1 is selected, the patient sees:

```
1.  PERFORMANCE ANXIETY

    WHAT YOU TELL YOURSELF
    WHEN YOU DON'T GET OR
```

```
KEEP ERECTIONS:

1. YOU MUST WHENEVER YOU
   HAVE SEX.

2. YOU HAVE TO IN ORDER
   TO HAVE INTERCOURSE.

3. YOU'RE A FAILURE
   UNLESS YOU DO.

4. YOU'LL NEVER HAVE
   THEM AGAIN.

5. YOU'RE THE ONLY MAN TO
   HAVE THIS PROBLEM.

                    PRESS 1.
```

The first two statements and their challenges read as follows:

```
1. YOU MUST HAVE ERECTIONS
   WHENEVER YOU HAVE SEX.

   WHY, JOE?
   NO SEXUAL SITUATION IS
   DEPENDENT ON YOUR
   PENIS' PERFORMANCE; NOT

   -KISSING,   -LICKING,
   -HUGGING,   -FINGERING,
   -TOUCHING,  -INTERCOURSE.

   RELAX AND ENJOY WHAT YOU
   ARE DOING.   REMEMBER,
   NO SEXUAL SITUATION IS
   DEPENDENT ON YOUR PENIS'
   PERFORMANCE!
                    PRESS 1.

2. YOU HAVE TO HAVE AN
   ERECTION TO HAVE INTER-
   COURSE.

   NOT TRUE - FOR YOU OR
   YOUR PARTNER. HANDICAPPED
```

```
MEN, MEN ON MEDICATION,
AND MEN RECOVERING FROM
ILLNESS, ACCIDENTS, AND
SURGERY KNOW BETTER.
INSERTING A SOFT PENIS
IN THE SIDE, OR ANY SIMI-
LAR POSITION WORKS. USING
FINGERS OR OTHER BODY
PARTS HELPS YOUR PARTNER
ALSO, JOE.

NO SEXUAL SITUATION IS
DEPENDENT ON YOUR PENIS'
PERFORMANCE.

                    PRESS 1.
```

After the patient sees the next three displays, completing Performance Anxiety, he presses 6.

```
ALL RIGHT, YOU HAVE BEGUN
DEALING WITH SOME OF THE
REASONS WHY YOU MAY NOT GET
ERECTIONS.

ALONG WITH SOME HELPFUL
ARGUMENTS AGAINST THOSE
REASONS.

NOW, JOE, CHECK YOUR-
SELF ON WHAT YOU'VE LEARNED
ABOUT BEING ANXIOUS WHEN
YOU'RE HAVING SEX.

                    PRESS 1.


        T OR F

1. BEING TIRED IS A VALID
   REASON FOR NOT GETTING
   AN ERECTION.

2. EVERY MAN HAS INAPPRO-
   PRIATELY GOTTEN SOFT AT
```

```
           ONE TIME OR ANOTHER.

       3.  NOT GETTING HARD YESTER-
           DAY DOESN'T MEAN YOU
           WON'T GET HARD TOMORROW.

       4.  INTERCOURSE IS ONLY ONE
           ASPECT OF SEX.

                      PRESS 1.




       IF YOU ANSWERED 'T' TO ALL
       FOUR OF THE QUESTIONS,
       YOU'RE READY TO MOVE
       ON, JOE.

       IF YOU WANT TO TAKE THE QUIZ
       AGAIN , JUST TO BE SURE,
       PRESS 3.

       IF YOU ANSWERED ANY OF THE
       QUESTIONS 'F', OR WANT TO
       GO OVER THIS SECTION AGAIN,
       PRESS 2.

       WHEN YOU'RE READY TO GO ON
       TO THE NEXT PART, PRESS 1.
```

Thus, he has dealt with the area of Performance Anxiety, and will move on through Relationship Problems and Sexual Guilts. Each category poses statements indicative of the category that most men tell themselves about their impotence. In context, these are followed by challenges and disputes to those statements. Finally, the patient (by name, remember) tests himself after completing the particular area.

Following Sexual Guilts is a "miscellaneous" category:

```
       OTHER ISSUES WHICH COULD
       PRECLUDE ERECTIONS

       1.  LACK OF SEXUAL DESIRE.

       2.  SEXUAL BOREDOM.

       3.  HOSTILE FEELINGS.
```

```
4. ANOTHER LOVER.

5. CONFUSED SEXUAL
   ORIENTATION.

6. EMOTIONAL DISTURBANCES.

                    PRESS 1.
```

As in the other categories, each of these statements gets its own review, complete with challenges and a quiz that offers the patient the choice of going back to the area again or moving forward.

When all these areas, challenges, quizzes, answers, and choices of instructions have been done, the final displays come on.

```
YOU'VE DONE REALLY WELL,
JOE; YOU'VE ABOUT CON-
CLUDED THE FIRST HALF OF
YOUR PROGRAM ON PSYCHO-
LOGICAL IMPOTENCE: THE
'ATTITUDE RESTRUCTURING'
PART.

YOU'VE SEEN MANY OF THE
THINGS THAT MEN TELL THEM-
SELVES WHEN THEY DON'T GET
ERECTIONS.

AND THE VALID ARGUMENTS
CHALLENGING AND DISPUTING
THEIR MYTHS, MISCONCEPTIONS,
AND MISUNDERSTANDINGS.

                    PRESS 1.


YOU CERTAINLY HAVE ALTERED
MANY OF YOUR OWN BY NOW,
HAVEN'T YOU, JOE?

AND EVERY TIME YOU DO, YOU
CONTINUE TO CHANGE YOUR
ATTITUDE.

THIS GOES A LONG WAY TOWARD
```

EFFECTIVELY DEALING WITH
YOUR IMPOTENCE PROBLEM
ITSELF... FROM A POSITION
OF STRENGTH.

                        PRESS 1.

THIS 'ATTITUDE RESTRUCTUR-
ING' IS ESSENTIAL TO THE
SUCCESSFUL COMPLETION OF THE
UPCOMING FINAL PORTION OF
YOUR PROGRAM, THE 'BEHAVIOR-
AL CHANGE', OR THERAPY PART.

                        PRESS 1.

BUT, JOE, IF YOU SEEM
TO HESITATE IN MAKING THE
CHANGES SUGGESTED HERE OR
RESIST LETTING GO OF FAULTY
THINKING, IT MAY HELP YOU TO
SEE SOME OF THE BELIEFS THAT
MAKE CHANGING DIFFICULT. ·

                        PRESS 1.

FOR EXAMPLE, YOU TELL
YOURSELF YOU HAVE NO CHOICE
BUT TO THINK OR BELIEVE THE
WAY YOU DO BECAUSE:

--YOU'VE ALWAYS DONE IT
  THIS WAY.

--YOU'RE NOT SURE THERE ARE
  OTHER WAYS TO THINK.

--PEOPLE UNDERSTAND IF YOU
  THINK THIS WAY.

--THAT'S THE WAY LIFE IS,
  AND YOU HAVE NO CHOICE
  ANYWAY.

                        PRESS 1.

```
BUT YOU DO HAVE A CHOICE,
JOE.

IF YOU CHOOSE TO CONTINUE
RESTRUCTURING YOUR ATTITUDE,
AND YOU ARE READY TO PROCEED
WITH THE THERAPY THAT WILL
HELP YOU REGAIN CONTROL OVER
YOUR ERECTIONS, PRESS 1.

IF YOU CHOOSE TO GO BACK AND
RE-STUDY ALL OR PART OF THE
PROGRAM TO BE BETTER PRE-
PARED FOR SUCCEEDING IN THE
THERAPY PART, PRESS 2.
```

Once the patient elects to move forward, he is confronted with this frame:

```
HI AGAIN, JOE, GLAD
TO HAVE YOU ABOARD!

IN THIS SECOND HALF OF YOUR
PROGRAM WE GET TO THE EXER-
CISES AND ASSIGNMENTS THAT
WILL OFFER PRACTICAL HELP IN
REGAINING YOUR CONFIDENCE
AND ABILITY TO HAVE ERECT-
IONS VIRTUALLY WHENEVER YOU
WANT THEM.

THIS PROGRAM WILL ALSO HELP
YOU TO BETTER HANDLE SITUA-
TIONS WHEN YOU MIGHT NOT GET
ERECTIONS.
```

You have seen approximately 20% of the first half of the psychological impotence program. Some of the comments from professionals who have attended the three "showings" of this program are:

● I felt locked in while seated in front of the screen, literally forced to work on my problem.

- I was a bit frightened at first, but got into it pretty soon and found myself really interested in moving forward. I liked retesting myself often.
- I thought I would skim over the reasons for a man not getting hard when he wanted to, but found myself going through it all carefully and wondering how I'd feel if it ever happened to me.
- It never occurred to me that what I told myself, how I felt about myself if I couldn't perform sexually, made any difference.
- At first I thought this would eliminate the need for sex therapists in time, but the more I saw of it, the more I could see how I could use it with my patients.

With respect to the people discussed in the opening case histories, all could make use of this program on their home computers in a variety of practical ways.

D. L., in going through the cognitive restructuring, will

- Find a source that will deal with most of his sexual confusion;
- Discover a great deal of background information on why many men become psychologically impotent;
- See some aspects of himself and his sexual history reflected in the information offered;
- Be encouraged to go deeper into any doubts he has about his masculinity;
- Role-play sessions with his computerized sex-counselor/therapist;
- Realize he has this additional resource and, with continuing effort, perhaps reconsider psychotherapy.

M. K., the wife, will:

- Learn about male sex problems, especially impotence;
- Better understand her role as partner in a relationship that has a sex problem;
- Hopefully, find encouragement to seek help with her husband to resolve their complaints.

R. K., the husband, will:

- Be able to get into a "private dialogue" with a knowledgeable and nonjudgmental source;
- Help integrate his sexuality into his whole persona;
- Gain insight and information into male sexual problems;
- Clear up some of his fear and confusion by offering challenges to his beliefs about sex and his problems;

- Hopefully, find encouragement to seek help together with his wife to resolve their sexual complaints.

P. N. will:

- Open up new avenues of pertinent information in a constructive way, about himself and impotence;
- Gain confidence in himself so as to seek active help with his problem;
- Find practical face-to-face ways to put his difficulty into a workable perspective;
- Discover enlightened alternatives that have a logical potential for success.

The future for therapeutic uses of home computers is, to me, here now; the scope of self-help through the uses of minis is boundless and endless.

Currently 38 additional programs are under development.* These range from sex education (ages 5 to 18) and sex therapy (other male problems, women's problems, desire problems, and couple's problems) to a host of other subjects particularly adaptable to cognitive therapy and the small computers. These include personal and self-motivational programs and are designed to be used either by oneself or with therapists as adjuncts to and backing up sound psychological principles.

NOTE

The equipment used includes the Texas Instruments 99/4A console and its disc controller and 1 disc drive plus Memory Expansion, RS232 interface and the Epson 80 printer. The programs are on diskette, utilizing the TI "Extended BASIC." Programs are also on IBM-PC and compatible equipment.

---

*Further information on these programs can be obtained by contacting the author.

45

The Word Processor as a Patient Education Tool in Psychotherapy

Danny Wedding, PhD

Many psychotherapists believe patient education to be a critical part of the therapeutic process. While other components may play an important role, essentially the therapeutic environment is one that allows the patient to try out a series of new behaviors, to learn that behavioral change is possible, to appreciate that often-feared behaviors do not result in disastrous consequences, and to practice these new behaviors in the presence of a supportive role-model who has presumably mastered the skills that the patient desires to learn. Behavior therapists, rational emotive therapists, reality therapists, and cognitive behavior therapists are all apt to conceptualize patient problems and the therapeutic process in terms of skill deficits and faulty cognitive patterns. Given this conceptual framework, new learning plays a vital role in virtually every therapeutic interaction.

While much of the learning that occurs in psychotherapy is experiential or vicarious, some is simply didactic. For example, the patient who presents with an unmanageable child may not know the rudiments of effective parenting or simple principles of behavior change. This information base is necessary if the patient is going to fully profit from either instruction or modeling. While the therapist can use therapy time to present this information, it is inefficient and costly. The therapy hour is clearly better spent with the patient actively involved, rather than sitting and absorbing information that is available from other sources.

Bibliotherapy offers a partial solution to the patient-education problem. However, often an entire book will not be germane to a particular problem or the material presented will only approximate the needs of the patient. In addition, particular books recommended by the therapist will often be out of stock and a delay of several weeks will occur before the book is received. In addition to slowing the learning process, this delay is unfortunate in that patients may lose much of the motivation that brought them to seek help in the first place. My experience has been that learning is optimized when the patient can begin at once to use bibliotherapy to integrate and consolidate information and experiences provided during the therapy hour.

As a partial solution to the limitations of bibliotherapy, I have begun to send out semipersonalized letters to many of the patients I see. Typically, the letters are mailed after the patient's third or fourth visit and outline my views on the particular problem presented by the patient. These letters reiterate and elaborate many of the points I have made up to that time in therapy; occasionally they will anticipate points I hope to make in the future. For example, with a patient who is learning to be increasingly assertive, I will review the basic components of an assertive response, discuss eye contact, posture, gestures, and voice level, and review a number of possible assertive options in the types of problem situations the patient has discussed with me in preceding therapy sessions. In the case of a maritally distressed couple trying to improve marital skills, I will usually discuss the importance of open communication, the importance of "I" statements, the dangers of labels, the problem of overgeneralization in communication, and the importance of utilizing "prime time" to enhance communication. While this information is available in other sources, a personal letter allows the therapist to offer tailor-made instructions and to delete information that may be nonrelevant or counterproductive. I have compiled a large number of descriptive paragraphs covering a variety of problem areas, e.g., sexual dysfunction, impaired communication, study skills, time management, and lack of assertion. These are stored on an office word processor, and my secretary and I both maintain a master list, with each paragraph numbered. After seeing a patient, I can simply jot down the patient's name along with the numbers and appropriate sequence of the information I wish to include. It is a relatively simple matter for the secretary to call up the necessary material and to have a personalized letter ready to be mailed the following day. The letter will typically arrive about three days after the therapy session and serves to both reinforce what is said in therapy and to increase compliance with any homework assignments they may have been given.

My overall experience with the system has been positive. Patients are pleased when they receive the letters and come into the office on their next visit eager to discuss both the content of the letter and their attempts to try out suggestions that were made. I will usually attempt to build on the basic information provided by the letter by recommending a variety of related books that present more detailed information about the problem confronting the patient. Without question, the use of the word processor to generate the semipersonalized letters has increased the effectiveness of the teaching I do and has allowed more time in each therapy hour to be devoted to individualized patient concerns.

The following is an example of a computerized personal letter from me to a husband and wife who are my patients.

November 8, 1982

Mr. and Mrs. John Doe
Route 1, Box XXX
Smithton, Va. 24354

Dear John and Jane:

I have been thinking about your case and decided to dictate some general remarks about communication. These are things that we have talked about in our sessions together; however, this is also information that you well might forget and therefore I wanted you to have this letter as a reminder. I hope you will find occasion to look over these comments frequently and try to adapt some of the recommendations I am going to make to your own style of interaction.

By this time you should be well on your way to developing a number of the nonverbal communication skills we discussed. This is why I have asked that you spend considerable time with simply touching or massaging each other. The point I want to make is that sexual communication does not necessarily involve intercourse. I want you to quite literally learn to "get in touch" with each other.

I also hope you, Jane, have thought about the problem of "mind-reading," which we discussed earlier. Oftentimes individuals will fail to assert themselves appropriately and then will feel hurt when their spouse or partner does not respond in a desired fashion. In general, I would like for you to avoid second-guessing what John is thinking or feeling. Clear communication requires that you be willing to ask and that John be willing to tell you exactly how he is feeling. In addition, you will want to avoid speaking for your partner. Phrases like "we want" or "we feel" are almost never true. It is far better to say, for example, "I'd like to go out and see a movie with you on Thursday and I think that John would enjoy it too, but I'll check with him and get back with you next week."

John, I hope you will also begin to think about the differences between your thoughts and feelings. It is a truism in working with couples that communication is more effective when it occurs in terms of *feelings* rather than thoughts. Beware especially of thoughts that misleadingly present themselves as feelings. For example, when you say "I feel that you're putting me down," you are actually expressing a thought and a value judgment. Perhaps it would be more effective to simply say, "I feel put down." This states your feelings precisely without becoming unduly cognitive and it does not assign blame.

As you continue to work on your relationship, I hope that you will both be very sensitive to *I statements* and that you will use these in lieu of *You messages*. The I statement implies a willingness to take responsibility for your own feelings. I believe this is essential, and I feel that it is important that you each realize that no one *makes* you feel anything. Although this will take some practice, I believe that you will find it tremendously facilitating as you try to work with each other more effectively. For example, saying "I feel unloved" is more likely to lead to a solution to your problem than is the statement: "*You* don't love me." Don't feel that you can never use the pronoun "you"; in fact, it may be very important when giving feedback. However, in general it is better to start off talking about your feelings and *then* to give the feedback; e.g., "I feel angry and frustrated when you. . . ."

I hope you will be able to work hard on avoiding labeling in your relationship. This is important because labels are conclusive and absolute and imply that change is unlikely. The person who is labeled *frigid* or *impotent* or *a slob* is likely to continue being frigid or impotent or a slob. However, you usually don't believe the truth of the label and in fact what you are desiring is not basic personality change (e.g., you don't really expect your wife/ husband to stop being a slob). Rather, you are hoping for a specific alteration of some behavioral pattern (e.g., putting away his or her socks and underwear after he or she undresses for bed in the evening). In addition, labels are often used not to provide information to your partner, but rather as a way of punishing him/her for his/her shortcomings.

There are other basic rules of communication that may be valuable to you, Jane. Beware of words that are absolute such as *always* and *never*. For example, to say to your partner "You always leave your socks on the floor" is probably not factual. In fact, John may well pick up his socks the majority of the time; it is the fact that he *sometimes* leaves his socks on the floor that is annoying to you. In general, you want your communication to be as accurate and as factual as possible. A related principle of communication is to always offer an alternative. For example, "Let's make love tomorrow morning" is a far more effective response than "I don't feel like it tonight."

I hope you will also begin to work on initiating any complaint or any discussion of a problem with a *positive* interaction. This is important to get your partner's attention and to insure that he or she is listening to what you have to say. In addition, it would be useful if you had a clear idea of where you want your interaction to go *before* you become involved in a discussion, debate, or argument. A few quiet minutes alone with your eyes closed, thinking about a positive end-point for the upcoming discussion may be useful. In addition, you want to make sure that all discussions occur on neutral ground. This is important because if you argue enough in a particular setting, the setting itself will become a conditioned stimulus, which will in the future elicit argumentative behavior. In addition, the very process of going to a neutral territory will allow the passions of the moment to subside and you are then far more likely to have a positive and effective argument. Finally, I would like you to be sure that you never fight in the bedroom; in particular, you want to avoid fighting in bed, an area that should be reserved for sleep and sexuality.

A final factor I would like you to consider is dealing with your relationship, insofar as possible, during your prime time. Prime time is that time of day when you feel best and when you are most alert. It is unfortunate in our society that oftentimes our personal and marital relationships get lower priority than such trivial matters as reading the newspaper or taking care of household chores. Sex is one example. Many people confine sexual activity to a time of night when they are sleepy and perhaps exhausted after a busy day. It may well be that night is your prime time; however, if it is not, consider working on your communication with each other during mutual prime time.

These general rules I have outlined are not absolutes—few things are—and you will have to adapt them to meet your personal needs. However, I hope you will think about these basic principles and, insofar as is possible, try to incorporate them into your patterns of interaction. With enough practice they will become habitual and I'm sure they will facilitate communication between the two of you.

I will continue to discuss these issues in my work with you and I hope that you will be sure to ask me to clarify any of this if it isn't clear or if you have any questions whatsoever.

I am looking forward to continuing to work with you and I hope that these tips will prove useful in our work together.

Very truly yours,

Danny Wedding, PhD
Assistant Professor of Medical Psychology
Licensed Clinical Psychologist

/wbd

46 | Automated Educational & Vocational Guidance System

Richard A. Murray, PhD

The proposed Educational & Vocational Guidance System is a coordinated arrangement of computer software, hardware, and firmware. The author has drawn from a wide range of publications and vendors concerned with microcomputer technology while conceptualizing and designing the system. It is expected that all people interested in education and work could benefit from using the proposed equipment and software.

The Automated Educational & Vocational Guidance System would permit both therapists and clients to use the power and speed of a microcomputer to organize and access information. The hardware and software that could be used as the basis for such a system is described. Its total cost would be less than $8,000.

The programs in the proposed system fall into two major sections. The first relates to the management of information; the second focuses on service to individuals. Using the Automated Educational & Vocational Guidance System, a record consisting of several variables could be developed for each client. The specific demographic variables selected for inclusion in the data base could be determined by the psychologist or psychiatrist. This would ensure that the collected information would be useful to the professional utilizing the data.

This system would also involve the collection and organization of and access to a vast amount of vocational and educational information. Presently, most of this information is organized and accessed by hand. Prior to the introduction of microcomputers, it was virtually impossible to keep abreast of current vocational and educational information needed to serve clients adequately. Telecommunication connections with existing data bases could enable access to automatically updated vocational and educational information, ensuring information provided to clients is current and complete. The system is also designed to offer exercises related to vocational exploration, and pre-employment and post-employment assistance. Clients could use the microcomputer to develop resumés, review vocational interests, study interviewing procedures, review their work-related values, and develop an understanding of what will be expected of them on the job during the first few weeks of work.

To paraphrase Freud, life is love and work. The Automated Educational & Vocational Guidance System (AE&VG) focuses on work-related concerns. Frequently, individuals seek professional assistance when planning their educational and vocational futures. To provide effective vocational and educational counseling, hundreds of hours are required to collect and organize related data. Some clients do not receive the guidance they require because professionals' time is so limited. This may be one reason why professionals seem to have attended to the world of work less than the world of love and interpersonal relationships. Without expert assistance, some individuals may be employed in positions that do not provide an opportunity for advancement or are not suited to their particular interests and abilities. In this paper, the hardware, software, and firmware of an automated educational and vocational guidance system that can readily be put together from products on the market will be described. The primary goal of this system is to improve the quality of educational and vocational counseling services provided by psychologists and psychiatrists.

During the initial phases of vocational and educational counseling, background information on clients, jobs, and educational opportunities is required. The mechanical task of obtaining information relating to the client's vocational interests, experience, and abilities must be performed. In addition, vast amounts of general educational and vocational information must be available. With the aid of a microcomputer, this background information can be accurately gathered with minimal effort. The professional would be freed from many routine clerical and information-gathering tasks and be in a position to focus on the more complex aspects of the individual's needs. The psychologist or psychiatrist would then be able to provide well-informed guidance and assistance, while saving valuable time.

The intent of this project is to offer the clinician a set of tools, including a microcomputer, to provide a complete vocational exploration and planning system. This system is directed toward realistic educational and vocational counseling, resulting in appropriate competitive employment for the client. The specific objectives of the system are to offer the following services:

1. Vocational exploration;
2. Vocational planning;
3. Interest inventory administration;
4. Work values review;
5. Interviewing and job-search guides;
6. Development of employment resumes; and
7. An evaluation of self-concept and work.

The vocational exploration and planning objectives could be met using a computer-based information system called *The Guidance Information System*. This data base includes a Career Information Delivery System accessed via a telecommunications link between an Apple computer and a Guidance Information System vendor. Such a vendor does exist. TSC, a Houghton Mifflin Company, provides a data base consisting of information related to occupations, two-year and four-year colleges, graduate and professional schools, and financial aids. The occupational information file contains 875 primary occupational listings, with reference to approximately 2,500 related jobs. The two-year-college information file and the four-year-college information file enable users to explore information about more than 3,300 colleges, universities, and technical institutions. The graduate and professional school information file contains information on over 1,500 graduate and professional institutions across the country. Finally, the financial aid information file contains information about national scholarship and financial aid programs worth millions of dollars. These files are continuously updated by the data base manager.

The system would also permit use of "stand-alone" computer-assisted instruction (CAI) packages. The Resumé Righter (sic), Job Readiness Software, and Basic Skills Work Series software are examples of currently available vocational software (see appendix at end of this chapter). The Resumé Righter (sic), provides step-by-step prompting, which builds the user's resumé. The program also keeps track of employers and job offers. The program disk comes with a free booklet, "Hints & Tips of Resumé Writing" by Catherine Winston. The Job Readiness and Basic Skills Work Series software packages consist of modules with the following titles:

1. How to get and hold a job
2. You can get the job
3. Self-concept and work
4. Earning money now; what you should know about insurance
5. First weeks of work
6. The interview.

New diagnostic tools and CAI programs related to vocational psychology are continuously being developed. Clients would be able to select from a variety of modules to meet their specific needs. Many of the CAI exercises will result in professional staff time saved, because the clients would be able to use the various modules semi-independently. The system should also include word-processing capabilities to expedite correspondence and report-preparation.

To the author's knowledge, a microcomputer-based career information system similar to the AE&VG has not previously been suggested. This may be because few individuals have a background in applied vocational and educational psychology and microcomputers to develop such a system. The author has ten years' experience providing counseling services and eight years' experience working with mainframe and microcomputers.

The AE&VG system is compatible with present Apple systems. The data-management section of the system requires development of data-collection procedures. A brief software routine could be developed to collect demographic data directly from clients, or the DBMaster program* can be used to record this information. When relevant variables are defined, staff members should be consulted to incorporate their unique data needs. Procedures should be followed to ensure confidentiality.

All hardware, software, and firmware needed for the system are currently available. A listing of the vendors is included for your reference (Table 47–1). Those who wish more detailed information on the

TABLE 47–1. Listing of Vendors

HARDWARE

Apple Computer, Inc.
10260 Bandley Drive
Cupertino, CA 95014
(408) 996–1010
(Apple & Disc II)

Sanyo Electric, Inc.
Communications Products
1200 West Artesia Boulevard
Compton, CA 90202
(Video monitor)

Epson America, Inc.
3415 Kashiwa Street
Torrance, CA 90505
(213) 539–9140
(Printer & card)

Videx, Inc.
897 N.W. Grant Avenue
Corvallis, OR 97330
(503) 758–0521
(80-column card)

Prometheus Products, Inc.
4509 Thompson Court
Fremont, CA 94538
(415) 791–0266
(Versacard 4 in 1)

R.H. Electronics, Inc.
566 Irelan, Bin P2
Buellton, CA 93427
(805) 688–2047
(Super Fan II)

D.C. Hayes Associates, Inc.
Microcomputer Products
10 Perimeter Park Drive
Atlanta, GA 30341
(404) 455–7663
(Micro Modem)

*The DBMaster program is a data base management software system developed by Stoneware Microcomputer Products, San Rafael, CA.

SOFTWARE

Stoneware Microcomputer Products
50 Belvedere Street
San Rafael, CA 94901
(415) 454–6500
(DBMaster-Data Management)

Sensible Software
6619 Perham Drive
Dept. P
West Bloomfield, MI 48033
(313) 399–8877
(Super Disc Copy 3)

Computer Solutions
6 Maize Place
Mansfield, Q. 4122
Australia
(Aust) (07) 349–9883
(International) (61) (7)349–9883
(Zardax Wordprocessor)

Hammett Microcomputer Division
Hammett Place
Box 545
Braintree, MA 02184
(617) 848–1000
(Job Readiness Software)

Matex Associates, Inc.
90 Cheery Street
Box 519
Johnstown, PA 15907
(Basic Skills Work Series)

SSM Microcomputer Products, Inc.
2190 Paragon Drive
San Jose, CA 95131
(408) 946–7400
(Telecommunications Software)

Acro-matic, Inc.
256 S.W. 5th Street
Boca Raton, FL 33432
(Resume Righter)

OTHER VENDORS

Cover Craft
P.O. Box 555
Amherst, NH 03031
(Dust cover)

TSC
A Houghton Mifflin Company
Box 683
Hanover, NH 03755
(The Guidance System)

Fiberbilt Cases
Ikelheimer-Ernst, Inc.
601 West 26th Street
New York, NY 10001
(212) 675–5820
(Computer printer & monitor cases)

Disks, ribbons, and paper:
contact your local computer store

specific equipment and software needed to implement the AE&VG system can write to the vendors. The estimated cost (as of November 1982) is $7,798.60 (Table 47–2). Specific details are included in the budget, which follows. Carrying cases were included in the budget, to make the complete system portable.

TABLE 47–2. Cost of the Automated Educational & Vocational Guidance System

Equipment Description (Itemized)	COSTS (as of Nov. 1982)
HARDWARE	
Apple II Plus 48K RAM (DOS 3.3)	$1530.00
Disc II Floppy Disc and Controller	$645.00
Disc II — Drive only	$525.00
Sanyo Video Monitor 12″ Green Screen	$299.00
Epson MX80F/T Printer	$645.00
Epson/Apple Interface Card and Cable	$100.00
Replacement Head for Epson Printer	$30.00
Videx Video Term 80 Column	$345.00
Prometheus Versacard (4 in 1)	$249.00
Super Fan II	$74.95
D.C. Hayes Micro Modem	379.00
SOFTWARE	
DBMaster (Data Management)	$229.00
Basic Skills Work Series	$205.00
Job Readiness Software	$225.00
Super Disc Copy 3	$30.00
Transend II Data Communications	$250.00
Zardax Wordprocessor	$295.00
Resume Righter	$24.95
SUPPLIES	
Floppy Disks (6 boxes)	$300.00
Ribbons for Epson Printer (4)	$48.00
OTHER EXPENSES	
Dust Cover for Apple II	$11.95
Fiberbilt Computer Case	$173.75
Fiberbilt Monitor and Printer Case	$275.00
Apple Service Agreement	$225.00
Occupational Info Data Base	$684.00
Total Operating Expenses	$7798.60

A Comparison
of the Effectiveness
# of Spoken, Written,
and Computer-Based
Instruction
(A Review)

Marc D. Schwartz, MD

omputer-person interaction is of interest to a number of researchers and practitioners. An interesting study carried out at the Beth Israel Hospital in Boston compares the computer's effectiveness in patient teaching with written materials or personal instruction.

The authors [Fisher et al.] note that "despite homage (paid) to the education of patients, instructional dialogue is difficult, time-consuming and expensive and often omitted from the practice of medicine. Some clinics use *written* instructions in an effort to provide accurate and inexpensive directions. In the absence of dialogue, however, it is difficult to respond to the needs of individual patients, and there is no assurance that the instructions will be read, understood, and followed. A digital computer, on the other hand, can interact directly with the patient, while providing instructional guidance in an accurate, consistent, and thorough manner."

In an attempt to compare different methods of instruction, a large group of young women were given computer, spoken, written, or no instructions for the collection of a clean-voided urine specimen. The measure of effectiveness of the instructions was the number of

"Collection of a Clean Voided Urine Specimen: A Comparison Among Spoken, Written, and Computer-Based Instruction," by L. A. Fisher, T. S. Johnson, D. Porter, H. L. Bleich, and W. V. Slack, appeared in the *American Journal of Public Health*, July 1977, *67*, 640–644. The above review of that article originally appeared in *Computers in Psychiatry/Psychology*, 1978, *1*(2), 9 and is reprinted by permission.

contaminating bacteria cultured from clean-catch urine subsequently collected. I found this a particularly elegant research design, since so little inference is necessary to judge the effectiveness of the difficult instructional method: the better each works, the fewer bacteria will be present.

The spoken instructions and written instructions were no mere straw persons for the computer. The individuals who gave the spoken instructions gave them in a well-organized, unhurried, personal way, encouraging questions and asking the patients to repeat the instructions so that points needing clarification could be identified.

Patients who received written instructions were asked to read them in the presence of an attendant, who encouraged questions and was available for discussion.

The computer instructions were given on a CRT and subjects responded on a typewriter-type keyboard. Since progress through the computer interview was contingent on the patient's answers, the machine could detect misunderstandings and respond appropriately to individual needs.

The results? "Total bacterial counts were lowest in urine cultured from members of the group receiving computer instruction." The computer took longer but was more thorough. Most of those exposed to personal instruction first liked it better. Most of those who had computer instruction first liked *it* better. The computer's novelty, anonymity, and patience appealed to some. The human's warmth, speed, and ability to individualize were attractive to others.

48 Computer-Assisted Instruction for the Private Practitioner

John P. Flynn, PhD
Terry Kuczeruk, MSW

Among the many potential uses of computing machinery in private practice, computer-assisted instruction (CAI) is perhaps one of the least visible forms of the technology. To be sure, many of the management information system possibilities, such as record-keeping, report-generation, and billing, are more immediately germane to operation of the enterprise. Also, some programs, such as client-administered tests or practitioner use of small statistical packages, are perhaps more likely candidates for practice technology. Computer-assisted instruction, as with teaching or training in many areas, is not likely to be a top priority. Nevertheless, CAI capability offers an opportunity to provide in-house or on-site training and, at the same time, the maximization of a practitioner's capacity. First, however, it would be useful to gain some understanding of what CAI is and from whence it has come.

COMPUTER-ASSISTED INSTRUCTION—ORIGINS

Computer-assisted instruction is nothing more than the planned and systematic utilization of computer machinery (e.g., microcomputers or mainframes) and procedures (e.g., software or courseware) for the purpose of achieving an educational or training goal. CAI is generally ori-

---

Much of the material utilized in this paper is extracted from a research project "Computer-Assisted Instruction as a Training Methodology for Child Placement Licensing Staff," conducted by a student-faculty group in the School of Social Work, Western Michigan University, Spring 1982. Project members were: Margaret Dokter, Dale R. Hein, Terry Kuczeruk, Kay Loftus, Jon Manby, Peter Matchinsky, Robert Monsma, James Muller, Michele Rutherford, and John Flynn (Project Director).

ented to an individual's convenience wherein the system is utilized in an interactive mode. There is, of course, the potential use of CAI in orientation of new staff, in training of existing office personnel to new procedures or methods, or in administering procedures to clients through a medium that provides immediate and explicit feedback. It also has potential for providing training to clients or patients in a mode that is highly individualized as to availability, repetitiousness, and the provision of feedback.

In 1954, B. F. Skinner adopted the idea of a teaching machine because he saw great potential in its development. Skinner regarded the machine as an excellent tutor for five reasons: (1) there was a constant interchange between the user and the program, thus making it possible for the user to remain alert and to sustain activity; (2) the machine, by virtue of its program, insisted that the user had to master a concept before moving on; (3) the machine presented only that material for which the user was ready; (4) the machine helped the user to respond correctly by hinting, prompting, and suggesting in an orderly presentation of frames; and (5) the use of feedback to shape behavior and maintain user interest reinforced correct responses (Collagon, 1976).

Skinner developed a linear teaching program composed of a small set of logical steps leading incrementally through the subject matter, a program based on his theory of operant conditioning. Such an approach, Skinner argued, increased the propensity for correct responses because the student's response is conditioned and reinforced by the previous frames. Two techniques serve to reinforce correct responses: orderly construction of the problem and the use of hinting, prompting, and suggesting (Collagon, 1976).

In the 1960s, Norman Crowder developed intrinsic or branching programmed instruction. Crowder argued that there were two shortcomings in a linear program. First, elimination of user error in instruction was both undesirable and impractical. Second, elimination of user error requires the program to be constructed with such small and simple steps that educational objectives will not be served. In short, Crowder saw in Skinner's approach too much busywork for the user (Collagon, 1976).

The intrinsic program consists of frames in the form of multiple-choice questions and answers. The user is presented with a problem or question having several possible answers. The user's answers can be anticipated and material prepared for them in advance can be employed, based on an answer to any particular question. If the user answers correctly, reinforcement is given for the correct answer. If the answer entered is incorrect, feedback is given to explain the error (Collagon, 1976).

Skinner and other proponents of the linear approach suggested that there are three dangers in intrinsic programming: (1) there is a danger of overloading the user with information; (2) not all incorrect answers can be anticipated; and (3) intrinsic programming provides less opportunity for meaningful error than does linear programming (Collagon, 1976).

The use of the computer to provide instructional content directly to the user has, in many ways, resolved this controversy. The CAI program offers the best of both approaches. It provides the user with information to be learned as well as feedback to specific responses. The experience for the user becomes more individualized and the interaction between the user and the machine becomes more humanlike. CAI, therefore, is the result of a marriage between the computer and programmed instruction (Collagon, 1976).

For large learning/teaching systems, an entire program of CAI-related programs can be developed, which will provide instructional management functions like storing user performance or scheduling user course selections. Computer-managed instruction (CMI) is more likely to be found in large training systems and is less likely to be needed by private practitioners.

The use of the computer as an instructional device is an outgrowth of the educational technology field. Educational technology employs a systems approach to instruction, which includes specific, measurable instructional objectives, diagnostic testing criteria for performance, and repeated redesign of curricula (Schoen, 1977). These are all characteristics that CAI has borrowed and employed and that should be carried over into CAI applications in private practice.

It is useful at this point to look at some of the advantages and disadvantages of computer-assisted instruction.

Advantages of CAI

1. Due to constant participation, the learner is active and attentive;
2. By being able to move privately at their own pace, gifted learners are not bound, slower learners are not rushed, and shy learners are not embarrassed by incorrect answers given in public;
3. The computer is impartial, patient, and objective;
4. The learner gets immediate feedback to answers given, enabling the learner to check progress and to produce responses that can be measured and evaluated;
5. The computer can secure, store, and process information about the participant's performance prior to and/or during instruction to determine subsequent activities in the learning situation;

6. Due to more immediate feedback, computers produce more efficient learning and perhaps more highly motivated learners than with traditional didactic methods;
7. The learner can make up work missed;
8. The computer can provide greater flexibility in scheduling learning programs than with traditional didactic methods;
9. It is possible for a few learners to take a programmed course, although there may be insufficient numbers to justify a conventional section;
10. Computers store large amounts of information and make it available to the learner more rapidly than any other medium;
11. Computers provide programmed control of several media, such as films, slides, television, and demonstration equipment;
12. Computers give the author an extremely convenient technique for designing and developing a course of instruction;
13. Computers provide a dynamic interaction between learner and instructional programmer not possible with most other media;
14. The computer can be used to achieve heretofore impossible versatility in branching and individualized instruction;
15. CAI forces or enables the author of CAI courseware to become cognizant of the instructional process;
16. Computers have the ability to simulate real-life situations;
17. CAI provides a variety of learning opportunities;
18. The responsibility for learning is placed directly on the individual; and
19. The learner becomes aware of modern technology and can develop a sense of control over his/her learning environment.

Disadvantages of CAI

1. In many programs the user's efficiency is dependent upon reading ability and comprehension;
2. The teaching program is only as good as the material that goes into it;
3. Programmed instruction insists on deep and intrinsic learner motivation;
4. Learner encouragement, inspiration, and stimulation becomes mechanical with machines;
5. Learners are unable to ask questions to clear up problems;
6. A learner cannot learn more than is programmed;
7. Good programming is time-consuming to prepare;
8. Hardware and the development of courseware are both costly investments;

9. There can be problems in finding personnel to develop course-ware; and
10. There remains a question of cost-effectiveness, i.e., are the outcomes worth the financial investment? (Collagon, 1976; Ingle, 1976).

ISSUES FOR PLANNING, RESEARCH, AND DEVELOPMENT

Necessity dictates that quality research and planning play a fundamental role in the development of the CAI system. The need for planning is a basic tenet of any kind of organizational project, whether it is computer-related or not. But the commitment in time, effort, and resources that is required to develop CAI mandates even greater care in planning than noncomputerized projects would require. Though the benefits of CAI can be great, the potential pitfalls, if unanticipated, can place the developer in circumstances worse than when it started.

Chris Dimas suggests that the first priority for CAI development is that an organization define and clarify the role it wishes CAI to perform in an educational program (Dimas, 1978). This should come in the form of a policy or purpose statement, the goal of which will be to give direction to all aspects of CAI development. For example: should CAI be treated as a supplement to a broader range of instructional methods, or should it become the sole means of instruction? An answer to a question of this type will determine many things, not the least of which is cost, as well as the type of hardware and courseware to acquire. The advantages of such policy statements cannot be overestimated.

Diane Essex and William Sorlie have provided an excellent list of recommendations for planning of CAI (Sorlie & Essex, 1979):

1. A six-month, funded start-up phase for planning and recruitment of developers is recommended. The task of defining the operational goals of the project must be completed early in this phase. If the private practitioner will not do the initial development work, personnel recruitment must be undertaken at this time. If the decision is made to use existing staff, they must be provided with any necessary training in computer usage and instructional methods.
2. The resources needed to meet the objectives of the project must be identified and provided. These include staff requirements, hardware requirements, and software requirements.
3. Courseware design must not only relate necessary concepts and

facts, but must also be presented in a useful and creative manner. Unless this occurs, the lessons will go unused and the hardware will collect dust in the equipment storeroom (Daneliuk & Wright, 1981). Planning must address these considerations.

4. Evaluation of the CAI project must be provided for from the very beginning. The evaluation must be both ongoing (formative) and end-product-directed (summative). This will provide flexibility to the project and will facilitate any necessary alternatives that may present themselves. Such evaluations should review all aspects of CAI development, ranging from costs to the adequacy of materials content.

Different practitioners will approach these issues and recommendations in ways unique to their particular circumstances. Both resources and needs will inevitably determine the nature of CAI design. Though the specifics may be different, this list does suggest the key elements for effective planning of CAI.

Carole Bagley supplies a list of specific characteristics that must be rank-ordered for selecting any CAI system (Bagley, 1979). Each characteristic is subject to one's rankings, which again depend on needs and resources. The characteristics to be ranked are presented as follows:

1. Cost of hardware;
2. Cost of software;
3. Cost of telephone communications, if any;
4. Cost of courseware not contained in the software costs;
5. Ease of student use;
6. Ease of author use;
7. Maximum capability for users;
8. Maximum capability for author use;
9. Message-sending capability between student and teacher; and
10. Whether or not to use an already existing administrative computer to deliver CAI (called "piggybacking") or to create CAI (called "authoring").

In the January 1979 issue of *Educational Technology*, Fred Splittberger developed a useful list of various CAI and CMI systems (Splittberger, 1979). Each system is presented with information about the system developer, system type (including a description of its basic components), services, and applicability to certain curricula and student types. This list is not an exhaustive one, though it does present information on some of the leading systems; as such it may be a helpful resource for some interested practitioners.

SELECTION OF APPROACH

Most private practitioners will likely rely on a personal computer or microcomputer for their various needs, including CAI if appropriate. Mainframe or time-sharing systems are not apt to be so attractive, particularly on a cost basis, though some networking and time-sharing arrangements are growing rapidly.

The personal computer, however, is a complete computer in itself and therefore does not suffer from the same disadvantages as the time-sharing systems. Personal computers have advantages of their own. The development of small integrated circuits has expanded the capability of personal computers and lowered their initial purchase price and maintenance costs (Joiner, Miller, & Silverstein, 1980). It is now possible to interlink microcomputers with major computer systems via telephone lines. In other words, microcomputers can have the additional capacity for acting as terminals. Also, Joiner suggests that the personal computer is much less mysterious to the user than large computers because of its compactness (Joiner, Miller, & Silverstein, 1980).

However, Joiner notes three disadvantages to the use of microcomputers: (1) there is a lack of CAI language for microcomputer application (although this deficiency is changing rapidly with authoring languages like PILOT); (2) microcomputers have a limited ability to perform repetitive calculations (though this limitation is disappearing); and (3) they have limited ability to store and recall large data files. Hard-disk storage has made an impact upon this problem. As mentioned earlier, engineering and marketing trends suggest that microcomputer capabilities will increase, while costs will decrease (Joiner, Miller, & Silverstein, 1980).

The prospective buyer of a personal computer must be aware of several things. Microcomputers sold as blank slates must be programmed from scratch (Joiner, Miller, & Silverstein, 1980). Telephone links to a large computer require acoustic couplers, which are devices necessary to permit signal passage between the two computers (Crease, 1977).

For best educational use, the video display unit (VDU) should be capable of showing alphanumeric and graphic information (Bork, 1979). The text display capacity (the number of characters that can be viewed on the screen at one time) must be ample, since a small text display is a definite handicap to the user (Bork, 1979). When accessing time-sharing computers, attention should be given to response time. CAI suffers if output is continually interrupted or if replies are slow in appearing (Crease, 1977). New hard disks for microcomputers can store up to 2,000,000 bytes and can access any point on a disk in a fraction of a second.

What does all this information imply? Bork writes:

> Going beyond this, we can ask whether [a personal computer] acting alone will be (particularly when one reaches large-scale production) an effective mechanism for developing the types of materials we are now considering. The answer is probably no. One needs many of the capabilities of a larger system in such activity. Hence, it is likely that development will take place in a distributed environment with both personal computers and a central machine. The central computer will be for massive storage of programs and other information for management, for early testing of the material, and for resources beyond the capabilities of individual machines. [Bork, 1979, p. 10]

The handling of CAI by a personal computer interfaced with a large-frame computer may be "the ideal situation" (Crease, 1977, p. 48).

The term *software* refers to the computer's programs and accompanying documentation. Software is stored in a secondary storage area (e.g., disks) when not being used. When the user requests a program, the computer reads the software into its main memory in order to use the program. A program is a series of instructions to a computer, which causes the computer to solve a problem or perform a task (Douglas & Edwards, 1979). CAI courseware is merely a particular type of computer program.

Seven modes of instructional use for computers exist: tutorial, drill and practice, problem-solving, gaming, simulation, inquiry, and dialogue. The tutorial mode presents facts, skills, and/or concepts to the learner for the first time. Its emphasis is on the educational material and it is sometimes designed to evaluate the user's response in order to modify the material to the user's level. In the drill-and-practice mode, an individualized routine is provided, which reviews and practices basic skills or concepts acquired through some separate instructional process. The user responds to questions concerning the skills or concepts, responses are evaluated, and immediate reinforcement or feedback is given concerning the correctness of those responses. The user of the problem-solving mode uses a computer language, such as BASIC, FORTRAN, or COBOL to instruct the computer in how he/she would solve a problem. In the gaming mode, the user learns gaming skills by interacting with the computer via a terminal. Each game operates upon specific rules, which are programmed into the computer and are presented to the user. In the simulation mode, the computer randomly selects "real-life" situations that reflect exigencies that the user must deal with. The inquiry mode, based on the user's need and interest, consists of a data base of information and strategy of accessing it in some logical pattern. The user searches the material, focusing on those elements that answer the criteria set forth in the data base. Finally, the usage-dialogue mode, in a highly developmental stage on the research frontier, allows the user to interact in the form of dialogue with the computer in the user's own language (Austin, 1978). The appropriate mode in the private practice situation would depend, of course, on the particular purposes or objectives of each CAI project.

A computer language is a language used to communicate with a computer. Assembly or machine language is a programming language written in binary, octal, or hexadecimal notation. Programs written in machine language do not need to be translated in order for the computer to execute its instructions because machine language is computer language. A general purpose or high-level language (such as BASIC, FORTRAN, PASCAL, etc.) is symbolic. The instructions to the computer are represented by words or mnemonic devices, which humans can understand. The translator, speaking both human and computer language, is the compiler.

Compiler language instructs a compiler to translate general-purpose language into machine language (Douglas, 1979). An author language, such as GNOSIS or PILOT, is a higher-level language than a general-purpose language. An authoring language is specially designed so that it contains instructions helpful to the courseware author and the instructional programmer. These languages are higher-level languages, since it would usually take several general-purpose language instructions to carry out a single authoring language instruction (Schuyler, 1979). Authoring languages are sometimes referred to as "user-friendly" (Leiblum, 1979, p. 8). Consequently, many private practitioners can more readily learn to "program" in authoring language than in the high-level popular symbolic languages.

An author who is anticipating that a learner will be using a terminal and large-frame computer to run a program is well-advised to use an authoring language to implement that CAI program. However, as noted above, there is a relative lack of authoring languages for microcomputer use (Joiner, Miller, & Silverstein, 1980), though some variations on the PILOT language for CAI are now coming out. As microcomputer systems increase in speed and storage capacities, one can expect to see a number of authoring languages available on each processor (Schuyler, 1979).

Authoring languages were created specifically for CAI use. BASIC is a comparatively limited and less effective language to use for CAI purposes. Since microcomputers are often a cost-saving option over the large-frame computer, and since investing in a terminal over a microcomputer could subsequently be a waste of resources if and when more authoring languages for microcomputer use are developed, the rapid rate of language development is a key issue here, since private practitioners are more likely to develop their own microcomputer uses.

Three essential characteristics of all programmed instruction identified in the history of CAI, are first, that there be an interaction between learner and material and immediate feedback, which informs the learner of the adequacy of her or his response. Second, the subject matter to be presented is composed in a programmatic format (i.e., as an ordered set of presentations and questions for the learner). Third, it is composed of a series of items referred to as frames (units of the program, which require a response from the learner). The information needed to correctly answer a given item must be contained either in that item, in the preceding items, or in both (Collagon, 1976).

Going a step beyond programmed instruction, the author of CAI courseware should become aware of the "systems approach" for designing instructional materials. This approach includes: (1) identification of educational needs; (2) behavioral objective formulation; (3) strategy selection and sequencing; (4) media selection; (5) instructional preparation; (6) evaluation of learning objectives and materials; and (7) reworking defective parts (Ingle & Musterman, 1979).

During the third phase, strategy selection and sequencing, the author must decide what instructional methods are important and how they are to be sequenced. The fifth phase, instructional preparation, refers to building the actual program. Once the final program has been tested during the sixth phase, evaluation of learning objectives and materials and defective parts must be identified and revised during the seventh phase, reworking defective parts, which may include re-evaluation and reworking of all system steps (Ingle & Musterman, 1979).

The purpose of courseware evaluation is simply to improve courseware and to establish its effectiveness. There are seven methods of evaluation commonly used (Crease, 1977):

1. Learner interviews;
2. Learner feedback sheets;
3. Pretests and posttests;
4. Questions within the program;
5. Computer monitoring (which records learner-controlled inputs as a function of time and produces them as a table for study);
6. Staff interviews; and
7. Close observation of package use (which enables an observer to record what the learner is saying as well as typing, giving insightful clues to weaknesses in the package).

There is no simple way of evaluating a CAI program. A general impression should be formed, based on several sources. Interviews should be the most influential sources of information. As the program stops changing rapidly, interviews should be replaced by learner feedback forms, which will maintain a check on the use of the program. Pretests and posttests are difficult to construct and may not be necessary to a complete evaluation. If they are used, they should be short so they will not inconvenience the learner, but they should be penetrating and pertinent to the program (Crease, 1977). Interestingly, the practitioner is in a unique position of being both provider and evaluator in this regard.

A person who is interested in developing CAI courseware should keep the following suggestions in mind:

1. Develop and keep long-range goals;
2. Be imaginative (don't be confined to what has been done);
3. Work with groups if possible;
4. Do not start at square one;
5. Consider pedagogical problems independently of programming problems;
6. Revise your program;
7. Avoid BASIC if possible; it is not good for complex materials;
8. Avoid today's minimal systems; and
9. Avoid tape-cassette-based systems. [Bork, 1979]

Courseware, then, is a specific type of computer program created for computer-assisted instruction use. Authoring languages were created specifically for writing CAI programs and therefore are the most efficient type of language to use in the courseware creation process. Courseware is created by a CAI staff and the issues involved in developing a CAI staff were cited above. Finally, it should be kept in mind that the authors of courseware should use the systems approach in the courseware creation process.

COSTS

Cost estimation for CAI is a very difficult topic to address (Spuck & Bozeman, 1978; Bozeman, 1979). Seltzer claims that employing the computer for instruction involves judgments based on the following three criteria: (1) if the computer provides a unique and effective approach to the instructional process, then it should be used regardless of the cost involved; (2) if the computer is a more efficient instructor than a traditional approach, and the cost of its use is minimal, then it should be used; and (3) if the cost of CAI is relatively high, while its effectiveness is only marginal, then the computer should not be used for instruction (Patrick & Stammers, 1977). These three broad criteria may provide practitioners with some direction in considering the cost of a CAI system. Having presented this very general approach to cost consideration, what kind of specificity can be extracted from the literature?

In particular, cost estimation of CAI must include hardware, software, courseware, logistics, telecommunications, personnel training, research and development issues, and any potential "hidden" costs. The emphasis placed on each issue will vary, depending on such things as the purpose of the CAI system, and how many of the costs have already been absorbed.

Hardware Costs

The cost of hardware is a question that can be framed in the context of the basic computer types, i.e., the mainframe or maxicomputer, the minicomputer, and the microcomputer. Daneliuk and Wright (1981) advise that prospective use of CAI hardware be determined only after research and evaluation comparing the cost of the mainframe, minicomputers, and microcomputers.

As a further guide to considering the hardware costs of microcomputers, the prospective purchasers should ask the following questions: (1) Will the microcomputer serve as a terminal in a time-sharing system? (2) How many microcomputers will be needed to adequately serve the projected level of use? (3) What is the anticipated life span of the hardware? And, finally, (4) How should the expenses be amortized? (Joiner, Miller, & Silverstein, 1980). These questions can also be rephrased to apply to the possible purchase of both the minicomputer and mainframe computer.

Software Costs

The hardware cost estimations for CAI are relatively easy in comparison to cost estimations for the other categories, though estimation of hardware cost is by no means simple. Relative to other aspects of computer systems, software expenses have been steadily increasing over the past 30 years. Software made up 15% of the total cost for a computer system in 1955. It rose to 75% in 1977 and projections for 1985 place it at 90% of the total cost (Schoech, 1982). There is no simple reason for this increase, but generally speaking, it is due to a decrease in hardware costs and a greater demand for a variety of software items (and, consequently, a greater reliance on personnel as opposed to machinery).

According to Schoech, there are three major sources of software: premanufactured software accompanying certain brands of hardware; in-house developed software; and professional software firms

(Schoech, 1982). Programs manufactured to accompany hardware are specifically designed for use with those particular computer systems. In-house programs are self-produced by an agency or organization. Professional software firms design programs contracted for by organizations or agencies. Choosing a source of hardware, it should be noted, is an important cost consideration for software as well and must inevitably be addressed when designing a CAI system. One word of warning: good-quality, premanufactured software for use in the human services is not readily available; consequently, practitioners must be wary of purchasing such products unless they are absolutely sure of acquiring what they need.

The in-house production of software involves cost considerations, primarily in terms of personnel. This is especially an issue when the practitioner does not have the time or resources to produce his or her own materials. Who will create the programs and write the lessons? Will training need to be provided for the personnel, and at what cost? How many hours will be required to develop lessons, and at what cost? If a programming consultant must be hired, how much will it cost? Hebenstreit speaks to some of these issues in his study on the costs of 10,000 microcomputers in French secondary schools. His findings revealed that 50% of the initial costs were for training the teachers in programming and 25% for hardware. Thereafter, 70% of the costs consisted of staffing, teacher training, and program writing. He estimates 100 to 300 hours are needed to develop one program (Hebenstreit, 1980).

The key question for the use of software provided by a professional firm is, "Can such a program be produced at less expense than an in-house program?" The evaluation of software cost is difficult to address and varies from unit to unit. Some underlying assumptions for software costs are suggested by Kearsley (1977). His list includes expenses for purchasing or renting the CAI system, course-authoring languages, graphics and/or audio software, and utility programs. Kearsley claims that these costs are frequently excluded from cost estimates, either because they are too difficult to project or because they are assumed to be negligible. Any assumption that these costs are negligible is not only unfounded, but also foolish.

Courseware and Other CAI Costs

Courseware, the instructional programs themselves, imply costs over and above that of the more generic category, software. Once the instructional program has been developed, it will periodically need revision, due to a number of circumstances. For example, new developments in the content field will outdate lessons. It is a serious mistake to assume that once a lesson is in place it will no longer need inputs of time, money, and energy. Another mistake is the omission of cost estimates for producing adjunct materials, such as manuals on computer operation or supplementary instructional materials (Kearsley, 1977).

The literature indicated that logistical questions and telecommunications are two other categories that must be factored into cost estimates for CAI. They are both topics often overlooked. "Telecommunication costs involve simply the transmission costs via voice-grade telephone lines, digital data networks, microwave, UHF television, or satellite transmission" (Kearsley, 1977, p. 101). If the use of telecommunications will be necessary, a practitioner must determine what services and equipment (modems, etc.) will be needed, as well as their cost.

The task of research must also be factored into cost estimations for CAI. Generation of user feedback, a vital part of the CAI development process, will produce costs; such things as design and implementation of questionnaires will mean additional expenses. Again, cost estimates should always be balanced against alternative modes of instruction (Kearsley, 1977).

Interagency or intra-agency distribution of cost is often employed by organizations utilizing CAI. In principle, this approach seems to have merit; however, in private practice this opportunity is not generally available. While practitioners could possibly share CAI materials, courseware is not easily transferred from system to system if two practitioners have different hardware. The lack of standardization of systems may require considerable writing and rewriting of courseware, even when transferring material to supposedly "identical" systems. Such problems can prove to be formidable barriers and may, in fact, effectively eliminate any hope of cost savings from a joint venture.

Hidden Costs

Finally, practitioners must be aware of an entire category of "hidden" costs. Often overlooked are the available service provisions from system manufacturers. What manufacturer services are available for the hardware? What will the cost be? Will service be readily available? Where is the service facility located? (Joiner, Miller, & Silverstein, 1980) Operating costs must also be considered. Further, all cost estimates must allow for the effects of monetary inflation. Though this list of "hidden" costs is not exhaustive, it does serve to alert the potential user of CAI to some possible unanticipated expenses.

In summary, the literature revealed cost estimations for CAI to be a difficult and complex task, but a task that must be accomplished to develop any CAI system. Costs can be divided into convenient categories: hardware, software, courseware, logistics and telecommunications, personnel, research and development, and potential "hidden" costs. If no other points are remembered, it is imperative to remember this: relative to all other costs of any computer project, software has been continually rising and makes up the majority of cost consideration.

HUMAN FACTORS

A practitioner contemplating the use of CAI must consider the human factors. Learner use and author use are the two main human factors identified in the literature. Learner use includes information on user characteristics, user personality characteristics, and recommendations to facilitate learner use. Author use includes information about CAI system capabilities requiring different levels of author skill and about how to utilize the author's creative abilities.

A good CAI system accounts for user characteristics by maximizing strengths and minimizing weaknesses. But no current CAI system has the sophistication to gather all the possible information on user characteristics to provide individualized instruction (McCann, 1981). Therefore, the gathering of such needed information becomes the responsibility of both the designers and implementers of the CAI system.

User characteristics consist of prior knowledge of materials content, and prior knowledge of the computer and the learner's visual, verbal, and mental abilities. If the user has little prior knowledge of the materials content, appropriate instructional support to provide help in answering content questions is needed; however, an advanced user would become bored with excessive support. If the user has prior knowledge of the computer, that user will tend to be less apprehensive of its use and therefore will make better use of CAI. If the user's visual and verbal abilities are poor, elaborate visual and verbal representations will need to be provided (Carrier, 1978). Individuals with high mental ability benefit more from CAI presentations that are "perceptually complex, of fixed pace, informationally laden, in multi-channel motion pictoral forms (movies and televisions)" than does the individual with low mental ability (McCann, 1981, p. 138).

It is important to consider three user personality characteristics: psychological factors, apprehension factors, and the degree of user motivation. Bozeman used Jungian concepts of perception and judgment in a study of the Wisconsin System for Instructional Management (WIS-SIM). He measured the following factors: apprehension toward use of human-machine systems; confidence in WIS-SIM; and perception of usefulness of WIS-SIM.

Bozeman found that extroverts more readily use the computer, because their main interest is in the external environment of people and things; consequently, they are more receptive to information, ideas, and concepts that may be learned from CAI. Introverts, on the other hand, are less receptive to external sources of information and concepts; and hence, are less likely to make effective use of CAI. Students with extrovert and cognitive tendencies had more confidence in the WIS-SIM than introvert and affective-oriented students. The extrovert/cognitive students found WIS-SIM more useful because, typically, they tend to be analytical and methodical and they respect that which is rational and objective. As a result of these findings, Bozeman suggests that CAI decisionmakers must have a more complete understanding of psychological types of learners for CAI use. This must include both research and implementation of the necessary information (Bozeman, 1978).

User apprehension is often a result of anxiety with the hardware. This anxiety stems from two sources: the rapidity with which the computer can perform its tasks, and its complexity and newness.

The user's degree of motivation is also an important factor to consider. Specifically, those individuals who want to work with people and have a high regard for interpersonal relationships may not be receptive to heavy doses of the computer (Carrier, 1978). Therefore, it may be reasonable to infer that those with a human-services perspective may not be totally receptive to CAI. It is alleged that CAI is both dehumanizing and impersonal. For example, Collagon suggests that student encouragement, inspiration, and stimulation become mechanical while using machines. Collagon suggests further that CAI leaves little room for creativity on the part of the student (Collagon, 1976). However, Magidson refutes these allegations by pointing to CAI's individual treatment of each student. He also points out CAI's capacity to provide a patient, tireless, and objective tutor, counselor, tester, and/or evaluator. CAI even tolerates alternative answers and solutions. Therefore, it is suggested the CAI be used in as personal a manner as possible to counter the allegation that CAI is dehumanizing and impersonal (Magidson, 1977).

Design of CAI lessons should facilitate use. This requires user input, feedback, and administrative support. If possible, material design features should consist of user-controlled options for replaying the text, reviewing the text, and choosing the text's route.

Materials design must be adaptive and responsive to the user. The sequence and style of material will also facilitate ease of use. Materials must be as interactive as possible. For example: lesson menus should be provided within a program allowing for choice of content. A lesson should provide prompts that hint at the correct answers, instead of responding with "No, try again." Questions should never be asked of the user unless information necessary to answer them is still on the terminal screen (Caldwell, 1980).

User input and feedback is also important. User input can be obtained by assessment of a needs questionnaire, feedback opportunities in the lessons themselves, and actively seeking feedback once the lessons are in use (Daneliuk & Wright, 1981).

Administrative support of CAI is vital to its use, because it encourages individuals to utilize it. Without administrative support, users may regard CAI unfavorably and therefore not utilize it (Spuck & Bozeman, 1978).

Ease of author use and system capabilities provided by certain programming languages is another important consideration for design and implementation of CAI. Authors of a CAI lesson should utilize their creative abilities within the lesson. They should remember that creativity must manifest itself within the materials in order to provide a positive opportunity for the user. CAI materials are an extension of the author's own personality (Collagon, 1976; Magidson, 1977).

To summarize: participant and author use are the two important points to remember for CAI systems. Participant use includes prior knowledge of content and computer use; visual, verbal, and mental abilities; and personality characteristics. Recommendations for materials design should consider user characteristics. Author use must balance CAI system capabilities with different levels of author skill and creativity.

ISSUES IN EVALUATION

A great deal of literature exists in the field concerning evaluation, most of which deals with the topic of efficacy; that is, whether or not CAI is effective as a teaching method over and above more traditional instructional methods. A smaller portion of the literature represents more formative kinds of evaluations; i.e., basic issues and facts for design and implementation of CAI.

Efficacy questions as presented in the literature, however, cannot be ignored. Sorlie and Essex assert that evaluation of CAI should be both formative and summative (Sorlie & Essex, 1979). Most certainly, it is vital to ask the question: "Is CAI an effective method of instruction?" Presumably, the decision to develop CAI must be based on, among other things, an affirmative answer to this question. We reviewed several relevant articles. Generally, most of the literature answers the above question in the affirmative: CAI *is* an effective teaching tool (Thomas, 1979; Smith & Von Feidt, 1979). David Thomas reviewed the effectiveness of CAI in secondary schools and found that it led to achievement levels equal to or higher than traditional instruction, as well as to favorable user attitudes, savings of time and, finally, comparable levels of learning retention and cost (Thomas, 1979). A five-year longitudinal study in the U.S. Navy was also favorable, though certain cautions are given (Misselt et al., 1980).

Other portions of the literature have suggested mixed results for CAI (Bagley & Klassen, 1979). A study of the use of CAI in Minnesota correctional facilities indicated no achievement or attitude increase that could be attributed to CAI; however, there were indications that CAI could be used to provide repetitious drill for low-ability students and that it increases motivation and problem-solving skills.

A small portion of the literature suggests the ineffectiveness of CAI. Edward Nelson presents the result of a program of individualized instruction in typing and shorthand classes. He suggests that, although CAI did reduce costs and did accommodate increased enrollments, it was not successful in terms of student achievement and faculty utilization (Nelson, 1978).

A number of other studies have indicated different effectiveness levels based on varying CAI systems, curricula, and student types (Splittberger, 1979). There are some suggestions that subjects allowing "high student discretion," such as humanities, are not subjects easily taught through CAI. On the other hand, subjects of "low student discretion," such as mathematics and the hard sciences, are more applicable to CAI.

Differing results concerning effectiveness of CAI are almost certainly reflections of the particular circumstances involved in the development of each system. There are a number of complex variables necessary to constitute a quality system; and in this light, it is no surprise that some systems fail to produce the expected results. At some point, the practitioner should undertake a study of the effectiveness of CAI. The results of such a study would be important feedback for possible system alteration. The importance of utilizing formative evaluations should be emphasized.

The methods of evaluation depend, of course, on the practitioner's particular needs and resources. Margaret Hazen argues that evaluation of CAI should be multimethod in nature (Hazen, 1980). She argues that evaluations should employ attitude questionnaires, interviews, archive research, observation, and experimental methods. Her article refers essentially to effectiveness evaluations, but does have relevance for formative approaches as well.

In a microcomputer CAI project in Canada, Daneliuk and Wright report that extensive use of discussion papers provided the essential evaluative method (Daneliuk & Wright, 1981). Project staff were required to submit discussion papers at predetermined stages of development and implementation. Papers were submitted by many participants and covered a broad range of topics.

To summarize: the literature suggested that evaluation of CAI should be both formative and summative. Effectiveness of CAI has been evaluated by many studies, most of which have indicated positive results. However, some literature did suggest mixed and negative results. Whether or not CAI is useful for a particular organization depends on many variables, and it can reasonably be asserted that effectiveness of a particular CAI system depends largely on the commitment of that organization to CAI. Finally, evaluations should utilize many methods and should be based on the essentials of CAI itself, the essentials that have constituted the content of this report. No evaluation of CAI can be considered adequate unless it has addressed as many of these issues as possible.

A TRIAL RUN

One experiment in determining the reaction of human-service workers to computer-assisted instruction was conducted with 29 social service workers who license homes for child welfare placement (Western Michigan University, 1982). Anticipating that human-service workers would tend to reject machine-related media in training, the research group was somewhat surprised. Regardless of age, professional experience, or experience with computers, the participants overwhelmingly indicated that the CAI experience was positive and that CAI would be a useful and practical supplement to their training. Incidentally, a vast majority of them went beyond minimal expectations for participation and voluntarily utilized the opportunity to interact with CAI. A large majority reported they felt in control of their progress and that the content and use of the method increased their knowledge base. Virtually all, though reporting considerable apprehension at the outset, reported little anxiety during or subsequent to the experience.

DISCUSSION AND IMPLICATIONS

On balance, computer-assisted instruction appears to offer something to the private practitioner. While the administration of test materials is the most obvious application, the CAI approach also holds promise for teaching a variety of substantive areas to clients, ranging from principles of good relationship behaviors through tutorial lessons, all the way to providing selected simulations in interpersonal conflict, for example. Then, of course, there are training and orientation possibilities for private practice groups, which find some considerable turnover in staff; CAI provides a uniform and consistent way to provide staff orientation and training.

One problem, however, is that CAI systems are often based on the assumption that a particular pool of users universally functions at the necessary or appropriate level to operate a computer terminal. It may just be that CAI is applicable to only a select population to be found in private practice; on the other hand, it may just mean that more orientation and training would necessarily be provided by a practitioner or his or her own staff. This, of course, would impact upon the cost of using CAI.

Then, too, there are other issues evolving around the matter of cost. On the face of it, it would appear that the potential uses of CAI by the private practitioner could be significantly more cost-effective than the traditional methods of administering client tests. First consideration in this item of cost is that the practitioner need not necessarily be present in a test administration based upon a CAI approach. Furthermore, there are automated methods of scoring some self-administered tests. On the other hand, CAI cannot be viewed as having universal applicability for all kinds of training or testing, and cost and effectiveness must be weighed and evaluated by each potential use.

In addition, there are other considerations of cost, such as the options related to independent microcomputing vs. the use of time-sharing through mainframe networks. This major decision is best made only after a careful analysis of all computing needs, such as uses for billing or record-keeping, in addition to CAI. System purchasers often make the mistake of purchasing a computer system with only immediate needs in mind. When developing a system, it is important to plan for the addition of features on into the future and, most ideally, to have an integrated and comprehensive view of overall computer system needs a priori. In this regard, CAI would be only one of many possible considerations in a computer system configuration. If the planned and proactive approach is taken, the costs of maintenance and purchase and/or development of new courseware (in the case of CAI) can be planned and managed by such foresight.

Perhaps the most significant issues for the use of CAI in private practice are to be found in the implications for the relationship between client or patient and the practitioner. There are, of course, limitations to the value of CAI in private practice. One set of limitations may have to do with cost; the other set surely has to do with relationships.

There is, quite naturally, some danger in dehumanizing the helping relationship through inappropriate use of CAI. However, the literature would appear to support the proposition that CAI, properly utilized, is anything but dehumanizing. It can be highly individualizing.

To be sure, a client's particular interaction with training or testing materials can be very idiosyncratic and a practitioner's subjective observations (e.g., the manifestations of stress during the CAI experience) are sometimes valuable. On the other hand, the potential elimination of the practitioner's biases may at times be just as beneficial to a helping relationship as is personal intervention. It appears that CAI has the capacity for limiting the amount of therapist bias sometimes associated with personally administered tests. Nevertheless, the issue of CAI and test administrator bias remains a matter for further research.

In summary, CAI has been an effective instrument in many areas of orientation, training, and testing. There are many reasons having to do with efficacy of the approach, cost-effectiveness, and perhaps even the appropriate exploitation of a new technology that may help to free the practitioner for practice.

REFERENCES

Austin, David. Computer assisted instruction. *Momentum,* 1978, *9*(2), 16–20.

Bagley, Carole. CAI update: So you want to do CAI? *NSPI Journal,* 1979, *18*(2), 35–36.

Bagley, Carole A., & Klasson, Daniel. Instructional computing in correctional institutions. *Educational Technology,* 1979, *19*(4), 37–40.

Bork, Alfred. The role of personal computer systems in education. *AEDS Journal,* 1979, *13*(1), 17–30.

Bozeman, William C. Human factors and considerations in the design of systems of computer managed instruction. *AEDS Journal,* 1978, *11*(4), 89–96.

Bozeman, William C. Computer managed instruction–Is it a system for your school? *Technological Horizons in Education,* 1979, *6*(4), 50–53.

Caldwell, Robert M. Guidelines for developing basic skills in instructional materials for use with microcomputer technology. *Educational Technology,* 1980, *20*(10), 7–12.

Carrier, Carol A. The role of learner characteristics in computer based instruction. *NSPI Journal,* 1978, *18*(5), 25–32.

Collagon, Robert B. A programming primer. *School Science and Mathematics,* 1976, *76*(5), 381–391.

Crease, Allan. Developing CAL for undergraduate science teaching. *Physics Education,* 1977, *12*(1), 48–51.

Daneliuk, Carl, & Wright, Annette. Instructional uses of micro-computers: The why, what, and how of the B.C. approach. *Education Canada,* 1981, *21*(3), 4–11.

Dimas, Chris. A strategy for developing CAI. *Educational Technology,* 1978, *18*(4), 26–29.

Douglas, Charles H., & Edwards, John S. A selected glossary of terms useful in dealing with computers. *Educational Technology,* 1979, *19*(10), 56–66.

Hazen, Margaret. An argument in favor of multi-method research and evaluation in CAI and CMI instruction. *AEDS Journal*, 1980, *13*(4), 275–284.

Hebenstreit, Jacques. 10,000 microcomputers for French secondary schools. *Computers*, 1980, *13*(7), 17–24.

Ingle, 1979 (ment p.13)

Ingle, Earl B., & Musterman, Richard E. CMI, CAI: What are they and what's in it for us?" *Kappa Delta Pi Record*, 1979, *13*(2), 46–48.

Joiner, Lee Marvin, Miller, Sidney R., & Silverstein, Burton S. Potential and limits of computers in school. *Educational Leadership*, 1980, *37*(6), 498–501.

Kearsley, Greg P. The cost of CAI: A matter of assumption. *AEDS Journal*, 1977, *10*(4), 100–112.

Leiblum, Mark D. Organizing for computer-assisted learning. *Educational Technology*, 1979, *19*(9), 7–10.

McCann, Patrick H. Learning strategies and computer-based instruction. *Computers and Education*, 1981, *5*(3), 133–140.

Magidson, Errol M. One more time: CAI is not dehumanizing. *Audiovisual Instruction*, 1977, *22*(8), 20–21.

Misselt, A. Lynn, et al. *Implementation and operation of computer-based education. MTC Report No. 25. Final Report*. Urbana: University of Illinois Computer-Based Education Research Lab., 1980, 48pp.

Nelson, Edward G. Individualized instruction: Another point of view. *Balance Sheet*, 1978, *60*(3), 122–125.

Patrick, John, & Stammers, Robert. Computer assisted learning and occupational training. *British Journal of Educational Technology*, 1977, *8*(3), 253–267.

Schoech, Dick. *Computer use in human services*. New York: Human Science Press, 1982.

Schoen, Harold L., & Hunt, Thomas C. The effect of technology on instruction: The literature of the last 20 years. *AEDS Journal*, 1977, *10*(3), 68–82.

Schuyler, Janis A. Programming languages for microprocessor courseware. *Educational Technology*, 1979, *19*(10), 29–35.

Smith, Joan McKeornan, & von Feidt, James R. A comparison of two media: CAI and instructional television. *Journal of Studies in Technical Careers*, 1979, *1*(2), 119–127.

Sorlie, William E., & Essex, Diane L. So you want to develop a computer-based instruction project? Some recommendations to consider first. *Educational Technology*, 1979, *19*(3), 53–57.

Splittberger, Fred L. Computer based instruction: a revolution in the making? *Educational Technology*, 1979, *19*(1), 20–26.

Spuck, Dennis W., & Bozeman, William C. Pilot test and evaluation of a system of computer-managed instruction. *AEDS Journal*, 1978, *12*(1), 31–41.

Thomas, David B. The effectiveness of computer-assisted instruction in secondary schools. *AEDS Journal*, 1979, *12*(3), 103–116.

Western Michigan University. *Computer-assisted instruction as a training methodology for child placement licensing staff*. Kalamazoo, Michigan: Western Michigan University School of Social Work, 1982, 97 pp.

PART XIII

Choosing a Computer

Part XIII addresses the question of what computer to buy and, more importantly, what software to buy. In this part, the authors present some of the considerations that are important in your purchasing decision. Remember, the most important question is not which computer should you buy, but how well does the software available for this computer meet your needs? The best computer in the world is useless to you if you cannot run the software you need on it.

The first chapter in the section presents the results of a survey done on the readers of the newsletter *Computers in Psychiatry/Psychology* in 1981. While the specific features and benefits of the computers being used have changed since the study was done, the general observations and experiences of the respondents remain relevant.

The remaining chapters in this part present the experiences and opinions of five clinicians, using different computers, each of whom is quite pleased with the system he is using. Once again, there is no intention here of promoting one or another system. The chapters should be read with an eye towards discovering the features and benefits, advantages and disadvantages, that you should consider in purchasing your own system.

Selecting a Computer for Use in the Practice of Psychiatry/ Psychology

Marc D. Schwartz, MD

During 1981 *Computers in Psychiatry/Psychology* conducted a survey of subscribers to determine more about their experience with computers. We were particularly interested in obtaining information that could help readers decide what computer, peripherals, and software to buy. Over fifty responses were received containing some very interesting observations.

The most commonly used computer was the Apple (28%), followed closely by the TRS-80 (25%). Far behind were the DEC (5%), Northstar (5%), Rockwell (3%), and Sol (no longer being manufactured, 3%). Twelve other computers were being used by one owner each.

Computers were most frequently used for text processing (37%), information systems (24%), and billing (16%). A relatively small percent of respondents were using a computer for testing purposes. Some were using their computers with modems for the Lithium Library, to exchange programs, and to transmit text and data. Others were using theirs for biofeedback, to maintain a problem-oriented record, for evoked potential studies, to work with DSM-III, and "to make money."

Hopes and dreams for computer use were much more diverse and included prosthetic devices for the handicapped, networking, analysis of practice data, career counseling, and personality simulations, to name but a few. Transforming computer dreams to reality is, as many have found, a difficult and often expensive process. A few, including the editor, have found computer work encompassing more of their time and effort, and they have changed the focus of their careers to pursue those interests.

The above article originally appeared in *Computers in Psychiatry/Psychology*, 1981, 3(5), 11–12, and is reprinted by permission.

It seemed particularly intriguing to compare experiences with the Apple and TRS-80, since these two computers accounted for more than half of the responses to the survey. Users were asked to rate their computers on four factors: reliability, versatility, service, and "overall." Ratings were from 1 (excellent) to 4 (poor). The Apple, along with Rockwell, received the highest average rating (1.2), followed by the Northstar (1.4). The DEC and TRS-80 scored about 1.8. Most Apple and TRS-80 respondents rated their computers 1 or 2 on most factors. Only one Apple owner gave his computer a 3 on reliability and repair. The TRS-80 received two 3s and one 4 for versatility. It also received two 3s and one 4 for repair.

Both Apple and TRS-80 had a majority of owners who liked their computers' software, peripherals, and local service. A few Apple owners liked the color graphics; a few TRS-80 owners liked its low cost. Also mentioned by various Apple owners were its portability, profitability (for the user), PASCAL programming capabilities, and the fact that Apple will stay in business for a while. Among the TRS-80 owners were those who liked the computer's dependability and the CP/M operating system, one which allows easy conversion of software from one make of computer to another.

What Apple owners didn't like was the 40-character screen line and its poor program editing and cursor control. What TRS-80 owners didn't like was the computer's poor graphics capability, "Radio Shack" (20% of TRS-80 respondents), slow number-crunching ability, limited disk capacity, and the fact that Radio Shack has limited the availability of TRS-80 peripherals by its policy of trying to monopolize that market.

Computers other than the Apple and TRS-80 were used by almost half of the respondents. Most commented quite favorably on their choice. The issues raised by their comments and those of Apple and TRS-80 users highlighted the kind of issues that should be considered by those planning to buy a new computer:

1. Is the size of the computer's memory and disk storage adequate for the user's specific needs?
2. Is there good software available for that computer?
3. Are there special software packages for psychiatrists/psychologists/social workers?
4. Will the company stay in business to provide support and repairs for your system?
5. Is there a user's group; a hotline?
6. Does the computer have multi-user capability?
7. Is the dealer competent, helpful, knowledgeable? (Get and call references.)
8. Is the documentation (manual) easy to read and understand? Is it helpful?

9. Does it run under CP/M?
10. Is repair service readily available?
11. Does it fit the budget? (Remember that good user software may cost about as much as the original hardware investment.)

Clearly, few readers will have identical needs. Buying a ticket on a 727 may be the perfect way for a person to fly if his/her interest is getting somewhere quickly and inexpensively. A single-engine one-seater, glider, or kit may be the perfect way to fly for another person who has another set of goals. Someone else's satisfaction or dissatisfaction is no guarantee of yours. Individual needs should be carefully matched with the computer's capabilities before deciding which computer to buy.

One last suggestion: if you are seriously interested in learning more about computer use, don't wait until you know everything or until the perfect low-cost computer comes along next year. Next year there will be an even better and cheaper one coming along the following year.

 # The Apple Contribution

Marvin W. Eidinger, Jr., PhD

I heard a story about Albert Einstein that I love to share. It was my good fortune to meet Norbert Einstein, Albert's cousin, many years ago. I had asked him if it was true that Albert Einstein was so advanced that he was always speaking beyond everyone's comprehension. In response he told me this story:

> One evening, shortly after his paper on relativity was published and before he was known in worldly circles, Einstein was sitting down for supper with his wife and his cousin, when there was a knock at the door. A handsome eleven-year-old boy stood at the doorway with his head somewhat bowed.
> "Dr. Einstein?"
> "Yes."
> "Dr. Einstein, my mom heard that you are very good at math. I'm terrible at math and in big trouble because of it. My mom thought you might help me with my math assignment."
> For the next four years, Einstein tutored the boy. Norbert Einstein related that the secret of true genius is the understanding of how the basics relate to the complex. Albert Einstein understood and could teach basic math because of his understanding of theoretical math.

The story of the Apple Computer is similar. Steven Jobs and Steven Wozniak, the creators of the Apple Computer, working with extremely sophisticated and complex microcircuitry, created a machine that operates simply. Their true genius lies not in the central processing unit (CPU, the heart) of the Apple Computer, but is reflected in how they arranged for those of us not technically adept enough to utilize a powerful computer.

Since 1975, Jobs and Wozniak have been designing and building computers that allow millions of creative minds—minds that lack computer expertise—to maximize data analyses, generate detailed high-

[Editor's note: The prices discussed in this chapter are as of 1982.]

resolution graphics, add, subtract, divide, and multiply with amazing speed.

The first Apple Computer manual—the infamous Red Book—was too simplistic and unchallenging for many in the computer business, who said "They're still programming in BASIC!" Yet, it opened the door to many nonprofessional programmers who had ideas for which computers were needed.

My first Apple Computer was an Apple II 16k unit that I hooked to my TV in 1977. (The "16k" means that my computer had 16,000 bytes, or storage units, of memory built into it.) The computer scoring and interpretation of the Minnesota Multiphasic Personality Inventory (MMPI) was my mission.

Shortly after I purchased the computer, Apple came out with their first "how-to-make-your-computer-work" manual. It was outstanding! From turning the switch "on" to pressing keys, the manual explained what had to be done and what the effect would be. The computer language was called *Integer BASIC*. One terrific quality Integer BASIC had was that only correctly worded programming statements would be accepted by the computer. For example, if an improper command to print the words "Good Morning" was given as part of a program (PRINT "GOOD MORNING—forgetting to put the second set of quotations following the word "morning"), the computer would reject the command and identify the problem (an attempt to enter this command into the computer memory would cause the computer to "beep" and print SYNTAX ERROR).

The Apple II was a big zero when it came to cutting back my workload; just to learn BASIC took real focus and created much frustration. Then I found out that the computer could easily write letters, do my income taxes (and keep track of the receipts), record addresses for mailing labels, run statistical data analyses, all with "canned," off-the-shelf software!

All my free time started to evaporate into endless hours of programming the Apple to do all kinds of projects that I would not have bothered with before. My wife began to complain that I spent too much time with the Apple and not enough with her—so I tried to program a cost-effectiveness report for her. All I really wanted was something to help me score and interpret the MMPI. I made thousands of programming errors. The programs were very lengthy and did not do much in the way of scoring the MMPI.

At the same time, I was becoming a programmer in BASIC—because the Apple would reject anything but decent programming statements. Soon I became obsessed with perfecting my programming techniques. The bookstores started stocking books on BASIC, and I found significant differences between Apple BASIC and other BASICs.

However, the books taught me how to think logically about solving problems.

Rarely were other BASIC programs of much use. The real contributions to my repertoire were from *Call-A.P.P.L.E.* (Apple Pugetsound Program Library Exchange), a club. The club published a one- or two-page mimeographed monthly newsletter with helpful hints and some moaning over the minuses of the Apple II. Early on, the members started to see Apple Computer, Inc. responding to our complaints and our inquiries. The club started a hotline that could be called during the day so that Apple would not have to answer some of the more "basic" questions about computer operation. Membership included doctors, lawyers, bricklayers, accountants, used car salesmen and, yes, some real live computer experts. If you had a question about using the Apple in a particular setting or about a programming problem, there was probably a member who could help out.

A much more advanced version of BASIC was released in 1978. Very few of the programming options offered on even sophisticated mainframe computers (found at universities and corporate headquarters) were not offered on Applesoft. Because Applesoft was much more sophisticated and "powerful," it would actually allow a programmer to input "incorrect" program instructions into a program without notifying the programmer. The reason for this is that in some cases those incorrect programming instructions might be all right. For example, the programmer was trying something fancy. From a beginner's point of view, this meant that the program might appear to be developing nicely when it was actually riddled with errors.

Of course all computer programs provide the computer programmer with one final check as to whether they were constructed correctly and effectively: they either run (producing the needed output) or they err (producing incorrect output or no output).

Even with the more advanced Applesoft, the computer would still allow for naivete. As the programmer is learning about BASIC and developing a program, he/she can "run" the program to find out how it is progressing. It may appear that that is not too significant, but on a mainframe computer, each run costs dollars.

Also, on a mainframe the run may take many hours, depending on how busy the computer is. The Apple II could run the same program several times during each minute. If an error is identified, the computer will display the location of the error and the type of error that was made. It can then be corrected and another run initiated. Most of my training in programming came from this "run—correct programming errors—run—correct programming errors—run . . ." system of program development.

Some level of programming expertise does seem to grow from all

this trial and error. The computer seems to provide immediate reinforcement for learning—the program works, you have mind over matter, you are IN CONTROL, the computer is your servant, YOU are the
boss. My ideas of what I should be doing with the Apple II seemed to
go on and on. I discovered that I could program for hours on end without tiring—in fact, programming was relaxing even when there was a
"bug" in the program and things were not going well.

From the MMPI programming, I learned to develop my own data
base system and search out particular data that met certain criteria. Of
course the "canned" software packages were becoming increasingly
available for the Apple II. At first they were very expensive; even the
quality game programs were about $100 each. Most of my efforts were
still directed toward the MMPI and developing my own BASIC programming.

The addition of the Apple Disk II was a tremendous step. For
years the Apple programmer had to load his or her program from a
cassette tape. The disk provided quick, reliable storage so that moving
from program to program could be done with ease. The disk unit used
floppy diskettes (about $5–6), which could be exchanged with other
programmers, and they each could hold many, many programs.

The disk system could also be used to store raw data. The programmer would store the data on a disk, and the computer program
would access the data for analyses. Although this process was possible
using the tape recorder, it was very time-consuming (several minutes
to load the data), and frequently there would be an error in the loading
and/or storing-data process, so some of the data would be lost forever.

The disk units also seemed to help proliferate software. The dras-
tic increase in microcomputer sales naturally helped, too. Prices fell.
The quality of the software increased at the same time. Off-the-shelf
software packages at the computer store were designed so well that it
became difficult to cause the program to "hang-up" on you or stall out.
The manuals were being rewritten for easier understanding and this,
too, increased sales. Many of the manuals were written with the assumption that you had not even read the Apple manual.

USING AN APPLE IN PRACTICE

Knowing how powerful the computer is (what the microcircuitry is capable of doing) helps to determine the potential of the software that
can be designed to fit the computer. Software is the computer program
that utilizes the computer's ability to add, subtract, display, or whatever. The Apple must have fairly powerful circuitry, as witnessed by
the more than 3,000 pieces of software that have been designed to
work with the Apple.

The next discussion will relate how an Apple Computer might be utilized in your practice and how it might improve your effectiveness and/or your business management by utilizing some of the software available for the Apple.

Starting Your Practice

The Apple Computer disk system comes with several short programs to demonstrate how to use the computer and the disk together. One of these programs is a short routine demonstrating how a data base system works. A data base is a systematic way of storing information. Your file cabinets contain records, and these records are in some kind of order so that you withdraw the information. The Apple can store information in a data base, making information retrieval a snap.

The short routine that comes with your Apple disk system allows you to store mailing labels. The phone book can provide the names of local professionals, such as physicians, attorneys, and psychologists in the community whom you would like to inform about your practice. The program will store the information needed to print the mailing label and then order the printer to print it.

Client Intake Information

Data base software packages have become so inexpensive that it is not worthwhile to try to make do with rather awkward Apple data base programs provided by Apple with their disk systems. Good quality data base systems are available for Apple computers starting at $80. With these data base systems, the programmer is only required to respond to the computer displays that ask about the information that is to be collected.

You might design your data base program to collect information on each new client: name, address, phone number, emergency phone number, presenting complaint, provisional diagnosis, initial treatment recommendation, and so on. You might order the printer to print copies of these computer records for your file cabinet. The information stored in this computer data base system could be used for announcements. The name and address records could be used for mailing labels to send out notifications of the change in your office hours. You might want to have the data base create mailing labels for only the attorneys to inform them about a new service you can provide the court.

Of course the data base could keep track of how many times a particular client has been seen by you; it contains billing information (fee/payment) related to the client. Some of the more advanced data base systems come with built-in word processing capability. With this powerful tool, you can use information about the client's billing history to send out billing statements, using a form letter.

The Checkbook

Several inexpensive programs are now available that can keep track of your checking account(s). Most can handle five checking accounts and up to 100 accounts that you bill to or are billed from. Some of these programs will actually type the check onto a preprinted check form used in your printer. You may also request to see a graphic display of where all the money is going!

Accounting

There are several excellent accounting packages available for the Apple. Most are expensive and are designed for a small company with 50 or more employees.

Income Tax

One of the most exciting areas of microcomputing is the quality and growth of the programs that do income tax accounting on an Apple Computer. Recent IRS rulings have authorized computer-generated income tax forms as being acceptable. Your software package should indicate that it creates acceptable forms. Most of the programs serving this function display a menu of the various IRS forms and ask you to choose one. The computer then cycles through each question on the form, memorizing your response. Some questions ask you for the total of some list of items (your receipts). Frequently, the income tax program can also be used as a data base to store such lists. An example may be helpful. If you have more than one income, the program could store information about each pay period (income, taxes paid, insurance information, tax-deductible contributions, etc.) and store the information for end-of-year use. The computer can then print out an itemized list of your income and expenses that your income tax forms are based on. The computer also exchanges totals between forms. If the 1040 form needs totals from the Schedule A, it receives the data and presents it on the screen. It then becomes possible to compare how various methods of deducting your expenses work at lowering your net taxable income. Several companies offer low-cost updates for their software, which reflect changes in the tax laws.

Electronic Spreadsheets

No one seems to have accurately predicted how quickly microcomputers would be accepted by the wide variety of professions that have in fact utilized this powerful tool. Electronic spreadsheets were computer programs designed to assist accountants with doing their ledgers on a microcomputer. Such programs combine the convenience and familiarity of a pocket calculator with the powerful memory and electronic screen capabilities of the Apple. In particular, a program called VisiCalc provides an easy method for the accountant to create a ledger on the Apple, and it clearly shows the items, debits, and credits. VisiCalc turned out to be the most cost-effective software package available for the Apple. This program can be used to store billing information, generate invoices, identify trends in certain accounts, store information about attendance records and grades, and run statistical analyses on data. I was able to program VisiCalc to score the MMPI. VisiCalc is an excellent tool to analyze stock market trends and for calculating moving averages. At the Hanford Nuclear Storage Site, Visi-Calc was used to create an economic model of nuclear waste disposal costs as well as to analyze various waste-storage methodologies. VisiCalc or a similar type of program should be included in the initial computer system package purchase.

Psychometrics

More and more programs are being developed to administer and score various psychological tests. Probably the most common test that has been computerized is the MMPI. Length of administration of the test can be reduced by as much as 60%, and test scoring can be reduced from 30 minutes to 90 seconds. Computers can also analyze a protocol according to hundreds of various research findings and calculate thousands of subscale outcomes in minutes. Most clinicians rarely have the time to examine a particular MMPI protocol with the detail that one of these programs can.

Biofeedback

There are several firms that have created software packages that interface the Apple with their biofeedback machines. The computer can track the process of the client and store information about performance for comparative analyses.

Word Processing

The Apple II is not designed to be a word processor. The keyboard is missing certain keys that make a word processor move paragraphs, indent, or whatever. However, there has been a flurry of creative word-processing programs that have ways to circumvent these obstacles. Some word-processing programs turn the Apple into a word-pro-

cessing system comparable to the $30,000 units. Professional corre-
spondence and report generation can easily be handled on the Apple.

Communications

A new area for the Apple computer is data communication over the
telephone. For several years now, hardware has been available to interface the Apple with large mainframe computers, using the telephone.
This was an expensive proposition—mainframe computing time is expensive. Recently, several banking institutions have designed systems
for customers to do their banking over the phone using an Apple.

Additionally, two large "networks" exist, Compuserve and The
Source, which provide for an Apple computer to tie into a large data
bank. These networks can be reached without calling long distance and
are fairly inexpensive. Such systems offer the opportunity to read from
various wire services, newspapers, popular magazines, and provide
for downloading of games and programming utilities—all over the
telephone.

CREATING AN APPLE SYSTEM

Apple Computer, Inc., offers computers, disk units, monitors, and
software. You may be asking these questions: What equipment is
needed to start? What software do I need to begin? What kind of
equipment is available for me to use in the practice of psychology or
psychiatry?

There are three essential elements of a good-quality computer system: high-quality hardware; appropriate software, which meets your
needs and experience level; and time—you will need plenty of time to
read the manuals and practice with your system.

Hardware

In general, I never buy "no-name" brand hardware. There are many
clone type computers, monitors, and disk units that look like Apple
Computer equipment, seem to act like it, yet are so much cheaper than
the real thing. The difference in cost can be eaten away if/when the
hardware fails and destroys part of your data base in the process or if it
takes a month to get it to the factory, fixed, and back with you again.

I believe in buying from a company with a good name and a good
history. The history of the company's supporting its products is crucial
in determining whether its "inexpensive" Apple accessory is truly inexpensive. During the early years of the Apple III production, Apple decided that the machine was not up to par, so they offered to buy back

the earlier versions of the Apple III from customers or upgrade the older Apple III with the newer, advanced electronics. That's class! Many of the software companies operate with that type of philosophy, too.

My recommendations will usually be limited to the brand of equipment and possibly the options to be included. Please recognize that I am also attempting to consider the cost restrictions most of us have to operate with. Therefore, many superior brands of equipment are not discussed, because I, for one, could not afford their luxury.

Negotiate the price of your equipment. Paying retail prices is easy, but some tact with your dealer will often result in a 10%–15% savings on a package deal. Most of the popular computer magazines run discount prices on software, which should save you 10%–40% on the cost of software. In the following discussion, relative dollar amounts are presented. It is assumed that you are willing to negotiate prices with your dealer; these numbers will assist with your expectations as to what is possible.

Computers. The best buy is the Apple IIe with 48k memory ($1,200–$1,400). This machine will allow you to do advanced BASIC programming and comes with many expansion slots so you can add to the machine needed peripherals (accessories, gadgets). It simply is not worth buying a smaller memory size or starting with the regular Apple II (with Integer BASIC). Most of the software available for the Apple II, which is written in BASIC, is written in Applesoft for 48k machines. The clone computers offer similar computing power, but they have not yet proven themselves as durable as the Apple II.

Monitors. A monitor is a televison without a channel selector. In fact it operates on a much lower frequency and presents a more stable image for the operator to look at. If you choose to use a TV, a RF Modulator will act as the interface between an Apple II and the TV. These units cost about $30. They are worth it if you will be using a color TV. However, if the computer will be used for programming and/or word processing, televisions usually present images that are more difficult on the programmer's eyes. The price of monitors makes them a good investment.

There are several good-quality monitors available, generating competition and lower prices. Those with green screens have been found to provide less eyestrain over many hours of programming. The Apple, Amdex, and NEC monitors ($135–$200) appear to present the best bets in price, quality of design, and serviceability. A 12-inch screen provides good character size on the screen.

Color monitors are nice additions, but most provide marginal quality presentation of lettering on the screen. If you will be doing lots of word processing and/or program development, stick with the green screens. One exception is the Amdex Color Monitor II ($925). This monitor seems to do everything well!

Disk Units. The Apple Computer Disk II ($550) seems to be the best investment. Other disk systems have not proven themselves, yet. The reliability of the Apple Disk II has been outstanding.

Printers. There are two major types of printers: Impact and dot-matrix. Your typewriter is an impact printer. The dot-matrix printers form letters out of dots. If the dots are close enough together, it is not too difficult to read the printouts. Some dot-matrix printers attempt to print over the spaces between the dots with dots, thus improving the quality of the printed character. The dot-matrix printers operate between two and six times faster than the impact printers.

The choice of printers should be based on how the printer will be used. It is important to get a wide carriage (if you can afford it) to handle the larger accounting problems you may be working. If most of your computer work will be related to word processing, go with the impact printers. Otherwise, the dot-matrix printers perform the most cost-effective printing.

The name brands for impact printing are Diablo, Transtar and C. Itoh ($1,550–$2,800). One deciding point may be the cost of ink ribbons and their availability. There are quite a few used heavy-duty word-processing printers on the market. These can be a real bargain and should not be overlooked. Check with a local word-processing sales organization and ask who is trying to get rid of their old equipment in order to purchase a new printer.

For dot-matrix printing, stick with an IDS, Epson, or C. Itoh printer ($545–$900) with graphics option ($100–$250 additional cost). These companies provide what appears to be the best options for expanding the use of your printer if your needs grow. Additionally, these printers tend to cost less to maintain and provide more easily understood manuals.

Special Additions. There are now hundreds of gadgets that you can attach to an Apple Computer. Most items are attached to the Apple in "peripheral slots" inside the Apple II. The circuit gets its power from the Apple II in that manner and the computer can interact quickly with the peripheral by just "addressing" that slot. The following represent items that might contribute, beyond the short-term pleasure of possessing them. They are listed in a priority of importance, reflecting not only their added cost, but the potential for making a real contribution to an Apple System.

Memory Expansion Card. The Apple thinks it's a 64k machine. A 48k Apple actually uses almost 64k of memory when one examines how the memory is "managed" within the hardware. There are several ways to get an Apple to act like it has much more than the standard

48k it comes with. Several companies are manufacturing expansion boards that plug into the Apple to add 16k, 32k, 64k, and more.

One additional nicety about such boards is the ability to have a "bilingual" Apple. The Apple can automatically load the BASIC language version, which is not in the main memory, into the expansion card. For example, if the computer is an Apple IIe, it comes with Applesoft BASIC in main memory. With an expansion card, Integer BASIC will automatically be loaded into the expansion card and available for your use. If you are a new programmer, learning BASIC with Integer BASIC is preferable to learning with Applesoft. My impression is that the Microsoft 16k expansion board ($165) is representative of the highest quality in design and manufacturing of such boards. However, for the same amount of money you may be able to purchase a Saturn Systems expansion board with twice the memory ($200). These two brands are your best bets.

Extra Disk Unit. Many of the new data base systems and some of the word-processing systems require two disk units. If you are developing software, the additional disk provides the ability to store your program on one disk with some programming utilities (which help with programming) on the other disk. My feeling is that the best investment in disk units is Apple Disk II ($485).

Keyboard Enhancer. The Apple II shift key does not operate like a typewriter shift key. The problem is in hardware design. There is a simple solution for this problem, which includes stringing wires within the Apple. However, Videx, Inc., provides an even better solution— the Keyboard Enhancer II ($130). This circuit board adds upper and lower case to your computer (the Apple II comes with only upper case), activates the shift key, and provides for the ability to program any key on the keyboard to do a little program that is specified. For example, you can program the keyboard to clear the screen and then display your most recent version of your program whenever you press the *"d"* key. Enhancing your keyboard in this way can provide for greater flexibility in programming and add to any word-processing program that you might purchase. The quality of Videx, Inc., products has been outstanding. Recently, they have significantly improved the quality of their manuals, so their products are better utilized.

80-Column Board. If you are doing word processing, you might consider the Videx 80-Column Board ($300) a good bet. Additionally, developing programs in the PASCAL language can be made easier with the 80-Column Board. The Videx Board seems to interfere less than some of its competitors with other peripheral boards inside the Apple and appears to be the easiest to install.

Cassette Tape Recorder. Built into each Apple II is the ability to upload a computer program from a cassette tape recorder. There are not many programs left that are sold on cassette tape when a diskette can be used instead. However, if you will be doing some programming and stretching your knowledge on the keyboard, a tape recorder should be sitting next to the computer.

There are some keyboard instructions that disable the disk units. No harm is done to the units, but your ability to store the program you have spent hours working on may be lost. One alternative is to shut the power "off" and "on" and reenter the entire program. The best alternative is to store the program on tape. Then you can get the disk unit working again by turning the computer "off" and then "on." Then it is possible to upload the program from the tape recorder onto the disk. Most cheap tape recorders will work fine. Stay away from expensive models because they tend to change the electronic signals from the computer and thus interfere with accurately storing your program.

Hard-Disk Systems. I am frequently asked if the prices on computers are still falling. The answer is *yes*, somewhat, but the price of disk storage is streaming towards the ground. The ability to store massive amounts of data is crucial for certain kinds of data management. The Apple can perform complex statistical and textual maneuvers; however, one needs the ability to provide the computer access to all the data that is to be considered. The Apple Disk II provides about 130k of storage. A hard-disk system can handle between 5 million and 20 million bytes of storage! Prices started at $5,000 last year for a 5-megabyte hard-disk system. Today's prices are closer to $1,000.

Instead of using a floppy diskette to store information, a hard-disk system uses a spinning drum. The drum is magnetized and keeps the information readily available to the computer upon request. A small hard disk is about equivalent to 35 regular disk units. The importance of this contribution is the ability to have your data base system store client information on one system as opposed to several diskettes. Backup data can be downloaded onto videotape for permanent storage with a few of the systems.

Corvus Systems makes an excellent hard-disk system for the Apple. In fact, I recommend their system over the Apple Hard Disk (Profile) for two important reasons: (1) Corvus provides a method of downloading (backing up) your data onto a videotape recorder and (2) the Corvus System has the ability to form networks so that up to 64 Apple Computers can share the same hard disk. Both of these features make the Corvus disk the better buy over the Profile. Stay clear of the other brands until they have had more experience creating products for the Apple.

Card Reader. Mountain Hardware, Inc., manufactures a high-speed card reader ($1,300) that interfaces well with the Apple. The unit reads punched cards or it can optically scan the mark-sense form for pencil-written responses.

Speech Synthesizer. The Echo II speech synthesizer by Street Electronics, Inc. ($200) generates excellent quality speech. Such accessories add flavor to your programming and sometimes generate quite a laugh. The manual for this item is very poor but, with some practice, I found that programming speech was not too difficult.

Modem. If you will be wanting to call up one of those big computers on the telephone, get the D. C. Hays Micromodem II system ($250). This company has created an excellent peripheral for interfacing the Apple II with nearly any mainframe computer.

Clock. A 24-hour clock ($127–$200) for the Apple is a peripheral that plugs into the Apple and can be "interrogated" as to what time it is. Three different companies make acceptable clocks: Thunderware, Mountain Hardware, and D. C. Hays. The last of these requires a separate interface card, but is also the classiest.

The Bare Bones System. If you are just starting out, plan to spend $2,900 or you will be frustrated until you do. The minimum system should consist of: Apple IIe with 48k memory, one Apple Disk II with controller, green screen monitor, dot-matrix printer with cable and interface card, and the VisiCalc software package. In fact you only need a computer with an RF Modulator and you are set . . . but unhappy. Think "power" when it comes to hardware.

Software

The emphasis here will be on "canned" programs that will add to your practice. Utility programs that help programmers will not be discussed, as they relate to experienced Apple users.

Electronic Spreadsheets. Personal Software, Inc., makes the VisiCalc software package ($185). There is no question that VisiCalc is the best buy in software for the Apple II. The manual is excellent, and the program itself is near foolproof. Other software companies have just not been able to beat the initial VisiCalc program. Recently, however, two new programs seem to be overshadowing the original VisiCalc. They are: the "advanced" version of VisiCalc ($400) by Personal Software and Microsoft's MultiPlan ($500).

Data Base Systems. There are good-quality data base systems ($80–$300) available for the Apple II that can handle most of the data storage that would come along in a practice. The secret to purchasing the best is to see which company will provide you technical support (over the telephone) if you get lost or confused and are concerned about losing all your data.

Two top brands of data base systems are Micro Lab (Data Factory, $280) and Stoneware (DB Master II, $170). Both companies provide excellent telephone support and their programming has been outstanding. The Micro Lab is somewhat of a favorite as the quality of their manuals has kept pace with the improvements in their data base. Both programs can interface with VisiCalc, so you can have the ability to display the data using a spreadsheet.

Graphics. Personal Software, Inc., has created VisiPlot/VisiTrend ($195) to utilize data from a VisiCalc tablet. In other words, you can download data from your VisiCalc tablet and upload it into VisiPlot/ VisiTrend for data analyses and graphic plotting. The graphic displays on the screens can be reproduced on most popular dot-matrix printers and a few impact printers. Software Publishing, Inc. makes GRAPH ($160), which can interface with VisiCalc and also run a plotter— generating hard-copy color plots, if you own a color plotter.

PASCAL. Apple has now made available its version ($200) of the UCSD PASCAL language. If you plan to do more than "light" programming, PASCAL is a must. The quality of your own programming, how readable your programs are, how efficient they are, and how easy they are to modify will all be enhanced by switching from BASIC to PASCAL. You must have an expansion card and two disks units to utilize PASCAL effectively.

Psychometrics. The author will demonstrate some prejudice here. After five years of development, PsiSoft ($400),* an MMPI scoring routine for the Apple II, is the best buy available. Most of the programs available for the Apple II do not score the protocol—they interpret it. The interpretations are short, one- or two-sentence paragraphs, making some basic analysis. PsiSoft accurately generates the raw, k-corrected, and t-scores for the basic clinical and validity scales. The program also analyzes the protocol against 35 subscales, the Megargee Offender Profile analysis, the Goldman analysis, and identifies the Welsh Code. The ability to store protocols on the disk is provided. Enhancements to be added later include: opscan protocol reading, Gilbertstat and Duker analysis, and statistical analysis of multiple protocols.

PUBLICATIONS

Reading really helps. I would like to identify certain periodicals and books that can help pick up the pace in understanding an Apple II and what it is capable of doing.

Periodicals

Softalk, by Softalk Publications, Inc., is published monthly. The emphasis is on software and software development. Each month there

---

*PsiSoft is available directly from the author of this chapter.

are columns on programming in BASIC and PASCAL, on new software that is coming out, on what is happening in the industry, and positive reviews of helpful and fun software.

Call-A.P.P.L.E., by Apple Pugetsound Program Library Exchange, is published monthly. This is the premier organization for supporting beginners in the Apple II. A wide variety of helpful utilities for programmers and discussions on how to enhance the capability of an Apple are included monthly. Programs are also offered for sale at a much reduced price; some are only available to members. A telephone hotline is also available to members experiencing problems with hardware and/or software.

Personal Computing, by Hayden Publishing Company, Inc., is published monthly. This periodical is written for a wider readership than the previous two magazines. I find most of the articles contribute little to help me with programming or understanding my Apple computer. However, companies seem to generate nice ads in this periodical, and, frankly, I buy this magazine to find out what is available in hardware and software.

Books

The Applesoft Tutorial, by Apple Computer, Inc., comes with the Apple II+. It is well worth reading this book cover to cover and performing the tasks as stated. If you have little or no experience with BASIC and programming, you will get some help here.

A Guide to Programming in Applesoft, by Bruce Presley, is an easy-to-read text on BASIC programming. Get this book if you are just starting out in computing.

Apple Machine Language, by Don and Kurt Inman, is a fun look at the language that the Apple Computer really uses, machine language. This text is a good introduction to programming in the assembly language, and text only requires that you have some understanding of BASIC.

Quality software usually come with quality manuals. These manuals provide excellent reading material to study whatever it is that you are planning for your computer.

SOME CONCLUDING REMARKS

An Apple computer can add significantly to the practice of psychology or psychiatry. The proliferation of personal computers has driven the prices downward for both hardware and software. Quality manuals allow beginners to perform sophisticated analyses and data management with very little computer experience.

An Evaluation of the Vector 2600 Computer and MicroPro Software

Lawrence G. Ritt, PhD

pproximately one year ago, I purchased a Vector computer and the following MicroPro software: WordStar, SpellStar, Mailmerge, DataStar, CalcStar, and SuperSort. This brief chapter will discuss my reasons for choosing this particular hardware/software combination and my user evaluations of these products.

THE VECTOR 2600

Prior to selecting the Vector 2600 computer, I devoted several weeks to reading manufacturers' materials and computer magazine reviews, visiting local dealers, and experiencing demonstrations of various hardware/software combinations.

Since my primary anticipated usage was word processing, I needed a good keyboard (the Vector's is similar to an IBM Selectric) and an 80-column screen so that an entire page width could be displayed without annoying scrolling. These requirements immediately ruled out the TRS-80 models I and III, and the "standard" Apple II. I also wanted a full 64K of onboard memory. (Although not available when I was originally shopping for a computer, the Osborne I is now offered with all of the above features plus WordStar, Mailmerge, MBASIC, and useful utility programs for less than $2,200. I recently purchased a fully equipped Osborne plus an $175 external monitor and find that it will do almost everything my Vector 2600 will do. Its only serious limitation is that its disk drives have approximately one-third

"An Evaluation of the Vector 2600 Computer and MicroPro Software" was originally published in *Computers in Psychiatry/Psychology*, 1983, 5(1), 13–15, and is reprinted by permission.

the storage capacity of the Vector 2600; the purchase of an "after-market" hard disk drive should alleviate this limitation.)

I wanted a system that would run some of the highly sophisticated business oriented CP/M software (including the MicroPro software); this ruled out the then new IBM Personal Computer (although it now has CP/M available). Since some of my anticipated data files were going to be quite large, I wanted a machine with high-capacity floppy disk drives. The Vector 2600's two 16-hard-sector double-sided quad density disks store 630K per drive; the low capacity offered by Xerox quickly eliminated that machine from consideration. Lastly, I demanded good local dealer support—a wise consideration, since there were some Vector/MicroPro interface "quirks" that required special installation patches—and some believable promise of quality aftersale service. Vector service is available through the TRW organization. My machine was purchased at a time when Vector offered nine months of free service through TRW, although that free offer has now been discontinued.

Unlike other companies (most notably, Xerox), who sold their machines with almost no "included" software, the Vector sale price included CP/M, two versions of MBASIC, the SCOPE program editor, RAID debugger, and such other useful aides as a sorting program and bad-disk reclaimer. When I compared prices for computers with essential software and operating systems, the Vector 2600, at $5,200, was quite competitive. Vector also offered a one-disk-drive version (Vector VIP) for $4,000, a dual 8-inch drive system (the Vector 2800) for $7,300, and a version with a single floppy drive/5-megabyte Winchester hard disk drive (Vector 3005) for $8,000. All of these units are currently available at discounts, since they are reportedly being replaced by the Vector Model 4 which will contain both 8-bit and 16-bit processors for increased speed, program options, and memory storage. The Vector Model 4 sells for under $5,000 with two floppy disk drives that are compatible with the Vector 2600 and for under $6,000 with a floppy disk drive and a 5-megabyte hard disk.

For the first year after purchase, I was extremely pleased with my choice of a Vector computer. Unfortunately, I have since experienced some serious "downtime" difficulties. On several occasions, the computer would fail, and it would take TRW several weeks to satisfactorily correct the problems. Other problems that have recently become obvious on my Vector 2600 include some unusual "bugs" in the Vector hardware that occasionally lead to "crashes" of MicroPro's WordStar software. These problems do not occur on most other computers running the same software. Appeals to the Vector Graphic Corporation for assistance in remedying these software and hardware problems have not—to date—been satisfactory.

Based on these recent negative experiences with Vector and my absolute satisfaction with my Osborne I computer, I suspect that if I were shopping for a computer today, I would rule out the Vector and purchase an Osborne instead.

Another major limitation of my system is that Vector is a relatively small company compared to Radio Shack, Apple, Osborne, and IBM, and consequently does not have the same range of machine-customized software as is available to the users of the other hardware. Although there are "bargains" in CP/M software, the catalog of available software is certainly more limited and generally more expensive than that available to TRS-80 and Apple computers. There is almost no test-administration or scoring software available for any CP/M system; users who need this application would be better advised to stick with Apple and the TRS-80.

MICROPRO SOFTWARE

WordStar is generally regarded as the most sophisticated and versatile word-processing software on the market. Although expensive ($495, with discounts available if you shop around), it has a marvelously complete onscreen "help menu", and other features as follows:

- Powerful editing commands that allow text to be deleted, moved, replaced, copied, and read from other files with ease;
- Wordwrap, which eliminates all need for carriage returns at the end of lines;
- Formatting options (page lengths, temporary paragraph indents, automatic line-centering, automatic page-numbering and "headers"/"footers";
- Semi-automatic hyphenating, justified or ragged right margins, microspace justification to evenly disburse extra spaces across a justified line, etc.;
- A wide range of print enhancements (bold print, underlining, subscripts and superscripts, variable character pitches, variable line-spacing in microspace increments, and the ability to change type styles within a given document as it prints);
- The ability to imbed directions within a file. (I use this feature to set up prompts for myself when I work on testing reports, social histories, and treatment summaries.)

It is also possible to write and edit source files (e.g., BASIC programs) using WordStar; I have found this feature very helpful in modifying programs for my own customized use. (For example, I was able to use the search/replace feature to modify statements throughout a lengthy BASIC program.) In short, WordStar is incredible!

When the Mailmerge option ($150) is added to WordStar, you greatly increase your data-handling and word-processing capabilities. Mailmerge is described as a file-merging tool. It allows you to insert variables from data files at specific places within a printed report with automatic rejustification of the output. Although I do not produce "boiler-plated" or "canned" reports, it would be very easy to set up a system for doing so with the WordStar/Mailmerge combination. For example, you could develop a large set of descriptive paragraphs that describe possible client conditions and then automatically insert the appropriate paragraph(s) at appropriate places to produce a complete individualized diagnostic report. The system is flexible enough to also allow individualized paragraphs and statements to be freely intermixed with "canned" paragraphs. Names, addresses, dates, and other client-specific data are automatically inserted at the proper places within the printed report.

Although not a true data-based management system, the DataStar ($350) and SuperSort ($250) combination allow the user to perform many DBM functions. These include data entry, retrieval, updating, sorting by key variables, and automatic field calculations. The user can also easily develop customized onscreen forms for data entry and retrieval using the DataStar form-generation program menu. For example, the clinician can develop a problem-oriented record format for onscreen presentation, enter or update information on specific clients, sort the data across files (e.g., all married clients between the ages of 20–35 with a given diagnosis and less than 5 treatment sessions), and than re-sort for such variables as treatment outcome. One of the great MicroPro features is the total compatibility of its component software packages; data files established by DataStar can be merged into reports, form letters, client billing statements, insurance claim reports, or mailing labels using WordStar with Mailmerge. I use these features to produce customized MMPI interpretive reports and have plans to use the combination to automate production of test data summaries (with appropriate research data footnotes) and to produce a simple filing and indexing system of resource and reference materials that currently reside in file cabinets and boxes all over my office.

MicroPro recently released a new software program, ReportStar, that will generate reports from DataStar records. When DataStar and ReportStar are combined, the combined package is called InfoStar. InfoStar is a true database management program that can be integrated with WordStar and Mailmerge to provide an almost infinite variety of formatted reports.

CalcStar is a very flexible spreadsheet program that will maintain and produce balance statements, general ledgers, patient statements, salary records, etc. Like DataStar, it has a menu for producing the data entry forms and is also fully interactive with WordStar. All of the currently available spreadsheet programs allow the use of "what if?" statements; CalcStar is no exception. Using this feature, one can immediately see the effect that changing one variable has on all dependent variables. For example, a clinician developing a proposed office operating budget can immediately see the effect on the total budget of changing such variables as number of employees (which affects salary, equipment and space needed, taxes and benefits paid, etc.), number of client contact hours anticipated, etc. If you tend to obsessively develop all types of "projections" using pad, pencil, and calculator, you'll find that programs like CalcStar make the obsessing almost painless (and infinitely less time-consuming).

The only disappointment in the MicroPro system is SpellStar ($250). This is a proofreading program that compares the words in a text file (letter, report, etc.) that you create against its 20,000-word dictionary, finds words that are not in that dictionary (or supplemental dictionaries that you can create with commonly used specialized words, names, etc.), and then "flags" the words on screen to allow you to make corrections (or add new words to the dictionaries). Compared to other proofreading programs that I have seen run, SpellStar has a number of shortcomings. It's slow, its dictionary does not contain many common, frequently used words, it responds to prefixes/suffixes as spelling errors, and it's no bargain when compared to some of the equivalent proofreading programs currently on the market (e.g., Spell, at $50).

The Cyborg
BioLab 21:
A Microcomputer
System
for Physiological
Data Acquisition
and Biofeedback

Danny Wedding, PhD

The advent of microcomputing has started a major revolution in the psychophysiological laboratory that has implications for both physiological research and patient care. Research that required on-line signal averaging once required minicomputers and fairly sophisticated engineering and programming in order to interface computer and polygraph equipment. However, the development of analog input capability for microcomputers and the ready availability of modular units and subroutine libraries have tremendously facilitated data acquisition and analysis; practicing clinicians now find it possible to collect data and to address research questions that once required the combined efforts of a multidisciplinary team. In addition, data can be selected and stored on each patient seen; it is possible to amass a significant data base for research purposes without significantly varying the clinical routine of the typical biofeedback laboratory.

Cyborg Corporation has taken an early lead in the area of computerized psychophysiological assessment. We have used three Cyborg BioLabs in the Department of Psychiatry and Behavioral Sciences at East Tennessee University for the past year; this chapter is a summary of our experience with the system.

The heart of the BioLab system is the Apple II computer with 64k memory. (An additional 16k of memory is available with the Apple Language Card.) The Apple was an excellent choice: it is more than adequate to handle the data-reduction needs of both the biofeedback clinician and the researcher; the popularity of the model makes servicing quite easy in virtually any location. In addition, the vast array of software available for the Apple can be used with the BioLab and, between patients, one can use the system for editing manuscripts, playing chess, or statistical analysis.

The Apple II and the BioLab hardware is housed in an attractive and durable white-and-gray modular rack with slots for eight individual units. The BioLab front is quite impressive, with a multitude of controls and dials; however, the system looks somewhat barren when it houses only the thermal, electromyogram (EMG), and audio modules (the basic clinical package recommended by Cyborg). It is not quite as attractively packaged as the hardwood Autogenics line; however, it does not require stacking of units and is quite space-efficient.

A wide variety of input and output modules are available, allowing the individual clinician or researcher to tailor a package to suit his or her current needs and to conveniently add modules as those needs change and as equipment funds become available. Each of our BioLabs is equipped with the following modules: thermal, electromyogram, electroencephalogram, R-P interval, an audio output module, and a general-purpose physiology module. Individual modules for assessing heart rate and electrodermal responding are also available.

The thermal input module (M120) is designed to assess peripheral skin temperature. Input can come from two separate thermal probes; these signals can be averaged or individually studied. One can sequentially study either signal during a single session; however, a second thermal unit will be required if it is necessary to simultaneously record skin temperature from two sites. Data can be recorded and presented in either degrees Fahrenheit or Centigrade. (Centigrade recording is necessary for scientific work; however, patients learning to control hand temperature almost inevitably prefer the Fahrenheit feedback mode). The module is designed to measure temperature in the range of 15°C–38°C (60°F–100°F), with resolution to .01 degree Fahrenheit. The unit is well-suited to the needs of the biofeedback clinician, who may be using thermal feedback to treat migraines or Raynaud's disease; however, because of the slow, tonic nature of the response, most patients will prefer the bar-graph feedback option (in lieu of the line graph mode, which displays change over time but which is not as sensitive to minute change and therefore not as appropriate as a feedback device). This problem is obviated when audio feedback is incorporated into the training session.

The Cyborg EMG (electromyogram) unit (M130) is designed for use in relaxation training (e.g., with muscle contraction headaches) and for neuromuscular re-education. It is possible to program the unit to operate in one of three selected ranges: 1–10, 1–100, and 10–1000 microvolts. Although settings for these specific ranges are built into the module itself, range is specified through software commands and the modular settings have no functional significance. Rear panel jacks allow for output of raw signal data. More meaningful data is available when this raw AC signal is converted to DC current. Cyborg has opted to use a root mean square (RMS) conversion instead of integral averaging, arguing convincingly that the former conversion produces a cleaner signal. In addition, Cyborg has built a pre-amplifier into the sensor apparatus that conducts the EMG signal from the patient to the module. This reduces the likelihood that a long cable will act as an antenna that will pick up interference and distort the actual EMG signal.

A number of sensor electrodes are available for use with the M150 module; however, only disk electrodes can be used and the module is not designed for use with needle electrodes of the type used in rehabilitation medicine. Although considerably more expensive, the use of Quick-Stick disposable sensor strips are extremely convenient for both the patient and the clinician and eliminate the need for cleaning the sensors after each use. In a clinical setting, the convenience clearly justifies the extra cost.

The M110 EEG module makes it possible to assess and feed back brainwave activity in the range of 5 to 17 hz (i.e., theta, alpha, and slow beta activity). However, only two bandpass widths are provided ($+1$ and $+2$ Hz). Although there are few clinical applications for EEG feedback, Cyborg has continued to market the module and it continues to be used, often inappropriately. Our own use of the module is restricted to research studies examining cerebral lateralization. Some preliminary studies have suggested that EEG normalization training may have some utility in the treatment of epilepsy; however, early results are very tentative and widespread clinical application is premature.

The Cyborg R-P interval module (M170) directly assesses pulse wave velocity (PWV) by measuring the latency, in milliseconds, between the R-wave on the EKG and the arrival of the cardiac pulse in the radial artery of the wrist. The radial pulse is measured with a cuff-mounted pressure sensor. The M170 can be used to directly assess heart rate (i.e., interbeat intervals), but its primary utility lies in the assessment of pulse transit time. The technique may have some value in the treatment of hypertensive patients insofar as PWV has been demonstrated to co-vary with blood pressure and, presumably, patients can learn to decrease both PWV and blood pressure. The primary advantage of the methodology is that it eliminates the need for a pressure cuff and allows for continuous monitoring. All other continuous monitoring methods are invasive and cumbersome. The major disadvantage of the R-P module lies in the fact that PWV correlates with systolic

pressure much more highly than with diastolic pressure. Unfortunately, it is diastolic pressure that is of more significance in many clinical situations. In addition, the pressure cuffs that are currently marketed are not sufficiently sensitive to pick up the radial pulse in many
patients and especially in the obese, who are more likely to be hypertensive.

The most sophisticated (and the most expensive) of the Cyborg
modules is the M150, a multipurpose input module that permits detection and amplification of skin potential response, galvanic skin response, single motor-unit activity, evoked potentials, vaginal blood
flow, pulse amplitude, EEG, EOG, EKG, EMG, blood volume, and res-
piration. The module is equipped with upper and lower frequency controls, five sensitivity settings, a balance control, a signal-inversion
switch, a 60-Hz notch filter, and an excitation current control. Although it is far more complicated than any of the other modules, anyone familiar with the operation of a standard polygraph should have
little difficulty in learning how to adapt the M150 to virtually any psychophysiological assessment need. In our laboratory we routinely use
the M150 to monitor skin potential responses while patients are engaged in biofeedback training.

Additional modules are available. These include the audio module
and interface modules for external equipment. The audio module provides feedback in the form of a tone that varies in pitch with changes
in an input signal. The audio module is standard equipment for most
clinical users, since relaxation training is frequently conducted with the
patient's eyes closed.

Two levels of software exist for the BioLab system. The first, Bio-
Text, is menu-driven and is exceedingly easy to learn, even for the
neophyte user. BioText is designed for use by clinicians who will be applying standard treatment protocols to particular patient groups and
for users who will not require the flexibility of a more extensive computer language. For more sophisticated users, a high-level extension to
Applesoft BASIC is available. This language, called BioSoft, adds 28 instructions to the Applesoft instruction set. By pre-interpreting all of its
commands, BioSoft permits fast sampling in a relatively simple command language. The addition of BioSoft requires an extra 2.5k of memory; however, this is little cost, given the extra flexibility of the language.

The Cyborg engineers and programmers have exploited the color
graphics capability of the Apple and the visual displays presented to
the patient are both colorful and well-planned. Up to four different
physiological parameters can be displayed simultaneously, each represented by a different color. Unfortunately, use of many common training times (e.g., 20 minutes) during feedback produces a truncated dis-

play in the line graph mode. While this is not a serious limitation, it is annoying and should be relatively easy for Cyborg to fix with minor software modifications.

The keyboard is a detached typewriter style ASCII unit, which is quite convenient to use. A separate keying system for entering numerical data would have been a useful addition, but isn't a requirement for most users. In addition, with a language card, MicroSoft BASIC, and a modem, all eight slots are full and there is some risk of overheating that could be avoided with the addition of a small fan.

The 13-inch color monitor that is provided with the basic system is adequate for biofeedback purposes, but the resolution is inadequate for text editing and any prolonged use will result in eyestrain.

Originally Cyborg marketed the Centronics 730 dot-matrix printer (80 columns) for day-to-day use along with the Trendcom 100 40-column graphic printer for printing patient graphs. The use of two separate printers was cumbersome at best and often a major nuisance. More recently, Cyborg has been including the Epson MX-80 as part of the BioLab package. This is a major improvement, insofar as the MX-80 will print both text and high-resolution graphics and will allow for both double-width and double-strike printing.

Much of the software that Cyborg sells along with the BioLab can be purchased for much less from private vendors. For example, the Apple Writer text-editing system, which we bought for $150, is available in a local computer store for half the price we paid. Likewise, the psychological testing package (designed by PsychSystems and marketed through a special arrangement with Cyborg) is extremely expensive ($1,500 plus royalty fees for each text administered), and I think stronger and far less expensive alternatives will be on the market by the time this book is published.

Despite my general enthusiasm for the BioLab system, it is important to note that the equipment is expensive. At this time (January 1983) the basic system starts at $6,700. The modules themselves are also expensive: EMG, $820; Thermal, $470; EEG, $680; R-P Interval, $1,000; Audio, $590; Psychophysiology, $1,250. These expenses are probably not justifiable unless the clinician is delivering biofeedback services on a daily basis. On the other hand, if the clinician has research interests in psychophysiology or if he or she has additional computer needs (patient billing, word processing, etc.), it may not be that much more expensive than a solitary microcomputer system, which would not provide the capacity for psychophysiological assessment and feedback.

In summary, Cyborg has developed an expensive but strong computerized system that is versatile enough to be adapted to the needs of both the researcher and the clinician. The system has served us well, and we are pleased with our choice. Most importantly, I believe that the widespread adoption of computerized assessment techniques will open new doors for applied research and permit us to more fully understand what biofeedback packages work, and for whom, and why.

From Mainframe to Mini to Micro: Efforts to Adapt Features from a Large Hospital System to Microcomputers

Douglas K. Gottfredson, PhD
Robert Wally Fort, BS

The Veterans Administration started using computers when the computer field was still in its infancy. At that time, computers were exceedingly expensive and very large. Consequently, strict guidelines were set for computer use. Any proposal for any computer application has to specify in great detail the requirements for equipment and exact performance specification, in addition to detailed cost analysis and proof of cost benefit. Approval for new applications, therefore, was very difficult to obtain. Because of the stringent policies, by the late 1970s the VA was considerably behind the private sector in the use of computers in medical settings. Fortunately, it was possible to use computers for research applications. In 1972, the Salt Lake VA received a research grant to demonstrate the use of computers in psychiatric assessment. The research project was under the direction of Thomas A. Williams, MD, assisted by James H. Johnson, PhD, and others. The project continued until 1977. Their work is reported in 25 journal articles and chapters in a number of books, for example, Williams, Johnson, and Bliss, 1975.

In 1978, the Veterans Administration began an effort to improve computer applications in medical care and catch up with technological developments. Because of its history of computer use, the Salt Lake VA Medical Center was selected as one of several sites to receive new computer equipment. In January of 1979, a DEC PDP 11/70 was installed. The PDP 11/70 uses the Massachusetts General Hospital Utility Multi-Programming System (MUMPS) language and operating system.

By April 30, 1979, the desired programs from the research project were all converted to run on the 11/70. In coordination with other VA Medical Centers with compatible equipment, we then proceeded to develop numerous computer applications for use throughout the medical center. A brief history of the development is given by the authors and others who have worked on the various projects (Gottfredson, Schmidt, Christensen, Beebe, & Fort, 1980). The computer applications were designed to provide support to clinicians, managers, and researchers, as reported by one of the authors during the Fifth Annual Symposium on Computer Applications in Medical Care (Gottfredson, 1981). Following the symposium, we received numerous requests for information about the computer system from all over the United States, Canada, and Australia. The development of the computer system occurred in the Veterans Administration and the software is, therefore, in the public domain. Upon request we have furnished portions of the software to individuals who have access to comparable computer equipment operating in MUMPS.

Although the software was developed in a government agency, the mental health part of the system includes approximately 80 psychological tests and about 20 interviews, many of which are copyrighted by various publishers. During the developmental process, we contacted the different publishers and were able to receive licenses or permission agreements to computer-administer, score, and interpret psychological tests for varying royalty fees, depending on test length, complexity of scoring, etc. When furnishing the software, we have requested evidence that the potential user has secured a license or permission agreement from the copyright holder and that the American Psychological Association standards for users of psychological tests are met.

Although the software has been demonstrated to be exportable, it was designed to run on a fairly large system. The Salt Lake System has a CPU with 384K bytes of MOS memory, and six disk drives with a combined storage of 616 megabytes. There are currently about 60 CRT terminals and 15 printers located throughout the medical center on the wards, in the pharmacy, the laboratory, admitting office, etc.; they support lab, medical, pharmacy, mental health, and administrative functions. We are expecting additional computer equipment to further enhance efficiency in providing medical care and all the supporting functions.

Many of the individuals and institutions requesting information about our computer system have asked about applications for microcomputers. Since the Veterans Administration is not in business to develop software, the authors decided to explore the feasibility of adapting some of the computer applications to microcomputers on their own time and with their own or other private resources. MUMPS is now available for microcomputers from a number of sources. We requested and received support for Apple-MUMPS from Micronetics Design Corporation, Inc.* We were interested in developing different systems for use on microcomputers with different memory and disk storage capacities. We started with an Apple II with 48K RAM memory and one floppy disk drive for 5½-inch single-density disks. By rewriting the programs to reduce their size, we have been able to put the necessary software and test information on one disk to administer, score, and print results from one to five different psychological tests. Each test could be administered any number of times. Since the test items are copyrighted, we requested and received permission from one copyright holder to develop and demonstrate the feasibility of computer administration and scoring of psychological tests on microcomputers. Upon approval of the various copyright holders, the disks could be distributed by them or by us, and they will receive royalty fees from sale of the disks. The disks will be prepared for a discrete number of administrations, after which the files containing the questions and scoring information will be automatically erased. The disks are copy-protected, so that additional disks cannot be made from the original disk supplied by the copyright holder. For the individual who has his own microcomputer, we anticipate that he or she will be able to enjoy computer administration, scoring, and interpretation at a much lower cost and more rapid turnaround time than would be needed for sending answer sheets to a computer scoring service. The present computer system will allow on-line administration or clerk entry of answers. With the addition of a card reader such as the Chatsworth, the tests can be group-administered and the scoring and interpretation completed in a matter of minutes after the conclusion of the testing.

The software for the Salt Lake computer includes an accounting system for payment of royalties. Requests for payment vouchers are sent to the copyright holders every quarter or semi-annually. We have also experimented with putting the psychological tests on microcomputers that have Corvus disk drives. The entire Salt Lake testing package can be put on a Corvus disk drive with a ten-megabyte capacity. This includes the accounting system for payment of royalty fees. The user who has a Corvus disk drive could then make an arrangement with the copyright holders similar to ours at the Salt Lake VA Medical Center.

The Salt Lake system includes Medical History Parts One, Two, and Three. Part One is a statement of the chief complaint, history of

---

*The Micronetics Design Corporation, Inc., may be contacted by writing to the Micronetics Design Corporation, Inc., 932 Hungerford Drive, Suite 11, Rockville, MD 19850.

the present illness, and medical history. This is completed on the computer as free-text entry, using a word-processor feature of the system. Part Two is an individual and family history of diseases, illnesses, etc. Part Three is a review of systems. The History Part Two and Part Three are completed on-line by the patient. The History Parts Two and Three can be included on a very small microcomputer system, such as the one previously described with 48K RAM memory and floppy disk drive. The History Part One could be included with any system that has word-processing capability. The Salt Lake system also includes a computer-prompted or computer-entered physical examination. The information is entered in approximately two to three minutes; the printout gives a summary of the abnormal findings first, followed by a complete description of the physical examination. The physical examination can also be adapted to either a small or larger microcomputer.

Software is also available for financial accounting for billing of individuals, third-party payers, etc., through Micronetics Design Corporation and others. With Corvus disk drive, the pharmacy package could also be made available for maintaining medication profiles on individuals, stock levels of various drugs, printing prescription labels and prescription information, etc. This project demonstrated the feasibility of implementing a wide number of computer applications in psychiatric, psychological, and medical settings.

REFERENCES

Gottfredson, D. K. A computer data base for clinicians, managers and researchers. In Henry G. Heffernan, S. J., ed., *Proceedings, The Fifth Annual Symposium on Computer Applications in Medical Care.* New York: IEEE Computer Society Press, 1981, 417–421.

Gottfredson D. K., Schmidt, L. J., Christensen, P. W., Beebe, B., & Fort, R. W. Computers in mental health treatment: The Salt Lake City VA Medical Center experience. *Computers in Psychiatry/Psychology,* 1980, 3(2), 5–8. [It also appears in Part I of this book—Ed.]

Williams, T. A., Johnson, J. H., & Bliss, E. L. A computer-assisted psychiatric assessment unit. *The American Journal of Psychiatry,* 1975, 132(10), 1074–1076.

PART XIV

Other Issues

The chapters of part XIV are a potpourri of topic touching on a number of computer applications and issues that do not fit comfortably into one category. They are included either because they represent important ideas, they present practical considerations, or they pose provocative questions about the use of the computer. The section starts with a description of the Lithium Information Center, a model of a computerized knowledge base in psychiatry. Such bases, with the proper financial support, can make vital, up-to-date information about a particular topic easily accessible to anyone with a means of connecting his or her computer to a telephone line.

Artificial intelligence seems to have an understandable fascination for most people concerned with how the human mind works. Its use in psychology and psychiatry is examined in the chapter by Gregory Freiherr.

Gary Tucker's and Stanley Rosenberg's work at Dartmouth exploring the characteristic verbal behaviors of schizophrenic patients is then reviewed. Will it be possible some day to automate diagnosis by having a computer analyze people's everyday speech? Or their brain waves? The next chapter takes a brief look at the very elementary but awe-inspiring studies by Donald York and Tom Jensen that use the computer to relate brain waves to micro-behavior as circumscribed as the utterance of a particular word.

Perhaps some day computers will even settle the question of whether or not there are really paranormal phenomena. For the time being, the computer may make its contribution by presenting information to subjects of studies of the paranormal in a reproducible and reliable manner. But then again, who will write the programs? The chapter by Dick Bierman looks at the use of personal computers for the study of paranormal phenomena.

For those with a practical bent, the section contains a chapter on the tax law of 1981 and the computer. (Maybe it's a deduction you didn't consider. But be sure to check with your tax adviser before doing anything rash. The law may have changed since the chapter was written.)

Part XIV concludes with some ideas about guidelines for user access to computerized patient records. While not attempting to spell out specific rules, the brief chapter at the end offers a useful approach for any group attempting to establish guidelines of its own.

54 The Lithium Information Center

The Lithium Information Center, founded in 1975 by Drs. James W. Jefferson and John H. Greist, now contains citations of over 7,500 references to the biological uses of lithium. The center is staffed by a full-time medical librarian and responded to more than 700 written and telephone requests for information in 1980. In addition, more than 35 sites have on-line access to the computer registry.

Under a grant from the National Library of Medicine, work is underway to develop synopses of approximately 500 subjects relevant to lithium and its medical uses. A lithium consultation computer program, which will provide clinicians with assistance in diagnosis and management of patients with lithium-responsive disorders, is also being prepared. Those interested in contacting the Lithium Information Center may do so by writing or calling Ms. Margaret Baudhuin at the Center for Health Sciences, 600 Highland Avenue, Madison, Wisconsin 53792, telephone (608) 263–6170.

This article originally appeared in *Computers in Psychiatry/Psychology*, 1981, 3(3), 8, and is reprinted by permission.

Artificial Intelligence in Psychology and Psychiatry

Gregory Freiherr

Most clinical and biochemical applications of AI [Artificial Intelligence] attempt to capture the effectiveness of human expertise without necessarily trying to model what goes on in the human mind. Many applications in psychology, however, are aimed specifically at constructing working models of human cognitive behavior. These systems are basically intended as research tools.

AI models of human cognition, including memory, inferential reasoning, language-processing, and problem-solving, are being assembled at Carnegie-Mellon University under the direction of Dr. John Anderson. Known as *Acquisition of Cognitive Procedures* and nicknamed *ACT*, the program is intended to represent the development and performance of decision-making. In essence, ACT is a basic research project in AI, containing a logic scheme that may be transferable to applications in specific areas in or outside of medicine.

"We hope that future versions of ACT will resemble very closely the process by which people learn to make decisions," Dr. Anderson says. "We could then apply this model of skill acquisition to such medical domains as diagnosis and scientific inference."

ACT's knowledge base consists of two components. One contains facts and serves as the program's memory—essentially a data base. The other is a set of rules used to make decisions based on what is contained in the memory.

As a result, new decision-making rules must be conceived and old ones modified on a continuing basis. Dr. Anderson and colleagues have built learning functions into the ACT program to accomplish this.

"Artificial Intelligence in Psychology and Psychiatry" is excerpted from "SUMEX-AIM and the Science Community: Seeds of Artificial Intelligence," in *The Seeds of Artificial Intelligence: SUMEX-AIM*, by Gregory Freiherr, Washington, DC: US Government Printing Office, 1980, pp. 54–55, 58–63.

New rules are automatically created; old rules are assessed, adjusted, combined, and sometimes thrown out.

A stumbling block in all learning systems is that rules commonly used in human decision-making often defy description, even by those who use them. Dr. Anderson says the system can create new rules only to the extent that people understand the skill to be acquired. Because this would leave gaping holes in the decision-making machinery, a fallback has been built in.

For relatively unstructured situations, ACT uses trial-and-error. The approach is an intelligent set of attempts to find the correct answer based on what has been learned by past mistakes. Tests of the system's ability to learn have been conducted. Recently the program was taught to generate and explain proofs in geometry, using some introductory exercises in high school textbooks. The system successfully created new decision-making rules and amended or discarded old ones. It also learned ways to reorganize its search for mathematical postulates so as to increase speed.

Although ACT is continually being revised, versions are "frozen" at various stages of development and made available to researchers throughout SUMEX-AIM.* One version has been applied by Drs. James G. Greeno and Alan M. Lesgold at the University of Pittsburgh to model the acquisition of reading and problem-solving skills. Entitled *Simulation of Cognitive Processes*, the project centers on modeling the processes involved in arithmetic and reading. These two skills were chosen because "they are very basic cognitive requirements for getting along in the world," Dr. Greeno says.

The project is founded on studies showing that various word-processing skills and arithmetic procedures are underdeveloped in children who do poorly in reading, mathematics, or both. Models are being developed to test this belief. One simulates the process of solving simple word problems. It is intended to determine the degree to which semantic and linguistic factors, rather than arithmetic knowledge, are responsible for children's difficulty in solving these problems at early grade levels.

"By providing a framework in which the effects of different levels of skill acquisition can be understood, we hope to provide criteria that will separate patients who have brain damage from those whose cognitive skills have developed poorly," Dr. Greeno says. "This is not something that we expect to result from our work in the immediate future. It is an example of what we hope to achieve."

---

*SUMEX-AIM is an acronym for the Stanford University Medical Experimental Computer for Artificial Intelligence in Medicine, a nationally shared computing resource devoted to designing AI applications for the biomedical sciences. SUMEX-AIM is funded by the National Institutes of Health Division of Research Resources, Biotechnology Resources Program.

The Higher Mental Functions project being conducted at the University of California, Los Angeles (UCLA) is devoted to researching personality problems, specifically paranoia and adult neuroses. Another segment of the project involves development of devices that will allow patients with language disorders, especially those who have suffered stroke, to speak. All three areas call for the development and use of AI programs.

Under the direction of Dr. Kenneth M. Colby, a psychiatrist at the UCLA Neuropsychiatric Institute, a computer simulation of paranoid thought processes is being constructed. Called *PARRY*, the simulation is used to test the consistency of a theory describing the pathology. PARRY also serves as a training device in teaching students or psychiatric residents about various aspects of paranoia. The program has proved its ability to do both.

Recently PARRY was interviewed by five psychiatrists via teletype. Each was granted two interviews. The psychiatrists were advised at the start that they would be communicating with either a patient or a computer. It was their task to distinguish the paranoid patient from the simulation. In the test, PARRY's responses matched those of the paranoid patient so closely that the psychiatrists could not tell the difference between the two.

Although the test does not prove that the theory on which PARRY relies is all-inclusive, it shows that the theory contains enough facets of the paranoid personality to confuse experts and to serve as a tool in teaching students about the pathology.

In using AI techniques to classify neuroses, Dr. Colby hopes to sharpen the rules that identify patients with different neuroses. He says the officially accepted means of classifying patients is unreliable.

"The idea is to find a better classification scheme, and one way is to find properties or characteristics of each neurosis," Dr. Colby says. "The scheme as it now exists depends on recognized signs and symptoms of the patient."

The program is being designed to work opposite to the way PARRY operates. Rather than interpreting questions presented by interviewers and returning paranoid answers, the AI program in neuroses must take neurotic answers and work backward to the underlying concepts or key ideas that distinguish the patient's pathology from those of other patients. These key ideas would then be clustered to form the profile of a certain type of patient, Dr. Colby says.

"A key idea for the profile of a depressive patient might be 'I am someone who should get more help.' In a normal person, the idea will surface again and again."

Seven expert psychiatrists and psychologists at the UCLA Neuropsychiatric Institute are collaborating on the neurosis project. At present the work is in the "exploratory pilot-study stage," Dr. Colby emphasizes. The program that will group key ideas into profiles is not yet written. But the application of AI to speech prosthesis has progressed to an advanced point.

In the past several years, Dr. Colby and colleagues have designed and constructed three speech devices, each composed of portable microprocessors and voice synthesizers. Patients use symbols that are translated by more than a thousand rules into verbal language.

One device is specially suited to patients who have suffered central brain damage due to stroke, tumor, or head trauma. Because these patients have difficulty remembering certain words, the device maintains a vocabulary important to the specific patient and helps the person by offering various candidates.

"A stroke patient might want to say 'chair,' but can't remember the word. But he does remember the word 'sit.' The program then generates a list of possible words, and the patient just has to hit the number of the right one," Dr. Colby says.

Devices for patients not so severely handicapped do not include this function. Such patients might be victims of cerebral palsy, Parkinsonism, laryngectomy, or might have tracheostomies. Their major problem is only speech and pronunciation.

The two types of devices, each no larger than a cosmetic case and weighing only 8 pounds, feature a large vocabulary of words, which can be constructed by using the English alphabet and a keyboard. The programs are used in microprocessors, but were developed and are being refined on the SUMEX computer. Of particular use, Dr. Colby says, is the extensive English dictionary that is available. He and colleagues have used the dictionary to write and test program rules. Memory and word-finding functions are also being refined through use of the computer dictionary.

Dr. Colby explains that rules of pronunciation for each letter of the alphabet are written into the program. The rules first identify the context in which the letter appears and then how the letter is pronounced in both usual and special cases. The electrical codes of the letters are assembled and passed on to a commercial voice synthesizer, which simulates the sounds of speech.

Patients hear the words first through a tiny earplug speaker, which gives them a chance to correct mistakes. Although words generated by the synthesizer are usually accurate, the process of communicating can be tedious for both sides of the conversation.

"If the patient is typing very slowly, the listener gets impatient," Dr. Colby says. "There's a solution, but it's even more complex than what we are working with now."

By using symbols that represent concepts rather than letters, basic ideas could be transformed into speech. For example, the concept of affection might be portrayed by a heart with an arrow pointing up. Unfortunately, the exact type of affection is not indicated by this symbol. As yet, a means to narrow concepts until they fit the context precisely is not available.

Despite the disadvantages of speech prosthesis devices now in use at the UCLA laboratory, they are a major aid for handicapped patients. "A speech prosthesis is a godsend," Dr. Colby says. "If you can't talk, life is hell. All the attempts to use teletypes have failed because people want to hear a voice. And because many of the patients who have speech problems are homebound, they do all their communication over the phone, and a teletype can't work in that case."

The three devices at UCLA have been used repeatedly by patients, and Dr. Colby says they are ready to be offered to a mass market, except for one stumbling block. The business world, at the present time, is not interested.

"In the sixties, you would find all kinds of people who wanted to invest in computers, but not today," he says. "We need a 'plunger' or a humanitarian willing to manufacture the devices."

Each speech prosthesis built from spare parts in the laboratory costs about $2,000. If mass produced, Dr. Colby says, the cost could drop as low as $500. But most large electronics firms are looking for broad markets, rather than specialized medical ones, Dr. Colby says. So he and his team are concentrating their efforts on refining and further developing the devices.

Dr. Colby consults with Drs. John Eulenberg and Carl V. Page, computer scientists at Michigan State University, who are now directing the COMMUNICATION ENHANCEMENT pilot project. Their goal also is to design intelligent speech prostheses for persons with severe communication handicaps. Proposed research includes the design of input devices that can be used by persons whose movement is greatly restricted, development of software for text-to-speech production, and production of a microcomputer-based portable speech prosthesis.

In 1978, project scientists designed and built a portable communication system for a 10-year-old boy with cerebral palsy who cannot speak or use his hands to write. Although only partially successful, the device influenced design of a lap-board communication aid, which was completed early in 1979. Called SAL (Semantically Accessible Language), it translates Bliss symbols into spoken language. The communication symbols, named after their inventor, C. K. Bliss, are used by people who have suffered brain damage. These symbols are interpreted by the semantic, nonverbal side of the brain.

When using the lap-board, patients choose symbols for various words. These are translated by a microcomputer into orthographic and phonetic strings, which are turned into sounds by a voice synthesizer and into typed words by a visual display unit. Grammar rules programmed into the computer guide the production of sentences.

"When a person makes the symbol for himself, it will come out either 'me' or 'I,' depending on whether it is the subject or object of the sentence," Dr. Page says. "These decisions are made by grammar rules contained in the program."

But vastly extending the intelligence of the program is necessary before project goals are met. "It is a very painful process to communicate with people afflicted by cerebral palsy. They're very, very slow. An enormous amount of concentration is required to make these symbols," Dr. Page says. "What we're really looking for is a means of communication that will give them the most output for whatever input they can provide. It has to do with finding the appropriate language or vocabulary to express thought. It's not just alphabetical letters; it's not words; and it's not grammar. It is some combination of these things. One approach is to build a very intelligent knowledge-based system, one that can infer what the person means with a minimum of input."

The complex cognitive processes that underlie text comprehension and planning are being explored in another project only recently accepted into the SUMEX-AIM community. Directed by Drs. Walter Kintsch and Peter G. Polson, the HIERARCHICAL MODELS OF HUMAN COGNITION project is partly focused on developing models of the processes people use to understand information and plan actions. Dr. Kintsch is studying the means by which people understand and summarize texts. He hopes to determine ways to improve the readability of texts. He believes that an explicit theory of normal comprehension might lead scientists to the factors that cause learning problems in children, as well as suggest ways to overcome these problems.

The other focus of the project, which is under Dr. Polson's direction, is modeling how people create plans and design complex systems. Specifically, Dr. Polson and colleagues are studying and comparing how experts and novices use their knowledge to design computer software. Given a coherent formulation of these processes, aids could be developed that would help people perform this task.

Using the framework provided by artificial intelligence, Dr. Charles F. Schmidt, a psychologist, and Dr. N. S. Sridharan, a computer scientist, both at Rutgers University, are refining a theory of human information-processing. Their goal is to define the way people assemble facts into a coherent, understandable pattern.

The program, called BELIEVER, is used to construct and test a psychological theory called BELIEF, which is intended to explain the process people use in understanding the observed actions of others. The scientists present situations to the computer and compare its interpretations with those of human subjects. If the two sets of interpretations match, the theory gains support. If they do not agree, the theory and the program may be altered, depending on the degree of contradiction.

Although descriptions fed into the computer are very precise, the BELIEF theory is composed entirely of general principles. The researchers hope to define the broad ideas that govern interpretation of actions, regardless of culture.

"BELIEVER is a framework in which to extend the theory. In that sense, the project is never-ending," Dr. Schmidt explains. "It's like reading books from a library. You expect to find answers, but you don't expect to run out of books."

At present many of the researchers in SUMEX-AIM design and build systems to suit their own specific needs. One side effect is a certain amount of duplication of effort. "The effort of such redevelopment is very large for such highly complex computer projects as the knowledge-based inference programs being developed in SUMEX-AIM," Dr. Feigenbaum says. "But we are taking important steps in sharing programs that already exist and learning to build future programs that can be more easily shared."

SUMEX-AIM community members have been successful at a type of community-building activity that has been called *"budding."* Projects intended for use in one area of medicine have provided the foundation to design systems aimed at others. For example, CASNET/Glaucoma has led to another project dealing with rheumatology. MYCIN, which was designed to assist in prescribing therapy for patients with infectious diseases, has spawned projects that have application to pharmacology (HEADMED) and pulmonary disease (PUFF/VM). Another example of sharing is the adaptation of ACT programs by Drs. Greeno and Lesgold to simulate the comprehension processes in children performing arithmetic and reading tasks.

According to Dr. Feigenbaum, a long-term goal of SUMEX-AIM is to develop program frameworks that can be applied more generally.

One effort in this direction is a system called *AGE* (Attempt to Generalize) being developed by Ms. H. Penny Nii and Dr. Feigenbaum. It is intended to "despecialize" software, making knowledge engineering more generally available to the scientific community.

"Projects in SUMEX-AIM such as DENDRAL, MYCIN, and MOLGEN have been creating intelligent agents to assist human problem-solving in task domains of medicine and biology," Ms. Nii says. "Without exception, the programs were handcrafted. This process takes many years, both for AI scientists and for experts in the field of collaboration."

AGE grew out of HEARSAY, a speech-understanding program

that envisioned a base containing knowledge of many different types. As a result, AGE is suited to the design of many different programs.

She hopes that the program will evolve someday into a means of building programs for widely differing purposes, thereby simplifying the process of writing software. A long-range goal, Ms. Nii says, is to allow researchers with only a rudimentary understanding of computer science to design specialized AI systems by using AGE. The program is now available on the SUMEX-AIM system and has been used to design several experimental programs. One of these is being developed as part of Drs. Kintsch and Polson's text comprehension project.

In another core research effort aimed at speeding the dissemination of information about AI techniques, Dr. Feigenbaum, Mr. Avron Barr, and colleagues are assembling a handbook of artificial intelligence. In final form, the handbook will contain some 200 articles covering the most important ideas, techniques, and systems developed during the past 20 years of AI research, Dr. Feigenbaum says. The articles, each about four pages long, will be written in language suited to the student of AI, as well as to professionals outside the field.

"Published research is not generally accessible to outsiders, and elementary textbooks are not nearly broad enough to be useful to scientists working in other disciplines who want to do something that requires knowledge of AI," Dr. Feigenbaum says. "The handbook will fill this gap."

Computerized Analysis of Verbal Behavior in Schizophrenia (A Review)

Marc D. Schwartz, MD

Classical linguistic hypotheses about schizophrenics have focused on the differences in the syntax of their speech and that of normal controls. For the most part the findings of these studies have been confusing and have had low rates of replicability. The authors of this study [Stanley Rosenberg and Gary Tucker] believe that it may be worthwhile to focus greater attention on the words spoken, that is, the lexical and semantic level of verbal behavior in schizophrenia, where more precise and quantifiable studies are possible.

Fairly extensive analyses of the verbal productions of schizophrenics have been carried out. They consistently report a decreased number of different words used in the verbal and written productions of schizophrenics and their use of relatively fewer adjectives. Structural or formal analyses of various kinds of thinking disorders, such as loose associations or overly abstract thinking, have indicated their greater frequency in schizophrenia, but their presence in speech is certainly not unique to this group. In another kind of study, more commonly done in laboratory settings than on clinical units, hypothesized defects such as attentional processes have been systematically examined in a laboratory or chronic ward. Once again, nothing has been demonstrated that is exclusive to schizophrenia.

In the study reviewed here, taped speech samples of a group of schizophrenics and nonschizophrenics were obtained in a standard 15-minute interview by an experienced psychiatrist who spoke only

"Verbal Behavior in Schizophrenia," by Stanley Rosenberg and Gary Tucker, appeared in *Archives of General Psychiatry*, November 1979, *36*, 1331–1337. The present review by Marc D. Schwartz of that article originally appeared in *Computers in Psychiatry/Psychology*, 1980, 3 (1), 5, 10, and is reprinted by permission.

when he thought it necessary to encourage the patient to continue talking. The tapes were transcribed and corrected by the interviewer prior to a content analysis. Approximately 600 words from each interview were placed into a computer for grouping into various thematic categories using the Harvard III Psychosocial Dictionary. This method allows 3,500 words (most words used in everyday speech) to be placed into 84 thematic categories, which have been specifically derived for their psychological and sociological significance. Using the Dartmouth Adaptation of the General Inquirer Computer Content Analysis Program, the authors were able to categorize over 90% of the words in the typescripts.

The thematic patterns of schizophrenics were found to deviate from both general and sex-specific concerns of nonschizophrenics. The themes that were found to characterize the schizophrenic patient were related to negativism, hostility, and somatic concerns, and were marked by a preoccupation with thought processes, communication, and nonpractical (artistic or academic) concerns. Schizophrenics also showed higher scores on themes of death, medicine/guidance, and cognitive disability. On the other hand, they scored lower on a factor that emphasized communication, pleasure, and sex.

The thematic differences became even more obvious when the study population was broken down into male and female groups. Male schizophrenics were most notable for their frequent use of artistic references at the time of admission, a use which decreased to nonschizophrenic levels when remission occurred. They also had higher scores on authority and power themes and lower ones on references to affection and natural objects.

Female schizophrenics were very high on the directing, guiding taking-over theme, one which is generally culturally reserved for men. Whether the authors believe such assertiveness in women is a sign of schizophrenia or whether they think assertive women experience so much societal pressure that they become vulnerable to breakdown is not clear. However, they do raise the related question of whether diagnosticians may discriminate against those who choose not to accept stereotyped sex roles by labeling them *schizophrenic*.

Computerized content-analysis can be an important tool in the understanding of verbal behavior. It focuses attention on the lexical dimension of speech in a way that the classical linguistic formulations do not. This may be very useful in delineating the verbal bases for differential diagnosis. Drs. Rosenberg and Tucker conclude that the conscious or subliminal apperception by clinicians may be far more influential in the diagnostic process than has been realized and is well worth further study.

57 Using the Computer to Read the Mind (A Review)

Marc D. Schwartz, MD

The February 16, 1979 issue of the JAMA describes a study reported at the 8th meeting of the Society of Neuroscience, in which computerized analyses of EEGs revealed message-specific patterns. "Electrical impulses were recorded from the left hemisphere in the Broca-Wernicke's area, the major speech center in the brain, during the second that preceded vocalization of short, simple words or nonsense syllables such as 'yes,' 'no,' 'eight,' 'ate,' and 'oot.' Each recording was stored in a computer, and recordings from 50 vocalizations were then combined to produce an averaged brain wave, called a *wave form*." Each syllable turns out to have a characteristic, identifiable wave form reproducible among people who speak the same language. The wave forms appear to be an electrical concomitant of the brain activity necessary for the accomplishment of the muscle movement that shapes speech.

What led the researchers to conclude the wave forms were related to muscle activity and not conceptual content? In one study, they found the wave form for "ate" and "eight" to be the same while those for "yes" and "*oui*" were different.

Could the EEG wave forms be artifacts of muscle activity involved in speech? This seems very unlikely in view of the facts that (1) the wave form always preceded any indication of muscle activity in the larynx and (2) the characteristic wave form could be produced by a person's merely thinking the syllable, without vocalizing anything. Having identified numerous word wave-forms, the authors of the study are programming a microprocessor that will be able to (gasp!) read people's minds. Or at least read syllables being thought therein.

There are many practical implications of this work. The authors are interested in exploring the technique for use in speech rehabilita-

"New Leads on Brain Functioning: How We Speak, Hear, and See," by Donald York and Tom Jensen, appeared in the *Journal of the American Medical Association*, February 16, 1979, 241 (7), 671. The present review by Marc D. Schwartz of that article originally appeared in *Computers in Psychiatry/Psychology*, 1979, 2 (1), 13, and is reprinted by permission.

tion (their field of specialization) and stuttering. They expressed concern in an interview that their technique might be abused by devising a cerebral lie detector which might be able to monitor a person's unspoken "yes/no" responses to questions.

The authors of this study, Donald York, PhD, and Tom Jensen, PhD, are at the University of Missouri, Columbia, Missouri, and are respectively in the fields of neurophysiology and speech pathology.

The Use of Personal Computers for the Study of Paranormal Phenomena

Dick J. Bierman, PhD

It may seem strange to say, but microcomputers are playing an ever-increasing role in such an exotic field as parapsychology—the scientific study of psychic phenomena. However, it is true. Paranormal phenomena such as telepathy, clairvoyance, and psychokinesis ("mind over matter") are studied experimentally by calculating the probability that the observed phenomena would have occurred by chance. By calculating how likely it is that the outcome of an experiment might have occurred by chance, we can also see how likely it is that it might have occurred not by chance, i.e., by some kind of paranormal effect.

In the early days of parapsychology, experiments were performed using cards or dice, but recently it has been found that microcomputers can be used far more effectively. Not only do they run experiments much more quickly, but they can keep their own records, so ruling out incorrect recording as a potential source of error.

At first glance one might think that the random function of most personal computers would be ideal for parapsychological work. In telepathy or clairvoyance, a target picture or symbol can be randomly selected by the computer and not displayed until after a guess has been recorded. In psychokinesis (PK) an attempt would be made to influence the random output of numbers, causing more of a chosen number or numbers to appear. However, in actual fact, the random function of almost all computers is only pseudo-random. Essentially the same numbers are produced in every random series, and only the entry point to those numbers may change. This not only means that no one

The Research Institute for Psi Phenomena and Physics, where Dr. Bierman works, functions as a kind of clearing house for information on software and hardware (Random Number Generators). The address is: RIPP, Alexanderkade 1, 1018CH Amsterdam, The Netherlands.

can be tested more than once, but it also introduces major statistical problems. For this reason, in parapsychology most microcomputers are harnessed to an additional piece of hardware called a random number generator (RNG). The total randomness of RNG's is derived from natural phenomena such as thermal noise or radioactive decay. (To be sure, this is not the only way to test paranormal abilities. One could, for example, try to test PK abilities by having the subject try to bend metal spoons. Although it is not known exactly how often spoons bend by chance, it seems to occur rather seldom and therefore such an occurrence at your "will" would be good proof of PK. However, it is generally observed that abilities of this magnitude are only present in a very few persons, if at all. Less spectacular subjects are easier to locate and are far more likely to be able to bring about minor and temporary changes in the effects of RNG's than permanent changes in cutlery.)

Another great advantage of the microcomputer is that it can provide instant and dramatic feedback to tell the subject how well he is doing. Some recent theoretical and experimental work has indicated that such feedback may be important in helping subjects to produce significant paranormal results. Rather than having to await the experimenter's dreary statistical analysis, the subject can watch his results being graphically illustrated on a CRT. They can appear in the form of a game, a race, or a spectacular display of colors. In fact, any game that involves chance (such as Conway's Game of Life, or even a form of Monopoly) could be adapted for use in parapsychological testing.

Although nearly all serious empirical research in parapsychology is directed towards the unraveling of the underlying processes, the very existence of the phenomena is not yet generally accepted in the scientific world. This discrepancy might be understood if one takes into account the notorious elusiveness of the psi phenomena, an elusiveness that has resulted in a complete failure to replicate the experimental findings independently. Most parapsychologists "explain" this failure by the assumption that in their experiments too many relevant variables are uncontrolled. Many outsiders, however, simply state that the elusiveness just reflects the fact that these phenomena are not real.

The use of microcomputers for the control of parapsychological experiments forces the experimenters to precisely specify and implement the experimental conditions in their software. This software is highly transportable, because the major parapsychological laboratories use similar microcomputers (there is even an APUG, Apple Psi User Group). And, what is more, even the skeptics, having access to a microcomputer, can independently try to replicate the reported results.

This development might therefore bring the desired across-laboratory replicability one step closer and thus result in the more general acceptance of the reality of psi phenomena.

Tax Tips for Computer Owners

Vernon K. Jacobs, CPA

There are a lot of things that you could do with a personal computer, but it's hard to be specific about how the computer will actually help you produce enough extra cash (after taxes) to pay for part, or all, of the cost. Whether you already own a computer or are just trying to find a good excuse to buy one, this chapter will show you how the new tax laws permit you to save enough income taxes to pay for twenty to sixty percent of the cost of a personal computer and possibly recover tax savings far in excess of the cost of the computer.

The tax laws do not permit you to deduct the cost of something that is a personal item—such as your clothing, food, a refrigerator, or a clothes washer. But if an item is purchased for use in a trade or a business (even a part-time business), it becomes deductible—over time if it will last more than a year. There are three major ways that you can deduct the cost of a computer on your tax return.

1. It's an ordinary and necessary expense of your trade and/or your business.
2. It's deductible as an employee business expense.
3. It's deductible as an expense of maintaining your investments.

First, the tax law will permit you to claim a deduction for the "ordinary and necessary" expenses of carrying on a trade or a business. The term "necessary" generally is used to mean that the expense is a normal and usual expense of the type of trade or business in which the taxpayer is engaged. The term "ordinary" usually means that the expense is not a capital expenditure like an automobile, shares of stock, or inventory. In other words, an expense is gone after it is paid for—there is nothing left to show for it. Equipment such as a computer must be capitalized (treated as a capital asset of the business) and depreciated over a period of three or five years. Therefore, the computer becomes deductible over the three or five year period rather than being

---

This chapter is excerpted from a longer report written by the author, entitled "Tax Breaks for Computer Buyers." The complete report is available from the author for $9.00.

deducted in one year. For equipment that is purchased in 1982 or 1983, up to $5,000 of the cost of business equipment can be deducted in a single year, but the cost in excess of that amount must be depreciated over a period of years. (Larger deductions are permitted after 1983.)

The second way to deduct the cost of your computer (if you are an employee) is to have it classed as an employee business expense. To do this, you must be able to show the IRS that having a computer is required by your employer as a condition of being employed. Using a personal car for business is often required for many types of jobs, but the employee may only depreciate the cost of the car to the extent that it is just used for his job. This same principle applies to deducting part of the costs of a home office when no other office facilities are available. Where a computer is deducted by an employee, only the time that the computer is used for business purposes is allowed as a tax deduction. That doesn't mean it must be used all the time for business. If it is used two hours per day for business and one hour per day for personal use, it would be appropriate to deduct two-thirds of the cost of the computer.

The third way to justify a deduction for a computer is to deduct it as an expense of managing your investments. The tax law permits investors to deduct the ordinary and necessary costs of managing or maintaining their investments. This generally requires that the investor already has some investments. Expenses associated with the acquisition of an investment are to be added to the cost of the investment— which means that the tax cost is only recoverable when the investment is sold.

One-Year, Three-Year, and Five-Year Deductions

Business equipment, such as computers, must be deducted over a period of years. Before 1981 the time period was based on the economic useful life of the equipment, and the law permitted the owner to claim a first-year deduction of 20% of the cost up to a maximum of $2,000 per year. The balance of the cost was to be deducted over a period of three, five, ten, or even thirty years—depending on the expected useful life of the equipment. The amount to be depreciated was limited to the expected loss in value. Therefore, any probable salvage or resale value was to be deducted from the cost to determine the amount that could be depreciated.

The tax law was changed drastically in October 1981, to require owners of business equipment to write off any equipment purchased after 1980 over prescribed periods of time. For computers, the time period is five years, unless the computer is being used for research and development purposes. If it is being used for these purposes, it can be written off over a three-year period. (Taxpayers may elect to write off the cost of their equipment over a longer period of time, but there are very few situations where that would be desirable.) The cost of equipment purchased and placed in service prior to 1981 will continue to be depreciated using the rules in effect when the equpiment was acquired. For equipment acquired in 1981, neither the 20% special depreciation available by prior law nor the full write off of the first $5,000 of equipment allowed by the 1981 tax law may be used.

For equipment acquired in 1982 or 1983, taxpayers may elect to deduct the first $5,000 worth of business equipment purchased and placed in service. Any equipment in excess of that amount is to be depreciated over the prescribed three-year or five-year period. For 1984 and 1985 the amount will increase to $7,500 per year. After 1985, the limit will be $10,000 per year. If the full write off is used, no investment credit (see comments below) will be available. For 1982, the five- or three-year depreciation option with the investment tax credit would be more profitable for most taxpayers. After 1982, the first-year 100% deduction of the first $5,000 of equipment purchased will be about equal in value to the combined effect of taking the tax credit and claiming depreciation. The full write-off option is not available for equipment owned as an investment. It is only available for those who are using the computer in a trade or business.

The 1981 law established fixed rates of depreciation that can be claimed for equipment with different cost recovery periods. The annual depreciation under these fixed rates is somewhat faster than just taking an equal amount each year—which is called the straight line method of depreciation. For equipment with a five-year recovery period, the depreciation in the first year is 15% of the cost, the second-year depreciation is 22% of the cost, and the depreciation in each of the next three years is 21% of the equipment cost. For property with a three-year recovery period, the depreciation rates are 25%, 38%, and 37% for the first, second, and third years. If straight line depreciation were chosen, the depreciation in the first few years would be slightly less.

Investment Tax Credits

Owners of equipment purchased for use in a trade or business or to be held for investment may claim a reduction on the amount of taxes due for up to 10% of the cost of the equipment. This reduction in taxes results from something called the investment tax credit. A deduction reduces your taxable income before your tax is computed. A credit reduces your tax after it is computed. If you owe $5,000 for federal income taxes (using a joint return for 1982), a deduction will save you about 29 percent of each dollar of deductions. A $1.00 tax credit will save you the full dollar in taxes. Thus, the tax credit has the same value as $3.45 of extra deductions—because 29% of $3.45 equals $1.00.

The investment tax credit is based on the cost of equipment purchased and placed in service for use in a business or held for investment. For computers with a five-year depreciation period, the tax credit will be 10% of the cost of the equipment—after deducting any trade-ins. If the computer is to be used for research and development and is being depreciated over a three-year period, the investment tax credit is limited to 6% of the cost.

The Tax Equity and Fiscal Responsibility Act of 1982 (TEFRA) modified the rules for claiming a tax credit. Basically, the new rules apply to equipment purchased after 1982 and require the buyer to choose between a smaller tax credit or a reduced amount of depreciation. If the maximum tax credit is claimed, half of the tax credit must be deducted from the cost of the property for purposes of future depreciation. The business owner can elect instead to depreciate the full cost of the equipment and to reduce the investment credit by two percentage points. Instead of taking a 10% tax credit, the credit would be limited to 8%. If the 6% credit were otherwise allowed, only 4% could be claimed in order to depreciate the full cost of the equipment. For the taxpayer in the 50% tax bracket, the effect is to reduce the tax benefit by 2.5% of the cost of the equipment—as compared to what it would have been before the 1982 changes in the law. For the investor in the 40% tax bracket, the new law will result in additional taxes of 2% of the cost of the equipment. Thus, on $10,000 of equipment, the extra taxes over a five-year period will be $250 or less, depending on your tax bracket.

If the reduced tax credit is not chosen, the cost of the equipment must be reduced by half of the tax credit for purposes of depreciation. For example, if a computer system cost $10,000, you could take the full 10% tax credit and depreciate only $9,500 over the next five years—or you could claim an 8% tax credit and depreciate the full $10,000 over the next five years. In table 59–1, an example of the 1982 rules and the two options available for 1983 for equipment costing $10,000 is shown. In this illustration, the taxpayer is in the 40% marginal tax bracket.

Although the dollar amount of the tax recovery from tax credits and depreciation are equal under either option for years after 1982, the first option offers a slight advantage in terms of how quickly you can get the cash tax benefits. However, if there are any limitations that might prevent you from being able to make full use of the tax credits, then you would want to use the second method. As pointed out earlier, the law also permits you to deduct the first $5,000 of equipment purchased in 1982 or 1983. However, no tax credit is permitted for the

TABLE 59–1. A Comparison of the 1982 Tax Credit
and Two 1983 Tax Law Options

	1982	1983(1)	1983(2)
Cost of equipment	$10,000	$10,000	$10,000
Tax credit at 10%	1,000	1,000	———
Reduced tax credit (8%)	———	———	800
Depreciable cost (basis)	10,000	9,500	10,000
Tax savings from depreciation at a 40% tax bracket	4,000	3,800	4,000
Tax savings from tax credit	1,000	1,000	800
Total tax savings/recovery	$ 5,000	$ 4,800	$ 4,800

amount of equipment that is fully deducted in the year of purchase. Before the changes introduced by the 1982 tax law (TEFRA), it was more profitable to depreciate the equipment over a five-year period in order to take the 10% tax credit. Now it would be better to take the full deduction for equipment purchased after 1982 and to depreciate only equipment purchased in excess of the amount that can be fully deducted.

Research and Development Tax Credits

A new type of tax credit was introduced by the Economic Recovery Tax Act of 1981 (the 1981 tax law or ERTA). This is the research and development (R&D) expense credit. To stimulate businesses to spend more money in research activities, the new law offers tax credits of 25% of the cost of R & D expenses in excess of the average cost for the prior three years. Where the average cost in the prior three years was less than half of the current year cost, then half of the current year cost will be used as the average research costs of the prior three years. My understanding of this new law is that depreciation expenses are not part of the costs that can be used to compute the total R & D expense. However, the law does appear to permit the cost of renting a computer as part of the expense that qualifies for the R & D tax credit.

Thus, it does not appear possible to claim the investment tax credit and the R & D tax credit on the same equipment. Given a choice between the R & D credit on rented equipment and the investment tax credit on purchased equipment, the R & D credit seems to be the better choice. The rules are very complex, and this is an oversimplification, but I feel it is a reasonably accurate explanation.

Companies that spend funds on research and experimentation efforts can also deduct the related costs in the year the funds are spent. Although investment partnerships can't take advantage of the R & D tax credit, upper bracket investors have been forming partnerships to perform research and development on new products and processes because they could deduct the full cost of the research efforts in the year of the investment, and the payback was usually in the form of a long-term capital gain. That means that only 40% of the resulting gain is taxable. Thus, if an R & D investment venture merely broke even, the investors would make a profit from the tax treatment of their income. The 1982 tax law (TEFRA) substantially reduced the appeal of the R & D investment partnership. The details are even more complicated than the information presented in the rest of this chapter and are beyond the scope here. Basically, business owners and investors must now decide whether to deduct R & D expenses in one year or to spread them over a period of ten years. If the one-year deduction is selected, then the difference between the total R & D expenses and the amount that would have been deducted if the costs had been allocated is to become part of a separate tax computation called the Alternative Minimum Tax (AMT).

Essentially, the AMT imposes a 20% tax on a taxpayer's deductions if those deductions result in a zero or a very low tax. The purpose is to prevent taxpayers from using tax deductions such as the R & D deduction to avoid taxes altogether. Because of this new provision, you should be sure to seek help from a tax advisor before the end of each year in order to plan your finances so that this alternative tax will not cause you to lose the benefit of some otherwise legitimate tax deductions or credits.

The tax laws and their interpretation change quickly. The information in this chapter may no longer be accurate by the time you read it. Please check with your accountant or lawyer for the most up-to-date information—ed.

60 | Guidelines for User Access to Computerized Patient Records (A Review)

Marc D. Schwartz, MD

---

ecent computer applications involving the traditional medical record have led to appropriate concerns over the potential misuse of information that is transferred outside the provider/patient relationship. In November 1976, the Committee on Standards of the Society for Computer Medicine initiated discussion about these concerns and reached a consensus regarding access by various parties to information basic to the medical record. Categories of information found in a record were established in order to determine the appropriateness of communicating that category of information to parties outside the immediate health care setting.

The committee recognized that there are many different users of the medical record whose access to medical information must be defined. In practice it does not appear that the blanket consent given by the patient is informed. The committee endeavored to adhere to the principles that only data of necessity should be transmitted and that any information that is released to responsible users should be in the patient's best interest and not bring harm to him or her.

Computerized medical records can include the capability of providing differential access to medical information dependent upon various user's predefined "need to know" and the computer's ability to synthesize elements from individual encounters to produce an electronically retrievable, up-to-date, medical-record summary.

The committee developed a set of matrices made up of rows of

The above is a synopsis by Marc D. Schwartz of an article written by Frederick Jelovsek, MD, and others in *Computer Magazine Newsletter,* which has ceased publication. The synopsis above originally appeared in *Computers in Psychiatry/Psychology* 1978, *1* (4), 8 and is reprinted by permission.

items (demographic, therapies, illnesses, test results, etc.) and columns of interested parties (medical provider, financial third parties, health care planners, clinical research and epidemiologists, quality controllers, medicolegal parties, and employer/school). Guidelines for permitting the release of items to interested parties were constructed. For example, financial third parties are not to be given information about race, home telephone numbers, past therapies, lab findings, etc. Health care planners are not to be given name, address, charges, name of provider, etc. Quality controllers are not to be given name, financial information, or medical information specified as confidential. And so on.

The committee hopes that computers can significantly improve the undesirable habit of merely copying whole or parts of medical records that convey both appropriate and inappropriate information to outside users. They hope also that these guidelines will contribute to planning in the area of privacy and confidentiality of medical information.

Computers in Mental Health: A Selected Bibliography

James L. Hedlund, PhD
Bruce W. Vieweg, MS

GENERAL REVIEWS

Crawford, J. L., Morgan, D. W., & Gianturco, D. T. *Progress in mental health information systems: Computer applications.* Cambridge, Mass. Ballinger, 1974.

Glueck, B. C., & Stroebel, C. F. Computers and clinical psychiatry. In H. I. Kaplan, A. M. Freedman, and B. J. Sadock (Eds.), *Comprehensive textbook of psychiatry* (Vol. 1, 3rd ed.). Baltimore: Williams and Wilkins, 1980.

Greist, J. H., & Klein, M. H. Computers in psychiatry. In A. Silvano and H. K. H. Brodie (Eds.), *American handbook of psychiatry.* New York: Basic Books, 1981.

Hedlund, J. L., Vieweg, B. W., Wood, J. B., Cho, D. W., Evenson, R. C., Hickman, C. V., & Holland, R. A. *Computers in mental health: A review and annotated bibliography* (NIMH Series FN No. 7; DHHS Pub. No. (ADM) 81-1090). Washington, D.C.: U.S. Government Printing Office, 1981.

Johnson, J. H. (Ed.). Computer technology and methodology in clinical psychology, psychiatry, and behavior medicine. *Behavior Research Methods and Instrumentation,* 1981, *13* (4), 389–636.

Sidowski, J. B., Johnson, J. H., & Williams, T. A. (Eds.). *Technology in mental health care delivery systems.* Norwood, N.J.: Ablex, 1980.

Spitzer, R. L., & Endicott, J. Computer applications in psychiatry. In D. A. Hamburg, & E. H. Brodie (Eds.), *American handbook of psychiatry: New psychiatric frontiers* (Vol. 6, 2nd ed.). New York: Basic Books, 1975.

GENERAL MENTAL HEALTH INFORMATION SYSTEMS*

Bank, R., & Needle, S. MSIS 2: The management information system for human services programs. In R. C. Insull, & J. H. Sumner (Eds.), *Proceedings of*

---

*See also the Community Mental Health Centers and Program Evaluation Sections of this bibliography.

the seventh annual MSIS national user's group conference. Orangeburg, N.Y.: Rockland Research Institute, 1982.

Bowers, G. E., & Bowers, M. R. *Cultivating client information systems* (Human Services Monograph Series, No. 5). Rockville, Md.: Project Share, 1977.

Chapman, R. L. *The design for management information systems for mental health organizations: A primer* (NIMH Series FN No. 5). Washington, D.C.: U.S. Government Printing Office, 1976.

Curriculum Development Project: *Information System Improvements for Mental Health Programs: Vol. I—Preparing for system improvement,* by L. Dreyer, N. Koroloff, & L. Bellerby (1979); *Vol. II—Planning information system improvements,* by L. Bellerby, N. Koroloff, & L. Dreyer (1979); *Vol. III—Managing the design of system improvements,* by L. Bellerby, L. Dreyer, & N. Koroloff (1980); *Vol. IV—Implementing information system improvements,* by L. Bellerby, L. Dreyer, & N. Koroloff (1981); and *Vol. V—Maintaining effective system performance,* by L. Bellerby, L. Dreyer, & N. Koroloff (1981). Portland, Oreg.: Regional Research Institute for Human Services.

Glueck, B. C. Computers at the Institute of Living. In J. L. Crawford, D. W. Morgan, & D. T. Gianturco (Eds.), *Progress in mental health information systems.* Cambridge, Mass.: Ballinger, 1974.

Hedlund, J. L., Sletten, I. W., Evenson, R. C., Altman, H., & Cho, D. W. Automated psychiatric information systems: A critical review of Missouri's Standard System of Psychiatry (SSOP). *Journal of Operational Psychiatry,* 1977, *8* (1), 5–26.

Hedlund, J. L., & Vieweg, B. W. Some utilization and maintenance issues with mental health information systems. In B. I. Blum (Ed.), *Proceedings of the sixth annual symposium on computer applications in medical care.* New York: Institute of Electrical and Electronics Engineers, 1982.

Hedlund, J. L., & Wurster, C. R. Computer applications in mental health management. In B. I. Blum (Ed.), *Proceedings of the sixth annual symposium on computer applications in medical care.* New York: Institute of Electrical and Electronics Engineers, 1982.

Laska, E. M., & Bank, R. (Eds.). *Safeguarding psychiatric privacy: Computer systems and their uses.* New York: John Wiley and Sons, 1975.

Laska, E. M., & Craig, T. J. (Eds.). Automated mental health information systems: Issues and options, and annotated bibliography. *International Journal of Mental Health,* 1982, *10* (4), 1–145.

Paton, J. A., & D'huyvetter, P. K. *Automated management informations systems for mental health agencies: A planning and acquisition guide* (NIMH Series FN No. 1; DHHS Pub. No. 80–797). Washington, D.C.: U.S. Government Printing Office, 1980.

Slavin, S. (Ed.). *Applying computers in social service and mental health agencies: A guide to selecting equipment, procedures and strategies.* New York: Haworth, 1981.

Taylor, J. B., & Gibbond, J. *Microcomputer applications in human services agencies* (Human Services Monograph Series, No. 16). Rockville, Md.: Project Share, 1980.

COMMUNITY MENTAL HEALTH CENTERS*

Elpers, J. R., & Chapman, R. L. Management information for mental health services. *Administration in Mental Health*, 1973, 12–25.

Giannetti, R. A., Johnson, J. H., & Williams, T. A. Computer technology in community mental health centers: Current status and future prospects. In F. H. Orthner (Ed.), *Proceedings of the second annual symposium on computer applications in medical care*. New York: Institute of Electrical and Electronics Engineers, 1978.

Gorodezky, M. J., & Hedlund, J. L. The developing role of computers in community mental health centers: Past experience and future trends. *Journal of Operational Psychiatry*, 1982, *13* (2), 94–99.

Hansen, K. E., Johnson, J. H., & Williams, T. A. Development of an on-line management information system for community mental health centers. *Behavior Research Methods and Instrumentation*, 1977, *9* (2), 139–143.

Hershey, J. C., & Moore, J. R. The use of an information system for community health services planning and management. *Medical Care*, 1975, *13* (2), 114–125.

Knesper, D. J., Quarton, G. C., Gorodezky, M. J., & Murray, C. W. A survey of the users of a working state mental health information system: Implications for the development of improved systems. In F. H. Orthner (Ed.), *Proceedings of the second annual symposium on computer applications in medical care*. New York: Institute of Electrical and Electronics Engineers, 1978.

Kupfer, D. J., Levine, M. S., & Nelson, J. A. *Mental health information systems: Design and implementation*. New York: Marcel Dekker, 1976.

Maypole, D. E. Developing a management information system in a rural community mental health center. *Administration in Mental Health*, 1978, *6* (1), 69–80.

Nelson, B. H., & Pecarchik, J. R. A computerized program audit for community mental health centers. *Community Mental Health Journal*, 1974, *10* (1), 102–110.

Paton, J. A., & Mayberry, D. Management information systems: Bringing the *M* and the *IS* together. In F. H. Orthner (Ed.), *Proceedings of the second annual symposium on computer applications in medical care*. New York: Institute of Electrical and Electronics Engineers, 1978.

Person, P. H. *A statistical information system for community mental health centers* (U.S. Public Health Service Pub. No. 1863). Washington, D.C.: U.S. Government Printing Office, 1969.

Sherman, P. S. A computerized CMHC clinical and management information system: Saga of a "mini" success. *Behavior Research Methods and Instrumentation*, 1981, *13*, 445–453.

St. Clair, C., Siegel, J., Caruso, R., & Spivack, G. Computerizing a mental health center information system. *Administration in Mental Health*, 1976, *4* (1), 10–18.

---

*See also the General Mental Health Information Systems and Program Evaluation sections of this bibliography.

Taube, C. A. (Ed.). *Community mental health center data systems: A description of existing programs* (U.S. Public Health Service Pub. No. 1990). Washington, D.C.: U.S. Government Printing Office, 1969.

Tippitt, J., Owens, R., & Frome, F. Indirect services and referral system for community mental health centers: Implementation and methods of measurement. *Community Mental Health Journal,* 1974, *10* (4), 450–465.

Wurster, C. R., & Goodman, J. D. NIMH prototype management information system for community mental health centers. In J. T. O'Neill (Ed.), *Proceedings of the fourth annual symposium on computer applications in medical care.* New York: Institute of Electrical and Electronics Engineers, 1980.

ALCOHOL PROGRAMS

Beresford, T., Low, D., Hal, R. C., Adduci, R., & Goggans, F. A computerized biochemical profile for detection of alcoholism. *Psychosomatics,* 1982, *23* (7), 713–720.

Elias, M. J., Dalton, J. H., Cobb, C. W., Lavoie, L., & Zlotlow, S. F. The use of computerized management information systems in evaluation. *Administration in Mental Health,* 1979, *7* (2), 148–161.

Evenson, R. C., Altman, H., Cho, D. W., & Montgomery, J. Development of an alcoholism severity scale via an iterative computer program for item analysis. *Quarterly Journal of Studies on Alcohol,* 1973, *34* (4), 1336–1341.

Lucus, R. W., Mullin, P. J., Luna, C. B., & McInroy, D. C. Psychiatrists and a computer as interrogators of patients with alcohol related illnesses: A comparison. *British Journal of Psychiatry,* 1977, *131,* 160–167.

Kadden, R., & Wetstone, S. Teaching coping skills to alcoholics using computer based education. In B. I. Blum (Ed.), *Proceedings of the sixth annual symposium on computer applications in medical care.* New York: Institute of Electrical and Electronics Engineers, 1982.

Matthews, D. B., & Miller, W. R. Estimating blood alcohol concentration: Two computer programs and their applications in therapy and research. *Addictive Behavior,* 1979, *4,* 55–60.

Morsicato, R. S. *A staff allocation model applied in a multimodal alcoholism rehabilitation facility.* Buffalo Research Institute on Alcoholism, 1980.

Parades, A. Management of alcoholism programs through a computerized information system. *Alcoholism,* 1977, *1* (4), 305–309.

DRUG ABUSE PROGRAMS

DeAngelis, G. G. Program-level evaluation using management information. *Addictive Diseases,* 1979, *3* (4), 555–561.

Levin, G., Hirsch, G., & Roberts, E. Narcotics and the community: A system simulation. *American Journal of Public Health,* 1972, *62* (6), 861–873.

Newman, R. G., & Cates, M. S. The New York City narcotics register: A case study. *American Journal of Public Health,* 1974, *64* (supplement), 24–28.

Schlenger, W. E. A systems approach to drug abuse users services. *Behavioral Science*, 1973, *18*, 137–147.

Sells, S. B., & Simpson, D. D. Implications for evaluation of dependency treatment based on data provided by a management information system. *Addictive Diseases*, 1979, *3* (4), 533–554.

Sells, D. B. The DARP research program and data systems. In S. B. Sells (Ed.), *The effectiveness of drug abuse treatment: Further studies of drug users, treatment typologies, and assessment of outcomes during treatment in DARP* (Vol. 3). Cambridge, Mass.: Ballinger, 1976.

Warner, A., & Dole, V. P. The operation of the data system in the methadone maintenance treatment program for heroin addiction. *American Journal of Public Health*, 1971, *61* (10), 2106–2114.

Wood, W., & Youatt, R. A computer feedback system for clinical research. *Computer Programs in Biomedicine*, 1979, *9*, 80–94.

Zalkind, D., Zelon, H., Moore, M., & Kaluzny, A. Planning for management information systems in drug treatment organizations. *International Journal of the Addictions*, 1979, *14* (2), 183–196.

MENTAL RETARDATION/DEVELOPMENTAL DISABILITIES

Crawford, J. L., Conklin, G. S., McMahon, D J., et al. An automated behavioral rehabilitation system for long term patients. In F. H. Orthner (Ed.), *Proceedings of the second annual symposium on computer applications in medical care*. New York: Institute of Electrical and Electronics Engineers, 1978.

Donohoe, J. F. Computer-based study of mental retardation. *Computers and Automation*, 1969, *18* (11), 50–52.

Gurthrie, D., Heighton, R., Keeran, C. V., & Payne, D. Data bases and the privacy rights of the mentally retarded: Report to the AAMD task force on data base confidentiality. *Mental Retardation*, 1976, *14*, 3–7.

Levy, J., & Pinder, S. Computer assisted management of state school waiting lists and admission procedures. *Mental Retardation*, 1971, *9* (5), 30–34.

Soforenko, A. Z. Computer aided client data programs. *Mental Retardation*, 1974, *12* (1), 40–41.

DIAGNOSIS*

Altman, H., Evenson, R. C., & Cho, D. W. New discriminant functions for computer diagnosis. *Multivariate Behavioral Research*, 1976, *11* (3), 367–376.

Benfari, R. C., & Leighton, A. H. PROBE: A computer instrument for field surveys of psychiatric disorder. *Archives of General Psychiatry*, 1970, *23*, 352–358.

Cassano, G. B., Castrogiovanni, P., & Conti, L. The computer diagnosis in a multicenter study of psychoactive agents. *Psychopharmacology Bulletin*, 1976, *12* (2), 22–24.

*See also the Prediction and Consultation section of this bibliography.

Erdman, H. P., Greist, J. H., Klein, M. H., Jefferson, J. W., Olson, W., & Salinger, R. Computer consultation for psychiatric diagnosis. In J. T. O'Neill (Ed.), *Proceedings of the fourth annual symposium on computer applications in medical care.* New York: Institute of Electrical and Electronics Engineers, 1980.

Fischer, M. Development and validity of a computerized method for diagnoses of functional psychoses (DIAX). *Acta Psychiatrica Scandinavica,* 1974, *50,* 243–288.

Fleiss, J. L., Spitzer, R. L., Cohen, J., & Endicott, J. Three computer diagnosis methods compared. *Archives of General Psychiatry,* 1972, *27,* 643–649.

Greist, J. H., & Klein, M. H. Computer programs for patients, clinicians, and researchers. In J. B. Sidowski, J. H. Johnson, & T. A. Williams (Eds.), *Technology in mental health care delivery systems.* Norwood, N.J.: Ablex, 1980.

Greist, J. H., Klein, M. H., & Erdman, H. P. Routine on-line psychiatric diagnosis by computer. *American Journal of Psychiatry,* 1976, *133* (12), 1405–1408.

Hedlund, J. L., Evenson, R. C., Sletten, I. W., & Cho, D. W. The computer and clinical prediction. In J. B. Sidowski, J. H. Johnson, & T. A. Williams (Eds.), *Technology in mental health care delivery systems.* Norwood, N.J.: Ablex, 1980.

Helzer, J. E., Robins, L. N., Croughan, J. L., & Welner, A. Reliability and procedural validity of the Renard Diagnostic Interview as used by physicians and lay interviewers. *Archives of General Psychiatry,* 1981, *38,* 393–398.

Hirschfeld, R., Spitzer, R. L., & Miller, R. G. Computer diagnosis in psychiatry: A Bayes approach. *Journal of Nervous and Mental Disease,* 1974, *158* (6), 399–407.

Johnson, J. H., Klingler, D. E., Giannetti, R. A., & Williams, T. A. The reliability of diagnosis by technician, computer and algorithm. *Journal of Clinical Psychology,* 1977, *36* (2), 447–451.

McDermott, P. A., & Hale, R. L. Validation of a systems-actuarial computer process for multidimensional classification of child psychopathology. *Journal of Clinical Psychology,* 1982, *38* (3), 477–486.

Overall, J. E. A configural analysis of psychiatric diagnostic stereotypes. *Behavioral Science,* 1963, *8* (3), 211–219.

Overall, J. E., & Higgins, C. W. An application of actuarial methods in psychiatric diagnosis. *Journal of Clinical Psychology,* 1977, *33* (4), 973–980.

Overall, J. E., & Hollister, L. E. Computer scoring of Research Diagnostic Criteria. *Psychopharmacology Bulletin,* 1979, *15* (2), 65–67.

Robins, L. N., Helzer, J. E., Croughan, J., & Ratcliff, K. S. National Institute of Mental Health Diagnostic Interview Schedule: Its history, characteristics, and validity. *Archives of General Psychiatry,* 1981, *38,* 381–389.

Singer, E., Cohen, S. M., Garfinkle, R., & Srole, L. Replicating psychiatric ratings through multiple regression analysis: The midtown Manhattan restudy. *Journal of Health and Social Behavior,* 1976, *17* (4), 376–387.

Sletten, I. W., Ulett, G. A., Altman, H., & Sundland, D. The Missouri Standard System of Psychiatry (SSOP): Computer generated diagnosis. *Archives of General Psychiatry,* 1970, *23* (1), 73–79.

Spitzer, R. L., & Endicott, J. DIAGNO: A computer program for psychiatric diagnosis utilizing the differential diagnostic procedure. *Archives of General Psychiatry*, 1968, *18*, 746–756.

Spitzer, R. L., & Endicott, J. DIAGNO II: Further developments in a computer program for psychiatric diagnosis. *American Journal of Psychiatry*, 1969, *125* (7 suppl), 12–21.

Spitzer, R. L., & Endicott, J. Computer diagnosis in automated recordkeeping systems: A study of clinical acceptability. In J. L. Crawford, D. W. Morgan, & D. T. Gianturco (Eds.), *Progress in mental health information systems: Computer applications*. Cambridge, Mass.: Ballinger, 1974.

Spitzer, R. L., Endicott, J., Cohen, J., & Fleiss, J. L. Constraints on the validity of computer diagnosis. *Archives of General Psychiatry*, 1974, *31* (2), 197–203.

Stroebel, C. F., & Glueck, B. C. The diagnostic process in psychiatry: Computer approaches. *Psychiatric Annals*, 1972, *2* (12), 58–77.

Wing, J. K., Cooper, J. E., & Sartorius, N. *Measurement and classification of psychiatric symptoms: An instruction manual for the PSE and CATEGO systems*. London: Cambridge University Press, 1974.

MENTAL STATUS

Donnelly, J., Rosenberg, M., & Fleeson, W. P. The evolution of the mental status—Past and future. *American Journal of Psychiatry*, 1970, *126* (7), 997–1002.

Meldman, M. J. Microcomputer technology for psychiatrists. In F. H. Orthner (Ed.), *Proceedings of the second annual symposium on computer applications in medical care*. New York: Institute of Electrical and Electronics Engineers, 1978.

Sletten, I. W., Ernhart, C. B., & Ulett, G. A. The Missouri automated mental status examination: Development, use and reliability. *Comprehensive Psychiatry*, 1970, *11* (4), 315–327.

Spitzer, R. L., & Endicott, J. An integrated group of forms for automated case records: A progress report. *Archives of General Psychiatry*, 1971, *24*, 540–547.

Spitzer, R. L., & Endicott, J. The Psychiatric Status Schedule: A technique for evaluating psychopathology and impairment in role functioning. *Archives of General Psychiatry*, 1970, *23*, 41–55.

Weitzel, W. D., Morgan, D. W., Guyden, T. E., & Robinson, J. A. Toward a more efficient mental status examination: Free-form or operationally defined. *Archives of General Psychiatry*, 1973, *28*, 215–218.

AUTOMATED NURSING NOTES

Evenson, R. C. *Missouri Inpatient Behavior Scale (MIBS)* (Manual). St. Louis, Mo.: Missouri Institute of Psychiatry, 1978.

Evenson, R. C. *Geriatric Profile* (Manual). St. Louis, Mo.: Missouri Institute of Psychiatry, 1976.

Glueck, B. C., Gullotta, G. P., & Ericson, R. P. Automation of behavior assessments: The computer-produced nursing note. In J. B. Sidowski, J. H. Johnson, & T. A. Williams (Eds.), *Technology in mental health care delivery systems.* Norwood, N.J.: Ablex, 1980.

Morgan, D. W., & Crawford, J. L. Some issues in computer applications. In J. L. Crawford, D. W. Morgan, & D. T. Gianturco (Eds.), *Progress in mental health information systems: Computer applications.* Cambridge, Mass.: Ballinger, 1974.

Morgan, D. W., Crawford, J. L., & Frenkel, S. I. An automated patient behavior checklist. *Journal of Applied Psychology,* 1973, *58* (3), 393–396.

Olsson, D. E. Automating nursing notes—First step in a computerized record system. *Hospitals,* 1969, *41,* 64; 69–70; 74; 76; 78.

Stein, R. F. An exploratory study in the development and use of automated nursing reports. *Nursing Research,* 1969, *18* (1), 14–21.

Willer, B., & Stasiak, E. Automated nursing notes in a psychiatric institution. *Journal of Psychiatric Nursing,* 1973, *11,* 27–29.

PSYCHOLOGICAL TESTING

Birtles, C. J., Sambrooks, J., MacCulloch, M. J., & Holland, P. An inexpensive computer assisted psychometric system. *Medical and Biological Engineering,* 1972, *10,* 145–152.

Elwood, D. L., & Clark, C. L. Computer administration of the Peabody Picture Vocabulary Test (PPVT). *Behavior Research Methods and Instrumentation,* 1978, *10* (1), 43–46.

Elwood, D. L., & Griffin, H. R. Individual intelligence testing with the examiner: Reliability of an automated method. *Journal of Consulting and Clinical Psychology,* 1972, *38* (1), 9–14.

Fowler, R. D. Automated psychological test interpretation: The status in 1972. *Psychiatric Annals, 1972, 2* (12), 10–28.

Fowler, R. D. Automated MMPI. In J. B. Sidowski, J. H. Johnson, & T. A. Williams (Eds.), *Technology in mental health care delivery systems.* Norwood, N.J.: Ablex, 1980.

Gedye, J. L., & Miller, E. Developments in automated testing systems. In P. Mittler (Ed.), *The psychological assessment of mental and physical handicaps.* London: Methuen and Co., 1970.

Heaton, R. K., Grant, I., Anthony, W. Z., & Lehman, R. A. A comparison of the clinical and automated interpretation of the Halstead-Reitan Battery. *Journal of Clinical Neuropsychology* 1981, *3* (2), 121–141.

Hopwood, J. H., Wei, K. H., & Yellin, A. M. A computerized method for generating the Rorschach's structural summary from the sequence of scores. *Journal of Personality Assessment,* 1981, *45* (2), 116–117.

Johnson, J. H., & Williams, T. A. The use of on-line computer technology in a mental health admitting system. *American Psychologist,* 1975, *30* (3), 388–390.

Johnson, J. H., & Williams, T. A. Using on-line computer technology to improve service response and decision-making effectiveness in a mental health admitting system. In J. B. Sidowski, J. H. Johnson, & T. A. Williams (Eds.), *Technology in mental health care delivery systems.* Norwood, N.J.: Ablex, 1980.

Klett, C. J., & Pumroy, D. K. Automated procedures in psychological assessment. In P. McReynolds (Ed.), *Advances in psychological assessment* (Vol. 2). Palo Alto, Calif.: Science and Behavior Books, 1971.

Lanyon, R. I., & Goodstein, L. D. Automated personality assessment. In R. I. Lanyon, & L. D. Goodstein, *Personality Assessment.* New York: John Wiley & Sons, 1982.

Lushene, R. E. Development of a psychological assessment system. In H. J. Heffernan (Ed.), *Proceedings of the fifth annual symposium on computer applications in medical care.* New York: Institute of Electrical and Electronics Engineers, 1981.

Paitich, D. A comprehensive automated psychological examination and report (CAPER). *Behavioral Science,* 1973, *18,* 131–136.

Piotrowski, Z. A. CPR: The psychological x-ray in mental disorders. In J. B. Sidowski, J. H. Johnson, & T. A. Williams (Eds.), *Technology in mental health care delivery systems.* Norwood, N.J.: Ablex, 1980.

Space, L. G. The computer as psychometrician. *Behavior Research Methods and Instrumentation,* 1981, *13* (4), 595–606.

SCREENING AND HISTORIES

Angle, H. V., Ellinwood, E. H., & Carroll, J. Computer interview problem assessment of psychiatric patients. In F. H. Orthner (Ed.), *Proceedings of the second annual symposium on computer applications in medical care.* New York: Institute of Electrical and Electronics Engineers, 1978.

Chun, R. W., Van Cura, L. J., Spencer, M., & Slack, W. V. Computer interviewing of patients with epilepsy. *Epilepsia,* 1976, *17* (4), 371–375.

Coddington, R. D., & King, T. L. Automated history taking in child psychiatry. *American Journal of Psychiatry,* 1972, *129* (3), 276–282.

Greist, J. H., & Klein, M. H. Computer programs for patients, clinicians, and researchers. In J. B. Sidowki, J. H. Johnson, & T. A. Williams (Eds.), *Technology in mental health care delivery systems.* Norwood, N.J.: Ablex 1980.

Greist, J. H., Klein, M. H., & Van Cura, L. J. A computer interview for psychiatric patient target symptoms. *Archives of General Psychiatry,* 1973, *29,* 247–253.

Johnson, J. H., & Williams, T. A. Using on-line computer technology to improve service response and decision-making effectiveness in a mental health admitting system. In J. B. Sidowski, J. H. Johnson, & T. A. Williams (Eds.), *Technology in mental health care delivery systems.* Norwood, N.J.: Ablex, 1980.

Maultsby, M. C., & Slack, W. V. A computer-based history system. *Archives of General Psychiatry,* 1971, *25,* 570–572.

Metz, J. R., Allen, C. M., Barr, G., & Shinefield, H. A. Pediatric screening examination for psychosocial problems. *Pediatrics* 1976, *58* (4), 595–606.

Skinner, H. A., & Allen, B. A. Does the computer make a difference? Computerized versus face-to-face versus self-report assessment of alcohol, drug, and tobacco use. *Journal of Consulting and Clinical Psychology,* 1983, *51* (2), 267–275.

Stillman, R., Roth, W. T., Colby, K. M., & Rosenbaum, C. P. An on-line computer system for initial psychiatric inventory. *American Journal of Psychiatry*, 1969, *127* (7 suppl.), 8–11.

PSYCHOTHERAPY

Colby, K. M. Computer psychotherapists. In J. B. Sidowski, J. H. Johnson, & T. A. Williams (Eds.), *Technology in mental health care delivery systems*. Norwood, N.J.: Ablex, 1980.

Colby, K. M., Watt, J. B., & Gilbert, J. P. A computer model of psychotherapy: Preliminary communication. *Journal of Nervous and Mental Disease*, 1966, *142* (2), 148–152.

Hilf, F. D., Colby, K. M., Smith, D. C., Wittner, W. K., & Hall, W. A. Machine mediated interviewing. *Journal of Nervous and Mental Disease*, 1971, *152* (4), 278–288.

Ruesch, J. Psychotherapy in the computer age. *Psychotherapy and Psychosomatics*, 1968, *16*, 32–46.

Starkweather, J. A., Kamp, M., & Monto, A. Psychiatric interview simulation by computer. *Methods of Information in Medicine*, 1967, *6* (1), 15–23.

Stodolsky, D. The computer as a psychotherapist. *International Journal of Man-Machine Studies*, 1970, *2*, 327–350.

BEHAVIOR THERAPY/BIOFEEDBACK

Carr, A. C., Ancill, R. J., Ghosh, A., & Margo, A. Direct assessment of depression by microcomputer. *Acta Psychiatrica Scandinavica*, 1981, *64*, 415–422.

Carr, A. C., & Ghosh, A. Accuracy of behavioral assessment by computer. *British Journal of Psychiatry*, in press.

Carr, A. C., & Ghosh, A. Response of phobic patients to direct computer assessment. *British Journal of Psychiatry*, in press.

Dolan, P. M., & Shapiro, D. Interactive assistance for biofeedback and psychophysiological research: Pragmatics of development. *Behavior Research Methods and Instrumentation*, 1981, *13* (3), 311–322.

Lang, P. J. Behavioral treatment and bio-behavioral assessment: Computer applications. In J. B. Sidowski, J. H. Johnson, & T. A. Williams (Eds.), *Technology in mental health care delivery systems*. Norwood, N.J.: Ablex, 1980.

Schneider, S. J., & Benya, A. Computerized direct mail in a behavior modification stop smoking clinic. In B. I. Blum (Ed.), *Proceedings of the sixth annual symposium on computer applications in medical care*. New York: Institute of Electrical and Electronics Engineers, 1982.

Selmi, P. M., Klein, M. H., Greist, J. H., Johnson, J. H., & Harris, W. G. An investigation of computer-assisted cognitive behavior therapy in the treatment of depression. *Behavior Research Methods and Instrumentation*, 1982, *14* (2), 181–185.

PROBLEM-ORIENTED MEDICAL RECORD AND TREATMENT PLANNING

Brunell, L. F. The "Basic ID": A model for a computerized assessment, treatment planning and evaluation system for use in a psychiatric hospital. *Dissertation Abstracts International*, 1978, *39* (1B), 370.

Craig, T. J., Volaski, V., DiStefano, O., Alexander, M. J., Kadyzewski, P., Crawford, J., & Richardson, M. A. Automating the treatment planning process: How? Why? For Whom? In B. I. Blum (Ed.), *Proceedings of the sixth annual symposium on computer applications in medical care*. New York: Institute of Electrical and Electronics Engineers, 1982.

Diamond, R. J., & Chapman, M. Development of a data system in a day treatment program. In B. I. Blum (Ed.), *Proceedings of the sixth annual symposium on computer applications in medical care*. New York: Institute of Electrical and Electronics Engineers, 1982.

Giannetti, R. A., Johnson, J. H., Williams, T. A., & McCusker, C. F. Development of an on-line problem oriented system for the evaluation of mental health treatment services. *Behavior Research Methods and Instrumentation*, 1977, *9* (2), 133–138.

Gifford, S., & Mayberry, D. An integrated system for computerized patient records. *Hospital and Community Psychiatry*, 1979, *30* (8), 532–535.

Grant, R. L., Mizner, G. L., Pfifferling, J. H., Sletten, I. W., & Thomas, J. L. The problem oriented system and automation. In *The problem-oriented record in psychiatry* (Task Force Report 12). Washington, D.C.: American Psychiatric Association, 1977.

Hay, W. M., Hay, L. R., Angle, H. V., & Ellinwood, E. H. Computerized behavioral assessment and the problem oriented record. *International Journal of Mental Health*, 1977, *6* (2), 49–63.

Honigfeld, G., Pulier, M., Laska, E. M., Kaufl, R., & Ziek, P. An approach to problem oriented psychiatric records. In J. L. Crawford, D. W. Morgan, & D. T. Gianturco (Eds.), *Progress in mental health information systems: Computer applications*. Cambridge, Mass.: Ballinger, 1974.

Longabaugh, R., Fowler, D. R., Stout, R., Kriebel, G. Validation of a problem-focused nomenclature. *Archives of General Psychiatry*, 1983, *40*, 453–461.

Meldman, M. J., McFarland, G., & Johnson, E. *The problem oriented index and treatment plans*. St. Louis, Mo.: C. V. Mosby, 1976.

Miller, G. H., & Willer, B. An information system for clinical recording, administrative decision making, evaluation and research. *Community Mental Health Journal*, 1977, *13* (2), 194–204.

Pulier, M. L., Honigfeld, G., & Laska, E. M. Problem orientation in psychiatry. In E. M. Laska, & R. Bank (Eds.), *Safeguarding psychiatric privacy: Computer systems and their uses*. New York: John Wiley and Sons, 1975.

Roberts, B. A computerized diagnostic evaluation of a psychiatric problem. *American Journal of Psychiatry*, 1980, *137* (1), 12–15.

Ryback, R., Stout, R. L., & Hedlund, J. L. Computerization and the POR. In R. S. Ryback, R. Longabaugh, & D. R. Fowler (Eds.), *The problem oriented rec-*

ord in psychiatry and mental health care (2nd ed.). New York: Grune and Stratton, 1981.

TREATMENT MONITORING

Barton, J. L. A study of the effect of computer feedback on polypharmacy. *Journal of Clinical Psychiatry*, 1978, *39* (9), 690–692.

Bower, A. C., & Richardson, D. H. A computer based data bank. *Mental Retardation*, 1975, *13*, 32–33.

Conklin, G. S., Craig, T. J., Vickers, R., McCleery, G., & Mehl, B. Of computers in medical care and quality assurance: Why do systems fail? And what can be done. In B. I. Blum (Ed.), *Proceedings of the sixth annual symposium on computer applications in medical care*. New York: Institute of Electrical and Electronics Engineers, 1982.

Craig, T. J., & Conklin, G. Clinical considerations in the introduction of a computerized drug ordering and exception system. In H. G. Heffernan (Ed.), *Proceedings of the fifth annual symposium on computer applications in medical care.* New York: Institute of Electrical and Electronics Engineers, 1981.

Greist, J. H., Klein, M. H., Gutman, A. S., & Van Cura, L. J. Computer measures of patient progress in psychotherapy. *Psychiatry Digest*, 1977, *38* (9), 23–30.

Heiser, J. G., & Brooks, R. E. Design considerations for a clinical psychopharmacology advisor. In F. H. Orthner (Ed.), *Proceedings of the second annual symposium on computer applications in medical care.* New York: Institute of Electrical and Electronics Engineers, 1978.

Laska, E. M. An automated review system for psychotropic drug orders. *Archives of General Psychiatry*, 1980, *37* (7), 824–827.

Laska, E. M., & Siegel, C. *Knowledge-based information systems in mental health* (Presented at the American Psychiatric Association Meeting, Chicago). Orangeburg, N.Y.: Rockland Research Institute, 1979.

Mittel, N. S., Gardner, G. H., & Rose, B. W. Computerized monitoring of psychotropic drug orders: Some trends and revelations. *Hospital and Community Psychiatry*, 1981, *32* (4), 277–278.

Schnitker, K., & Boeker, K. Assuring accountability in residential self-help skills programs. *Mental Retardation*, 1978, *16* (4), 300–307.

Sorrell, S. P., Greist, J. H., Klein, M. H., Johnson, J. H., & Harris, W. G. Enhancement of adherence to tricyclic antidepressants by computerized supervision. *Behavior Research Methods and Instrumentation*, 1982, *14* (2), 176–180.

Strobel, C. F., & Glueck, B. C. Computer derived global judgments in psychiatry. *American Journal of Psychiatry*, 1970, *126* (8), 1057–1066.

Tupin, J. P., Overall, J. E., McKinley, C. K., Dreisbach, L. K., & Patrick, J. H. Computer monitoring and analysis of a psychiatric treatment program. *Mental Health*, 1967, *51* (3), 414–418.

Wilson, N. C., & Mumpower, J. L. Automated evaluation of goal attainment ratings. *Hospital and Community Psychiatry*, 1975, *26* (3), 163–164.

Winick, W. An automated system for reviewing patient care. *Hospital and Community Psychiatry*, 1972, *23* (4), 115–117.

PREDICTION AND CONSULTATION*

Glueck, B. C., & Strobel, C. F. The computer and the clinical decision process. *American Journal of Psychiatry*, 1969, *125* (7), 2–7.

Greist, J. H., Gustafson, D. H., Strauss, F. F., Rowse, G. L., Laughren, T. P., & Chiles, J. A. Computer interview for suicide risk prediction. *American Journal of Psychiatry*, 1973, *130* (12), 1327–1332.

Greist, J. H., Gustafson, D. H., Strauss, F. F., Rowse, G. L., Laughren, T. P., & Chiles, J. A. Suicide risk prediction: A new approach. *Suicide and Life Threatening Behavior*, 1974, *4* (4), 212–223.

Greist, J. H., Klein, M. H., Erdman, H. P., & Jefferson, J. Clinical computers in mental health. In B. I. Blum (Ed.), *Proceedings of the sixth annual symposium on computer applications in medical care*. New York: Institute of Electrical and Electronics Engineers, 1982.

Hedlund, J. L., Evenson, R. C., Sletten, I. W., & Cho, D. W. The computer and clinical prediction. In J. B. Sidowski, J. H. Johnson, and T. A. Williams (Eds.), *Technology in mental health care delivery systems*. Norwood, N.J.: Ablex, 1980.

Overall, J. E. The Brief Psychiatric Rating Scale in psychopharmacology research. *Modern Problems in Pharmacopsychiatry*, 1974, *7*, 67–78.

Overall, J. E., & Henry, B. W. Decisions about drug therapy: III. Selection of treatment for psychiatric inpatients. *Archives of General Psychiatry*, 1972, *28*, 81–89.

Overall, J. E., Henry, B. W., Markett, J. R., & Emken, R. L. Decisions about drug therapy: I. Prescriptions for adult psychiatric outpatients. *Archives of General Psychiatry*, 1972, *26*, 140–145.

Stroebel, C. F., & Glueck, B. C. Computer derived global judgments in psychiatry. *American Journal of Psychiatry*, 1970, *126* (8), 1057–1066.

PROGRAM EVALUATION AND QUALITY ASSURANCE*

Attkisson, C. C., McIntyre, M. H., Hargreaves, W. A., Harris, M. R., & Ochberg, F. M. A working model for mental health program evaluation. *American Journal of Orthopsychiatry*, 1974, *44* (5), 741–753.

Black, G. C. Evaluating management information systems: A protocol for automated peer review systems. In J. T. O'Neill (Ed.), *Proceedings of the fourth annual symposium on computer applications in medical care*. New York: Institute of Electrical and Electronics Engineers, 1980.

Block, W. E. Applying utilization review procedures in a community mental health center. *Hospital and Community Psychiatry*, 1975, *26* (6), 358–360.

*See also the Diagnosis and Treatment Monitoring sections in this bibliography.

Bloom, B. L. Human accountability in a community mental health center: Report of an automated system. *Community Mental Health Journal*, 1972, *8* (4), 251–260.

Cameron, J. C. Using a computer profile to assess quality of care in a psychiatric hospital. *Hospital and Community Psychiatry*, 1976, *27* (9), 623.

Evenson, R. C. Program evaluation using an automated data base. *Hospital and Community Psychiatry*, 1974, *25* (2), 80–83.

Evenson, R. C., Sletten, I. W., Hedlund, J. L., & Faintich, D. M. CAPS: An automated evaluation system. *American Journal of Psychiatry*, 1974, *131* (5), 531–534.

Fiester, A. R., & Fort, D. J. A method of evaluating the impact of services at a comprehensive community mental health center. *American Journal of Community Psychology*, 1978, *6* (3), 291–302.

Fishman, D. B. A computerized, cost-effectiveness methodology for community mental health centers. In J. B. Sidowski, J. H. Johnson, and T. A. Williams, (Eds.), *Technology in mental health care delivery systems*. Norwood, N.J.: Ablex, 1980.

Harman, C. E., & Meinhardt, K. A computer system for treatment evaluation at the community mental health center. *American Journal of Public Health*, 1972, *62* (12), 1596–1601.

Helmick, E., Miller, S. I., Nutting, P., Shorr, G., & Berg, L. A monitoring and evaluation plan for alcoholism programs. *British Journal of Addiction*, 1976, *71*, 39–43.

Huber, G. A., Wolfe, H., & Hardwick, C. P. Evaluating computerized screening as an aid to utilization review. *Inquiry*, 1974, *11* (3), 188–195.

Kaplan, J. M., & Smith, W. G. An evaluation program for a regional mental health center. In J. L. Crawford, D. W. Morgan, & D. T. Gianturco (Eds.), *Progress in mental health information systems: Computer applications*. Cambridge, Mass.: Ballinger, 1974.

Maguire, L. Peer review in community mental health. *Community Mental Health Journal*, 1978, *14* (3), 190–199.

Meredith, J. A Markovian analysis of a geriatric ward. *Management Science*, 1973, *19* (6), 604–612.

Meredith, J. Program evaluation in a hospital for mentally retarded persons. *American Journal of Mental Deficiency*, 1974, *78* (4), 471–481.

Miller, R. R., Black, G. C., Ertel, P. Y., & Ogram, G. F. Psychiatric peer review: The Ohio system. *American Journal of Psychiatry*, 1974, *131* (12), 1367–1370.

Murtaugh, C., Siegel, C., Fischer, S., Alexander, M. J., & Craig, T. J. Computers and quality of care. In B. I. Blum (Ed.), *Proceedings of the sixth annual symposium on computer applications in medical care*. New York: Institute of Electrical and Electronics Engineers, 1982.

Riedel, D., Brenner, M. H., Brauer, L., et al. Psychiatric utilization review as patient care evaluation. *American Journal of Public Health*, 1972, *62* (9), 1222–1228.

Riedel, D. C., Tischler, G. L., & Myers, J. K. *Psychiatric care evaluation in mental health programs.* Cambridge, Mass.: Ballinger, 1974.

Siegel, C., & Goodman, A. Evaluating the attainment of process objectives of community mental health centers using MSIS. In E. M. Laska, & R. Bank (Eds.), *Safeguarding psychiatric privacy: Computer systems and their uses.* New York: John Wiley and Sons, 1975.

Siegel, C., & Goodman, A. An evaluative paradigm for community mental health centers using an automated data system. *Community Mental Health Journal,* 1976, 12 (2), 215–227.

St. John, D. B., Dobin, D. R., & Flashner, B. A. An automated system for the regulation and medical review of long-term care facilities and patients. *American Journal of Public Health,* 1973, 63 (7), 619–630.

Thompson, K. S., & Cheng, E. H. A computer package to facilitate compliance with utilization review requirements. *Hospital and Community Psychiatry,* 1976, 27 (9), 653–656.

Tischler, G. L. The use of MSIS in program evaluation. In E. M. Laska, & R. Bank (Eds.), *Safeguarding psychiatric privacy: Computer systems and their uses.* New York: John Wiley and Sons, 1975.

Wolfe, P. C., & Haveliwala, Y. A model for program evaluation in a unitized setting. *Hospital and Community Psychiatry,* 1976, 27 (9), 647–649.

Index